MW01518361

T Cell Regulation in Allergy, Asthma and Atopic Skin Diseases

Chemical Immunology and Allergy

Vol. 94

Series Editors

Johannes Ring Munich
Kurt Blaser Davos
Monique Capron Lille
Judah A. Denburg Hamilton
Stephen T. Holgate Southampton
Gianni Marone Naples
Hirohisa Saito Tokyo

T Cell Regulation in Allergy, Asthma and Atopic Skin Diseases

Volume Editor

Kurt Blaser Davos

39 figures, 8 in color, and 11 tables, 2008

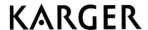

Basel · Freiburg · Paris · London · New York · Bangalore ·
Bangkok · Shanghai · Singapore · Tokyo · Sydney

Chemical Immunology and Allergy
Formerly published as 'Progress in Allergy' (Founded 1939),
continued 1990–2002 as 'Chemical Immunology'
Edited by Paul Kallós 1939–1988, Byron H. Waksman 1962–2002

Prof. Dr. Kurt Blaser
Obere Strasse 71
CH–7270 Davos (Switzerland)
E-Mail kblaser@siaf.uzh.ch

Bibliographic Indices. This publication is listed in bibliographic services, including Current Contents® and Index Medicus.

© Copyright 2008 by S. Karger AG, P.O. Box, CH–4009 Basel (Switzerland)
www.karger.com
Printed in Switzerland on acid-free and non-aging paper (ISO 9706) by Reinhardt Druck, Basel
ISSN 1660–2242
ISBN 978–3–8055–8628–3

Contents

29 Interaction of Regulatory T Cells with Antigen-Presenting Cells in Health and Disease

Mahnke, K.; Ring, S.; Bedke, T.; Karakhanova, S.; Enk, A.H. (Heidelberg)

40 Mucosal Regulatory T Cells in Airway Hyperresponsiveness

Strickland, D.H.; Wikstrom, M.E.; Turner, D.J.; Holt, P.G. (Perth)

48 Natural Killer Cells in Allergic Inflammation

Erten, G.; Aktas, E.; Deniz, G. (Istanbul)

58 Mast Cells and Mast Cell-Derived Factors in the Regulation of Allergic Sensitization

Taube, C.; Stassen, M. (Mainz)

189 Lung Dendritic Cells: Targets for Therapy in Allergic Disease

Lambrecht, B.N. (Ghent/Rotterdam); Hammad, H. (Ghent)

201 Antigen-Based Therapies Targeting the Expansion of Regulatory T Cells in Autoimmune and Allergic Disease

Leech, M.D.; Anderton, S.M. (Edinburgh)

211 Stem Cell Transplantation in Genetically Linked Regulatory T-Cell Disorders

Shenoy, S. (St. Louis, Mo.)

Preface
Role of T-Cell Subtypes in Allergic Inflammations

Allergic diseases are immune reactions which represent the currently best knowledge of cellular and molecular mechanisms, generating and regulating different clinical manifestations at different organs. The knowledge on the immunological background of allergy meets the current state of the art in immunology and immune-related inflammatory guises. One reason for this is the knowledge and accessibility of the ultimate trigger of the disease, the allergen, which can relatively easily be determined and produced in pure form. This and other typical properties of allergy provide a most suitable disease model for the study of specific immune responses. It has definitely overcome the state where allergy was defined as equal to serum-IgE antibody content and the knowledge on the disease has escaped the state of simple IgE antibody measure. Allergic diseases have their origin in a deregulated immunity to exogenous molecules, being harmless as such, facilitated mostly by a preferential genetical constitution. Thus, in normal immunity to allergen mostly IgG4 antibodies are elicited, which can block the allergen and do not display Fc-related antibody functions, such as binding complement or Fc receptors on effector cells. The regulation of both normal and allergic immunity is fully T-cell-dependent and relies exclusively on the activation and action of different subtypes of T cells and their products, which in consequence activate and direct the entire network of immune and involved tissue cells.

Allergic inflammations are induced by increasingly generated Th2 cells, which dominantly secrete IL-4, IL-13 and IL-5 cytokines, triggering IgE antibodies and prolonging eosinophilic granulocyte survival. Interestingly it appeared that inhibited apoptosis by IL-5/GM-CSF and not extensive production of eosinophils is the cause of eosinophilia. While allergy initially depends on Th2 cells, Th1 cells producing TNF and IFN-γ, and which are induced at a later stage by bacterial or viral superinfections and superantigenic activation, are involved in the chronic progression of the disease. Both TNF and IFN-γ are able to induce death receptors on tissue cells and thus, together with other ligands, induce tissue cell death, such as bronchial epithelial and smooth muscle cells and keratinocytes in skin diseases. Activated effector T cells are directed by tissue-selective homing receptors and attracted by the aid of different chemokines. This basic knowledge could be generated only after recombinant cytokines became available after 1980.

It is established today that a set of T-regulatory cells (Tregs) as well as other T-cell subtypes are

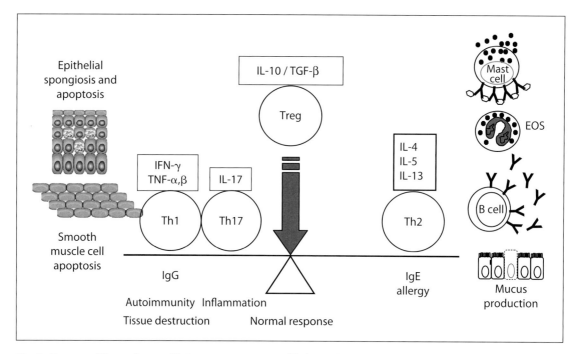

Fig. 1. Tregs equilibrate the specific immune response and balance the entire network of T and B cells and effector cells of allergy during activation.

involved in the mechanisms and regulation of allergic inflammations and that the interaction with tissue cells and effector cells plays an important role in the chronicity of the disease; Treg cells regulate the immune response to foreign triggers and participate in the maintenance of peripheral and central tolerance. Of decisive importance in immune response regulation to allergens and other specific triggers are functional Tregs (fig. 1). However, different functional Treg populations, such as CD4+CD25^{high} Tregs, Tr1, Th3 lymphocytes and NK cells exist, which can be distinguished by different cytokine profiles and marker expression. Tregs in allergy are highly activated, CD25+ peripheral T cells, which require continuous activation. TGF-β promotes the development of CD4+CD25^{high} FOXP3+ Tregs from naive CD4+ T cells. They are allergen-specific T cells, displaying immune suppressive functions, which are mediated by their IL-10 and/or TGF-β secretion. Thus, Tregs secreting these suppressive

cytokines are true regulatory cells in that they suppress effector cells of allergy and IgE production by B cells, while they activate blocking antibodies of IgG4 and IgA type and promote development of Tregs from naive T-cell populations (fig. 2). At initiation they express the transcription factor FOXP3 (forkhead box protein 3), while Th2 cells express GATA3 and Th1 cells, T-BET (fig. 3). Peripheral Tregs, like Th1 and Th2, represent an independent T-cell lineage, developing from naive T cells after activation by allergen and DC contact, with the aid of TGF-β. They cannot develop from Th2 cells, e.g. in specific immunotherapy. Moreover, FOXP3 and Treg development is suppressed by GATA3 and IL-4, and therefore after activation of Th2 cells. Accordingly, it is difficult to skew an established allergic or atopic state into a Treg-equilibrated normal immune state. This is probably the reason for the long immunization procedure required for successful allergen-specific immunotherapy, although Tregs are induced by

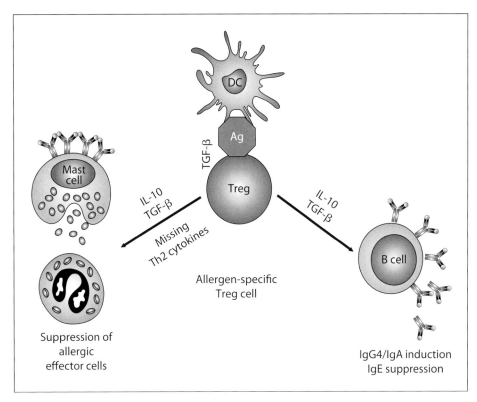

Fig. 2. Counter-regulatory effects of antigen-specific Treg cells in a peripheral immune response to allergen.

high allergen doses within a short time after the first immunization (2–3 days). Tregs are required in sufficient numbers proportional to the specific Th effector cells and their suppressive function depends exclusively on their numbers in relation to the effector T cells.

An important T-cell subtype in chronic allergic responses are the Th17 cells, being defined by their IL-17 production. The Th17 subset is distinct from the Th1, Th2 and Tregs. They are important players in chronic inflammatory responses such as allergy and autoimmunity, organ transplantation and tumor development. Differentiation of Th17 is initiated by TGF-β in combination with IL-6. Also IL-21, highly expressed by mouse Th17 cells, potently induces Th17 differentiation and suppresses FOXP3, the nuclear factor for Treg differentiation. The Th17 differentiation is initiated by

the orphan nuclear receptor RORγt, for humans termed RORC2. Th17 cells induce and amplify the inflammatory IL-1β and TNF-α response. Without the influence of these proinflammatory cytokines, IL-23 mainly from activated dendritic cells expands and stabilizes the Th17 population. In humans, Th17 cells are suppressed by IL-12, in the mouse, Th17 differentiation is inhibited by IFN-γ. GM-CSF is a crucial factor for granulocyte development and survival and development of organ-related autoimmune diseases. Innate GM-CSF induces IL-6 responses and generation of pathological Th17. TGF-β promotes the development of CD4+CD25^{high}+FOXP3+ Tregs from naive CD4+ T cells. The balance between Th17 and Tregs is regulated by IL-2, which displays differential effects on the two T-cell lineages. Treg cells increase under the influence of IL-2, whereas

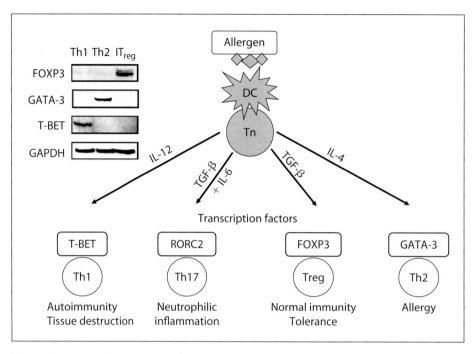

Fig. 3. Distinct cytokines generate the transcription factors required for development of the different functional effector T-cell phenotypes.

Th17 cell numbers are reduced and IL-2 neutralization boosts the Th17 differentiation. Both Th1 and Th2 differentiation depends on the strength of T-cell receptor activation and co-stimulatory interaction. Th17 cells require higher antigen doses for differentiation by enhancing IL-6 production and CD40L expression on dendritic cells. A lack of CD40-CD40L interaction leads to impaired Th17 production and autoimmunity. Thus, GM-CSF, antigen dose, and CD40-CD40L interaction regulate the IL-6 production, a key cytokine for Th17 development. A better understanding of transcriptional regulation of the different cell types and its relation to the inflammatory disease will provide further insight into the regulatory events involved in immune regulation of these chronic inflammatory diseases.

The present edition of 'Molecular Immunology' on 'T-Cell Regulation in Allergy, Asthma and Atopic Skin Diseases' provides the latest overview on the regulatory mechanisms by T lymphocytes and their subtypes in the organ-related allergic manifestations and specific treatments of the diseases. The issue is divided into three parts, the first part providing a modern view of the immunoregulatory processes in allergic inflammations. In particular, the development and the role of Treg cells in the induction of peripheral tolerance to allergens and the function of the Th17 cells in chronic inflammatory processes are described. In addition, the regulatory role of NK cells and the feedback interactions by activated mast cells, a major effector cell of the allergic reaction, are considered.

The second part describes the regulation and immunological events in different allergic diseases, such as asthma and atopic skin diseases, in parasite infection and delayed-type hypersensitivity. Special attention is paid to mucosal tolerance, which is important in many respects including also oral immunotherapy and tolerance induction. Finally, a most important part is devoted to the clinical consequences of the current immunological knowledge on T-cell regulation in novel therapeutic interventions. For almost 100 years it could not be demonstrated whether the effects of specific allergen immunizations rely on true immunological mechanisms or not. Thus, the demonstration of the immunological mechanism in allergen-specific immunotherapy, including the role of peripheral Tregs and their secreted suppressive cytokines, was a decisive step in both the understanding of the immunological background of this allergen-specific treatment and in allergic diseases in general. For a long time, and against clear facts, it was originally believed that specific allergen treatment should skew a Th2 into a Th1 response, which is clearly not the case since both extremes reflect pathogenic situations. From the understanding of mechanisms in allergen-specific

immunotherapy, the knowledge of peripheral tolerance induction and the importance of the allergen-specific Treg cells have mostly appeared.

While on the one hand the aspects of Tregs and tolerance induction in allergen-specific immunotherapy and different procedures of vaccination are described, one chapter is added which describes future possibilities of stem cell transplantation in genetically linked disorders.

Thus, based on the role of different subpopulations of T cells activated by allergen and their cytokine production and interaction with effector and tissue cells, leading to different allergic manifestations, this book provides a modern overview on the T-cell-dependent immunoregulatory events in allergic inflammations and their clinical and therapeutic applications.

Kurt Blaser, Prof. PhD
Davos, August 2008

Blaser K (ed): T Cell Regulation in Allergy, Asthma and Atopic Skin Diseases.
Chem Immunol Allergy. Basel, Karger, 2008, vol 94, pp 1–7

Th17 and Treg Cells Innovate the Th1/Th2 Concept and Allergy Research

C.B. Schmidt-Weber

Allergy and Clinical Immunology, Imperial College London, London, UK

Abstract

Allergic reactions are caused by harmless allergens, which are recognized by the specific immune system. Allergen-specific T cells are assumed to play a key role in the sensitization phase and in immunological memory. Current immunological concepts suggest that asymptomatic T-cell memory cells also exist, tagging the allergen as harmless and preventing an inappropriate response and thus allergic symptoms. Proinflammatory T cells mediate allergic inflammation by exceeding the induction of IgE and competing with other T-cell subsets. Therefore, molecular mechanisms leading to pro- or anti-inflammatory T-cell memory cells appear as the key mechanism in allergy.   Copyright © 2008 S. Karger AG, Basel

The dichotomic Th1/Th2 paradigm has dominated our view of allergy pathogenesis and has produced important concepts such as the hygiene hypothesis. Multiple studies could demonstrate the validity of this system, while it left open issues. The discovery of new T-cell subsets changed our cellular perspective, while a new work hypothesis on T-cell differentiation remains to be reformulated. Allergen-specific immune responses are dependent on B and T cells which encounter allergens as a whole by the immunoglobulin receptors or are presented by dendritic cells/B cells as peptide by the T-cell receptor. The IgE production of B cells requires the help of IL-4-producing Th2-type T cells to switch from IgM towards IgE. In contrast to B cells, T cells do not have direct allergen contact and therefore their function with the immune system is much more difficult to understand than the Ig-producing B cells. The Th1/Th2 paradigm was based on two T-cell subsets with the memory fraction of T cells, one IFN-γ-secreting Th1 and a Th2 subset characteristic for IL-4-secreting cells. Th1 and Th2 cells differentiate from antigen-inexperienced naive T cells, which polarize upon initial antigen challenge to Th1 or Th2 cells, but do not form mixed phenotypes. Since Th2 cells are critically important for the IgE switch of B cells, it was hypothesized that Th2 cells are important for humoral responses as observed in IgE-dominated allergic disease and are in competitive balance with Th1 cells, as observed in infections. Because of the competitive and exclusive mechanism of differentiation, which polarizes T-cell responses towards a discrete phenotype, it was hypothesized that allergen immunization along Th1 pathways could deviate allergen-specific responses away from Th2 phenotype and thus generate an allergen tolerance by immune deviation. Similarly, the hygienic conditions in a westernized lifestyle were suggested to limit Th1

Table 1. Overview of T-cell phenotypes, their induction pathway and their function

Phenoytpe		Induced in serum-free conditions in vitro by	Lineage supporting transcription factor	Products	Function
Th1		IL-12, anti-IL-4	T-BET	IFN-γ	MHC-II regulation on macrophages and Dc's, induced T-Bet (infections)
Th2		IL-4, anti-IL-12	GATA-3, GFI-1, c-Maf	IL-4, IL-5, IL-9 IL-13, IL-31	B-cell support towards IgE expression, GATA-3 induction, eosinophils support, tissue regulation, e.g. remodeling (allergies and parasitic infections)
Th17		TGF-β & IL-6 or IL-1β, anti-IL-4, anti-IL-12	RORC2	IL-17, IL-22, TNF-α	Induction of G-CSF, IL-6, IL-8, neutrophilic inflammation (acute inflammation, arthritis, acute neutrophilic asthma)
Treg	iTreg	TGF-β, anti-IL-4, anti-IL-12	FOXP3 (transient)	CD25^{high}, contact-dependent (TGF-β?)	Suppression of effector T cells and co-stimulatory capacity of DC's (asymptomatic responses)
	nTreg	Thymus-derived	FOXP3 (constitutive)	CD25^{high}, contact-dependent (TGF-β?)	Suppression of effector T cells and co-stimulatory capacity of DC's (autoimmunity)
	Tr1	IL-10?, ICOS, pDC	?	IL-10	Suppressive on cytokine production and co-stimulation, supports IgG4 (induced in immunotherapy)

reactions, which in turn gives space for more Th2 reactions. Regulatory T (Treg) cells and Th17 cells are more recently discovered subsets which have not yet found entry into these concepts and are likely to modify or change our view of immunological reactions in allergy (table 1).

General Role of T Cells in the Immune System

To establish new paradigms or to modify the Th1/Th2 paradigm, it is important to consider the function of the new subsets: Treg cells control or suppress effector T cells, most likely by a process involving antigen-presenting cells, while Th17 cells are important for neutrophilic inflammation by interacting with structural cells to induce IL-6 and IL-8 expression or by increasing the lifetime of neutrophils in the tissue. This spectrum of functions highlights on the one hand the great importance of T cells in control of immune tolerance and on the other hand the capacity of T cells to translate the immunological memory into the tissue-endogenous defense/regulation capacities (fig. 1). The tissue-interactive nature was also shown for Th2 cells, which interact not only with

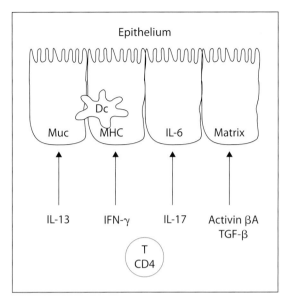

Fig. 1. Interrelationships of tissue cells with T cells, where T cells translate the immunological memory into tissue.

immune competent cells such as eosinophils (IL-5 [1, 2]), but also with structural cells such as smooth muscle (IL-9 [3]) and epithelial cells as well as keratinocytes (IL-13 [4, 5]). Interestingly, the more recently discovered cytokine IL-31 is also believed to be a Th2 cytokine and is received by monocytes and epithelial cells (IL-31 [6, 7]). Furthermore, it has been suggested that IL-31 could play a role in supporting nerve ends and regulate itch in atopic dermatitis [8, 9].

Beside the well-established role of Th2 cells in allergy, it also became clear that not only Th2, but also Th1 cells can contribute to allergic pathology, specifically in atopic dermatitis such as in acute lesional skin [10], where IFN-γ is known to induce cell death in keratinocytes causing the spongiform pathology observed in atopic dermatitis [11].

Treg Cells and Their Importance in Allergy

Treg cells are capable of suppressing effector cells and are therefore likely to play an important role in allergen tolerance by harnessing allergen-induced inflammation in early processes such as allergen sensibilization [12]. To rule out their contribution in allergic responses it is important to distinguish at least two different kinds of Treg cells: the thymus-derived, so-called natural Treg cells, which constitutively express high CD25 as well as intranuclear FOXP3 and Tr1 cells, which are characterized by IL-10 expression. Of note in human cells, IL-10 is not a Th2 cytokine, but also co-expressed by Th1 cells [13].

Tr1 cells are of particular importance for translational medicine, as they were found to be induced in specific immunotherapy and are thought to be part of the mechanism which re-induces allergen tolerance. The importance of IL-10 is also evidenced by the observation that healthy individuals have a higher frequency of allergen-specific, IL-10-producing T cells than allergic patients [14], which supports the idea that specific immunotherapy restores allergen tolerance. Recently, CD25, FOXP3+ and allergen (house dust mite, HDM) specific T cells were also characterized and shown to inhibit HDM-specific responses, while in vitro expanded clones of atopic and healthy donors did not differ in their suppressive capacity [15]. Thus it is currently not clear whether Treg cells play a causative role in allergic disease, while it is anticipated that they are fundamentally important in allergen tolerance in disease and therapy.

Effector T cells are suppressed by Treg cells in an antigen-specific manner and since antigen-specific activation of T cells are mediated by an MHCII-dependent mechanism, it is likely that the suppression process also involves dendritic cells. This could in fact be demonstrated in recent publications [16–18]. Interestingly, Treg cells also act outside the triangle of Treg-Teff and DCs, as they were shown to interact with neutrophils [19], B cells and NK or NKT cells [20], confirming the instructional character of Treg cells. The suppression process is a cell-contact-dependent mechanism and requires the activation of the Treg by the p38

MAP-, AKT- and p110 δ-phosphoinositide 3-kinase elements [21–23]. The Treg cells themselves silence their own cytokine expression by interaction of the FOXP3 transcription factor [24] with the activation/calcium-induced factor NFAT [25] and AML1/Runx1 [26] and also the expression of an E3 ubiquitin ligase (GRAIL) [27] and cAMP production [28]. These mechanisms mediate an anergic phenotype and suppressive T-cell phenotype. The target T cells are cell surface-contacted by the Treg cell with surface receptors, including LAG-3 [29, 30] and CTLA-4, of which the latter potentially boosts the activity of membrane-bound TGF-β [31–33]. To be biologically active, TGF-β needs to be proteolytically cleaved and present in a surface-bound condition [33], probably as part of the immunological synapse. In fact, TGF-β receptors were found in activation/contact zones of non-T cells and are raft resident [34]. This special subcellular, multigene scenery may explain how soluble and ubiquitous mediators such as TGF-β mediate antigen-specific suppression.

Th17 Cells – Proinflammatory Cousins of Treg Cells?

Th17 cells were recently discovered to constitute a separate subset, which plays an inflammation-driving role in arthritis, while Th1 cell are not observed to be critical for tissue changes in the joint [35–37]. However, in acute inflammation in the lung, Th17 were also shown to be relevant [38–40]. Th17 cells secrete IL-17 (or IL-17A), IL-17F, IL-6, TNF-α and IL-22 [36, 37, 41–43]. IL-17 is important in G-CSF induction, which promotes granulopoiesis [44, 45] and therefore is important for homeostasis of neutrophils. It also induces CXC chemokines (e.g. IL-8), which attracts neutrophils and enhances neutrophil survival [40] leading to neutrophilic inflammation [46, 47]. Interestingly, IL-17 also interacts with tissue cells, such as fibroblasts [48–51], epithelial cells [31, 52–56], smooth muscle cells [57] and

chondrocytes [58], induces proinflammatory cytokines, chemokines, and modulates matrix-relevant genes, underlining the important role for the instruction of tissue cells. IL-17 also activates macrophages [40, 59, 60] and neutrophils [38]. IL-17 acts in synergy with other cytokines, such as IL-6 to induce MUC5B and MUC5AC [31], or together with IL-1 and TNF-α to enhance VEGF expression [61]. This principle of co-induction is an important scheme in biology as it integrates cytokine-induced factors with factors of the innate immune system to reach activation thresholds for fundamental processes such as mucus secretion or angiogenesis.

Origin of T-Cell Phenotypes

The recently discovered T-cell subsets originate in naive, antigen-inexperienced precursor T cells and interestingly, both require TGF-β to be induced. While Treg cells require TGF-β only, the Th17 subset needs additional IL-6 or IL-1β. Recent studies showed that human T cells do not require TGF-β for T-cell differentiation, however the respective studies used TGF-β-containing serum, while serum-free conditions require TGF-β [unpubl. results]. It is thus remarkable that TGF-β can drive very diverse T-cell phenotypes, making it a 'jack of all trades' [62] and extending the long list of TGF-β functions. It is therefore important for our understanding of this gene how it modulates T-cell differentiation and which genes are made accessible by TGF-β-'flavored' immune responses. A key feature of this process is the polarization of a phenotype, which involves the competition of certain lineage-specific transcription factors, such as T-bet (Th1) and GATA-3 (Th2). T-BET interferes directly and blocks GATA-3 to bind its targets [63]. This process can be influenced by TGF-β, which is known to suppress GATA-3 as well as T-BET expression.

The balance of T-cell phenotypes at the initiation and during the course of disease determines the pathogenic features. The T cells carry the acquired phenotype into the tissue under the control of the antigen specificity and translate this antigen-associated information into the tissues, which in turn become immunoactive by secretion of chemokines, acute phase cytokines and other mediators of inflammation. We anticipate that immunotolerance is also linked to the tissue response, either directly or with the help of environment-sensing dendritic cells.

Future and Perspective

The newly discovered T-cell subsets are an important step regarding our attempts to translate immunology into clinically relevant therapeutic strategies to control disease. The example of Th17 cells highlights the specific, probably timely restricted window of action, which these cells occupy in pathology in inflammatory disease. Immunologic treatment must be specified on the current disease status. This implies that future anti-T-cell treatments must be patient-tailored and based on a solid set of biomarkers defining the individual immunological disease status.

Acknowledgements

Supported by the Swiss National Science Foundation Grant No. 310000-112329, 3200B0-105865, Bonizzi-Theler Foundation Zurich, The Swiss Life Foundation Zurich, Switzerland.

References

1 Dibbert B, Daigle I, Braun D, Schranz C, Weber M, Blaser K, Zangemeister-Wittke U, Akbar AN, Simon HU: Role for Bcl-xL in delayed eosinophil apoptosis mediated by granulocyte-macrophage colony-stimulating factor and interleukin-5. Blood 1998;92:778–783.

2 Simon HU, Plotz SG, Simon D, Dummer R, Blaser K: Clinical and immunological features of patients with interleukin-5-producing T cell clones and eosinophilia. Int Arch Allergy Immunol 2001;124:242–245.

3 Gounni AS, Hamid Q, Rahman SM, Hoeck J, Yang J, Shan L: IL-9-mediated induction of eotaxin1/CCL11 in human airway smooth muscle cells. J Immunol 2004;173:2771–2779.

4 Laoukili J, Perret E, Willems T, Minty A, Parthoens E, Houcine O, Coste A, Jorissen M, Marano F, Caput D, Tournier F: IL-13 alters mucociliary differentiation and ciliary beating of human respiratory epithelial cells. J Clin Invest 2001;108:1817–1824.

5 Deshpande DA, Dogan S, Walseth TF, Miller SM, Amrani Y, Panettieri RA, Kannan MS: Modulation of calcium signaling by interleukin-13 in human airway smooth muscle: role of CD38/cyclic adenosine diphosphate ribose pathway. Am J Respir Cell Mol Biol 2004;31:36–42.

6 Dillon SR, Sprecher C, Hammond A, Bilsborough J, Rosenfeld-Franklin M, Presnell SR, Haugen HS, Maurer M, Harder B, Johnston J, Bort S, Mudri S, Kuijper JL, Bukowski T, Shea P, Dong DL, Dasovich M, Grant FJ, Lockwood L, Levin SD, LeCiel C, Waggie K, Day H, Topouzis S, Kramer J, Kuestner R, Chen Z, Foster D, Parrish-Novak J, Gross JA: Interleukin 31, a cytokine produced by activated T cells, induces dermatitis in mice. Nat Immunol 2004;5:752–760.

7 Chattopadhyay S, Tracy E, Liang P, Robledo O, Rose-John S, Baumann H: Interleukin-31 and oncostatin-M mediate distinct signaling reactions and response patterns in lung epithelial cells. J Biol Chem 2007;282: 3014–3026.

8 Takaoka A, Arai I, Sugimoto M, Honma Y, Futaki N, Nakamura A, Nakaike S: Involvement of IL-31 on scratching behavior in NC/Nga mice with atopic-like dermatitis. Exp Dermatol 2006;15:161–167.

9 Takaoka A, Arai I, Sugimoto M, Yamaguchi A, Tanaka M, Nakaike S: Expression of IL-31 gene transcripts in NC/Nga mice with atopic dermatitis. Eur J Pharmacol 2005;516:180–181.

10 Grewe M, Bruijnzeel-Koomen CA, Schopf E, Thepen T, Langeveld-Wildschut AG, Ruzicka T, Krutmann J: A role for Th1 and Th2 cells in the immunopathogenesis of atopic dermatitis. Immunol Today 1998;19:359–361.

11 Trautmann A, Akdis M, Kleemann D, Altznauer F, Simon HU, Graeve T, Noll M, Brocker EB, Blaser K, Akdis CA: T cell-mediated Fas-induced keratinocyte apoptosis plays a key pathogenetic role in eczematous dermatitis. J Clin Invest 2000;106:25–35.

12 Schmidt-Weber CB, Blaser K: Regulation and role of transforming growth factor-beta in immune tolerance induction and inflammation. Curr Opin Immunol 2004;16:709–716.

13 Del Prete G, De Carli M, Almerigogna F, Giudizi MG, Biagiotti R, Romagnani S: Human IL-10 is produced by both type 1 helper (Th1) and type 2 helper (Th2) T cell clones and inhibits their antigen-specific proliferation and cytokine production. J Immunol 1993;150:353–360.

14 Akdis M, Verhagen J, Taylor A, Karamloo F, Karagiannidis C, Crameri R, Thunberg S, Deniz G, Valenta R, Fiebig H, Kegel C, Disch R, Schmidt-Weber CB, Blaser K, Akdis CA: Immune responses in healthy and allergic individuals are characterized by a fine balance between allergen-specific T regulatory 1 and T helper 2 cells. J Exp Med 2004;199:1567–1575.

15 Maggi L, Santarlasci V, Liotta F, Frosali F, Angeli R, Cosmi L, Maggi E, Romagnani S, Annunziato F: Demonstration of circulating allergen-specific CD4+CD25highFoxp3+ T-regulatory cells in both nonatopic and atopic individuals. J Allergy Clin Immunol 2007;120:429–436.

16 Cederbom L, Hall H, Ivars F: CD4+CD25+ regulatory T cells down-regulate co-stimulatory molecules on antigen-presenting cells. Eur J Immunol 2000;30:1538–1543.

17 Fallarino F, Grohmann U, Hwang KW, Orabona C, Vacca C, Bianchi R, Belladonna ML, Fioretti MC, Alegre ML, Puccetti P: Modulation of tryptophan catabolism by regulatory T cells. Nat Immunol 2003;4:1206–1212.

18 Misra N, Bayry J, Lacroix-Desmazes S, Kazatchkine MD, Kaveri SV: Cutting edge: human CD4+CD25+ T cells restrain the maturation and antigen-presenting function of dendritic cells. J Immunol 2004;172:4676–4680.

19 Lewkowicz P, Lewkowicz N, Sasiak A, Tchorzewski H: Lipopolysaccharide-activated CD4+CD25+ T regulatory cells inhibit neutrophil function and promote their apoptosis and death. J Immunol 2006;177:7155–7163.

20 Barao I, Hanash AM, Hallett W, Welniak LA, Sun K, Redelman D, Blazar BR, Levy RB, Murphy WJ: Suppression of natural killer cell-mediated bone marrow cell rejection by CD4+CD25+ regulatory T cells. Proc Natl Acad Sci USA 2006;103:5460–5465.

21 Adler HS, Kubsch S, Graulich E, Ludwig S, Knop J, Steinbrink K: Activation of MAP kinase p38 is critical for the cell-cycle-controlled suppressor function of regulatory T cells. Blood 2007;109:4351–4359.

22 Crellin NK, Garcia RV, Levings MK: Altered activation of AKT is required for the suppressive function of human CD4+CD25+ T regulatory cells. Blood 2007;109:2014–2022.

23 Patton DT, Garden OA, Pearce WP, Clough LE, Monk CR, Leung E, Rowan WC, Sancho S, Walke LS, Vanhaesebroeck B, Okkenhaug K: Cutting edge: the phosphoinositide 3-kinase p110 delta is critical for the function of CD4+CD25+Foxp3+ regulatory T cells. J Immunol 2006;177:6598–6602.

24 Lopes JE, Torgerson TR, Schubert LA, Anover SD, Ocheltree EL, Ochs HD, Ziegler SF: Analysis of FOXP3 reveals multiple domains required for its function as a transcriptional repressor. J Immunol 2006;177:3133–3142.

25 Wu Y, Borde M, Heissmeyer V, Feuerer M, Lapan AD, Stroud JC, Bates DL, Guo L, Han A, Ziegler SF, Mathis D, Benoist C, Chen L, Rao A: FOXP3 controls regulatory T cell function through cooperation with NFAT. Cell 2006;126:375–387.

26 Ono M, Yaguchi H, Ohkura N, Kitabayashi I, Nagamura Y, Nomura T, Miyachi Y, Tsukada T, Sakaguchi S: Foxp3 controls regulatory T-cell function by interacting with AML1/Runx1. Nature 2007;446:685–689.

27 Mackenzie DA, Schartner J, Lin J, Timmel A, Jennens-Clough M, Fathman CG, Seroogy CM: GRAIL is up-regulated in CD4+ CD25+ T regulatory cells and is sufficient for conversion of T cells to a regulatory phenotype. J Biol Chem 2007;282:9696–9702.

28 Vendetti S, Patrizio M, Riccomi A, De Magistris MT: Human CD4+ T lymphocytes with increased intracellular cAMP levels exert regulatory functions by releasing extracellular cAMP. J Leukoc Biol 2006;80:880–888.

29 Huang CT, Workman CJ, Flies D, Pan X, Marson AL, Zhou G, Hipkiss EL, Ravi S, Kowalski J, Levitsky HI, Powell JD, Pardoll DM, Drake CG, Vignali DA: Role of LAG-3 in regulatory T cells. Immunity 2004;21:503–513.

30 Macon-Lemaitre L, Triebel F: The negative regulatory function of the lymphocyte-activation gene-3 co-receptor (CD223) on human T cells. Immunology 2005;115:170–178.

31 Chen Y, Thai P, Zhao YH, Ho YS, DeSouza MM, Wu R: Stimulation of airway mucin gene expression by interleukin (IL)-17 through IL-6 paracrine/autocrine loop. J Biol Chem 2003;278:17036–17043.

32 Tang Q, Boden EK, Henriksen KJ, Bour-Jordan H, Bi M, Bluestone JA: Distinct roles of CTLA-4 and TGF-beta in CD4+CD25+ regulatory T cell function. Eur J Immunol 2004;34:2996–3005.

33 Oida T, Xu L, Weiner HL, Kitani A, Strober W: TGF-beta-mediated suppression by CD4+CD25+ T cells is facilitated by CTLA-4 signaling. J Immunol 2006;177:2331–2339.

34 Zhang XL, Topley N, Ito T, Phillips A: Interleukin-6 regulation of transforming growth factor (TGF)-beta receptor compartmentalization and turnover enhances TGF-beta1 signaling. J Biol Chem 2005;280:12239–12245.

35 Nakae S, Saijo S, Horai R, Sudo K, Mori S, Iwakura Y: IL-17 production from activated T cells is required for the spontaneous development of destructive arthritis in mice deficient in IL-1 receptor antagonist. Proc Natl Acad Sci USA 2003;100:5986–5990.

36 Harrington LE, Hatton RD, Mangan PR, Turner H, Murphy TL, Murphy KM, Weaver CT: Interleukin 17-producing CD4+ effector T cells develop via a lineage distinct from the T helper type 1 and 2 lineages. Nat Immunol 2005;6: 1123–1132.

37 Park H, Li Z, Yang XO, Chang SH, Nurieva R, Wang YH, Wang Y, Hood L, Zhu Z, Tian Q, Dong C: A distinct lineage of CD4 T cells regulates tissue inflammation by producing interleukin 17. Nat Immunol 2005;6:1133–1141.

38 Hoshino H, Laan M, Sjostrand M, Lotvall J, Skoogh BE, Linden A: Increased elastase and myeloperoxidase activity associated with neutrophil recruitment by IL-17 in airways in vivo. J Allergy Clin Immunol 2000;105:143–149.

39 Hashimoto T, Akiyama K, Kobayashi N, Mori A: Comparison of IL-17 production by helper T cells among atopic and nonatopic asthmatics and control subjects. Int Arch Allergy Immunol 2005;137(suppl 1):51–54.

40 Sergejeva S, Ivanov S, Lotvall J, Linden A: Interleukin-17 as a recruitment and survival factor for airway macrophages in allergic airway inflammation. Am J Respir Cell Mol Biol 2005;33:248–253.

Schmidt-Weber

41 Mangan PR, Harrington LE, O'Quinn DB, Helms WS, Bullard DC, Elson CO, Hatton RD, Wahl SM, Schoeb TR, Weaver CT: Transforming growth factor-beta induces development of the T(H)17 lineage. Nature 2006;441: 231–234.

42 Chung Y, Yang X, Chang SH, Ma L, Tian Q, Dong C: Expression and regulation of IL-22 in the IL-17-producing CD4+ T lymphocytes. Cell Res 2006;16:902–907.

43 Zheng Y, Danilenko DM, Valdez P, Kasman I, Eastham-Anderson J, Wu J, Ouyang W: Interleukin-22, a T(H)17 cytokine, mediates IL-23-induced dermal inflammation and acanthosis. Nature 2007;445:648–651.

44 Cai XY, Gommoll CPJ, Justice L, Narula SK, Fine JS: Regulation of granulocyte colony-stimulating factor gene expression by interleukin-17. Immunol Lett 1998;62:51–58.

45 Forlow SB, Schurr JR, Kolls JK, Bagby GJ, Schwarzenberger PO, Ley K: Increased granulopoiesis through interleukin-17 and granulocyte colony-stimulating factor in leukocyte adhesion molecule-deficient mice. Blood 2001;98:3309–3314.

46 Laan M, Cui ZH, Hoshino H, Lotvall J, Sjostrand M, Gruenert DC, Skoogh BE, Linden A: Neutrophil recruitment by human IL-17 via C-X-C chemokine release in the airways. J Immunol 1999;162:2347–2352.

47 Linden A, Adachi M: Neutrophilic airway inflammation and IL-17. Allergy 2002;57:769–775.

48 Koenders MI, Kolls JK, Oppers-Walgreen B, van den Bersselaar L, Joosten LA, Schurr JR, Schwarzenberger P, van den Berg WB, Lubberts E: Interleukin-17 receptor deficiency results in impaired synovial expression of interleukin-1 and matrix metalloproteinases 3, 9, and 13 and prevents cartilage destruction during chronic reactivated streptococcal cell wall-induced arthritis. Arthritis Rheum 2005;52:3239–3247.

49 Yao Z, Painter SL, Fanslow WC, Ulrich D, Macduff BM, Spriggs MK, Armitage RJ: Human IL-17: a novel cytokine derived from T cells. J Immunol 1995;155:5483–5486.

50 Kehlen A, Pachnio A, Thiele K, Langner J: Gene expression induced by interleukin-17 in fibroblast-like synoviocytes of patients with rheumatoid arthritis: upregulation of hyaluronan-binding protein TSG-6. Arthritis Res Ther 2003;5:R186–R192.

51 Chabaud M, Garnero P, Dayer JM, Guerne PA, Fossiez F, Miossec P: Contribution of interleukin 17 to synovium matrix destruction in rheumatoid arthritis. Cytokine 2000;12:1092–1099.

52 Van den Berg A, Kuiper M, Snoek M, Timens W, Postma DS, Jansen HM, Lutter R: Interleukin-17 induces hyperresponsive interleukin-8 and interleukin-6 production to tumor necrosis factor-alpha in structural lung cells. Am J Respir Cell Mol Biol 2005;33:97–104.

53 Jones CE, Chan K: Interleukin-17 stimulates the expression of interleukin-8, growth-related oncogene-alpha, and granulocyte-colony-stimulating factor by human airway epithelial cells. Am J Respir Cell Mol Biol 2002;26:748–753.

54 Kao CY, Huang F, Chen Y, Thai P, Wachi S, Kim C, Tam L, Wu R: Up-regulation of CC chemokine ligand 20 expression in human airway epithelium by IL-17 through a JAK-independent but MEK/NF-kappaB-dependent signaling pathway. J Immunol 2005;175: 6676–6685.

55 Awane M, Andres PG, Li DJ, Reinecker HC: NF-kappa B-inducing kinase is a common mediator of IL-17-, TNF-alpha-, and IL-1 beta-induced chemokine promoter activation in intestinal epithelial cells. J Immunol 1999;162:5337–5344.

56 Andoh A, Takaya H, Makino J, Sato H, Bamba S, Araki Y, Hata K, Shimada M, Okuno T, Fujiyama Y, Bamba T: Cooperation of interleukin-17 and interferon-gamma on chemokine secretion in human fetal intestinal epithelial cells. Clin Exp Immunol 2001;125:56–63.

57 Rahman MS, Yang J, Shan LY, Unruh H, Yang X, Halayko AJ, Gounni AS: IL-17R activation of human airway smooth muscle cells induces CXCL-8 production via a transcriptional-dependent mechanism. Clin Immunol 2005;115:268–276.

58 Lubberts E, Joosten LA, van de Loo FA, van den Gersselaar LA, van den Berg WB: Reduction of interleukin-17-induced inhibition of chondrocyte proteoglycan synthesis in intact murine articular cartilage by interleukin-4. Arthritis Rheum 2000;43:1300–1306.

59 Jovanovic DV, Di Battista JA, Martel-Pelletier J, Jolicoeur FC, He Y, Zhang M, Mineau F, Pelletier JP: IL-17 stimulates the production and expression of proinflammatory cytokines, IL-beta and TNF-alpha, by human macrophages. J Immunol 1998;160:3513–3521.

60 Jovanovic DV, Martel-Pelletier J, Di Battista JA, Mineau F, Jolicoeur FC, Benderdour M, Pelletier JP: Stimulation of 92-kd gelatinase (matrix metalloproteinase 9) production by interleukin-17 in human monocyte/macrophages: a possible role in rheumatoid arthritis. Arthritis Rheum 2000;43:1134–1144.

61 Honorati MC, Cattini L, Facchini A: IL-17, IL-1beta and TNF-alpha stimulate VEGF production by dedifferentiated chondrocytes. Osteoarthritis Cartilage 2004;12:683–691.

62 Veldhoen M, Stockinger B: TGFbeta1, a 'Jack of all trades': the link with proinflammatory IL-17-producing T cells. Trends Immunol 2006;27:358–361.

63 Hwang ES, Szabo SJ, Schwartzberg PL, Glimcher LH: T helper cell fate specified by kinase-mediated interaction of T-bet with GATA-3. Science 2005;307:430–433.

C.B. Schmidt-Weber
Allergy and Clinical Immunology, Imperial College London
South Kensington Campus, Sir Alexander Fleming Building, Room 365
Exhibition Road, London SW7 2AZ (UK)
Tel. +44 20 7594 9276, E-Mail c.schmidt-weber@imperial.ac.uk

Blaser K (ed): T Cell Regulation in Allergy, Asthma and Atopic Skin Diseases.
Chem Immunol Allergy. Basel, Karger, 2008, vol 94, pp 8–15

Regulatory T Cells and Antigen-Specific Tolerance

Karsten Kretschmer · Irina Apostolou · Panos Verginis · Harald von Boehmer

Harvard Medical School, Dana-Farber Cancer Institute, Boston, Mass., USA

Abstract

Foxp3-expressing regulatory T cells (Tregs) have an essential function of preventing autoimmune disease in man and mouse. Foxp3 binds to forkhead motifs of about 1,100 genes and the strength of binding increases upon PMA/ionomycin stimulation. In Foxp3-expressing T-cell hybridomas, Foxp3 promoter binding does not lead to activation or suppression of genes which becomes only visible after T-cell activation. These findings are in line with observations by others that Foxp3 exerts important functions through association with T-cell receptor (TCR)-dependent transcription factors in a DNA-binding complex. Tregs can be generated when developing T cells encounter TCR agonist ligands in the thymus. This process requires costimulatory signals. In contrast, extrathymic conversion of naive T cells into Tregs is inhibited by costimulation. In fact, DC-derived retinoic acid (RA) helps the conversion process by counteracting the negative impact of costimulation. Since AP-1 is produced after costimulation and appears to interfere with Foxp3-NFAT transcription complexes, it is of interest to note that RA interferes with AP-1-dependent transcription. Thus, RA may interfere with the negative impact of costimulation on Treg conversion by interfering with the generation and/or function of AP-1.

Copyright © 2008 S. Karger AG, Basel

Cellular therapy employing Foxp3-expressing regulatory T cells (Tregs) holds the promise to replace and/or supplement indiscriminatory immunosuppression by drugs. In order to achieve this goal in the clinic, we need to learn more about the generation, lifestyle and function of Tregs. One way to generate Tregs of any desired antigen specificity is the retroviral introduction of the Foxp3 gene into activated CD4 T cells. Foxp3 is a transcriptional repressor and activator that interferes with T-cell receptor (TCR)-dependent activation of genes and may exert its effect, at least in part, by compromising NFAT-dependent gene activation. Another way of generating Tregs extrathymically in vivo is the introduction of low amounts of peptides under subimmunogenic conditions. Such artificially induced Tregs have a long lifespan in the absence of the inducing antigen and can thus mediate antigen-specific tolerance. Antigen specificity of Treg-mediated immunosuppression is due to effective co-recruitment and expression of Tregs and T-effector cells to antigen-draining lymph nodes and sites of inflammation such that Tregs effectively suppress neighboring effector T cells at early or late stages of their differentiation. The latter allows for interference with already established unwanted immunity and may thus be employed to treat rather than prevent unwanted immune reactions.

Characteristics of Regulatory T Cells

Recent years have seen rapid progress in the characterization of Tregs. There is not one particular cell surface marker that defines Tregs but the CD25 surface molecule is at least expressed on the vast majority of cells that express the Foxp3 transcription factor, which has become a signature gene expressed in Tregs. The recognition that CD25+ cells are enriched in Tregs has thus contributed considerably to establishing their role in suppressing activation and function of other lymphocytes [1]. In the mean time, other molecules such as neuropilin-1 [2], CD103 [3], GPR83 [4], GITR [5] and CTL-A4 [6] have been shown to have a characteristic expression profile in Tregs and thus can be helpful in achieving optimal purification in combination with the CD25 marker. Recent evidence shows that CD4+CD25+ Tregs are IL-7R-negative in contrast to CD4+CD25+ cells that just represent activated T cells without obvious regulatory function [7]. Intracellular staining by Foxp3 antibodies represents a useful means to identify Tregs in various tissues [8] and in the mean time various Foxp3 reporter mice [9, 10] have become available which allow functional purification of Foxp3-expressing cells. While Foxp3 expression represents a good signature for Tregs, it can have its drawbacks because Foxp3 can be transiently expressed in activated T cells that, however, do not qualify as stable Tregs [8].

A variety of studies indicate that stable Foxp3 expression is sufficient to confer a regulatory T-cell phenotype to CD4 T cells [11–13]. Thus, retroviral Foxp3 transduction is a valuable means to endow antigen-specific T cells with a regulatory phenotype. This represents an important tool because, unlike the in vitro expansion [14, 15] of Tregs preformed in vivo, it allows to produce Tregs of any desired specificity.

Recent data suggest that Foxp3 can interact with NFAT to regulate gene expression such as downregulation of the IL-2 gene and upregulation of CTL-A4 and CD25 molecules [16]. It is presently not clear whether all Foxp3-dependent gene regulation involves NFAT and whether NFAT plays a crucial role in the generation of Tregs. It has become clear from the combined analysis of Foxp3 binding and genome-wide gene expression, however, that Foxp3 is an activator and a repressor that silences genes that are normally activated after T-cell stimulation, especially genes associated with TCR signaling [17]. This fact may contribute to the relatively poor response of Tregs in response to antigenic stimulation in vitro while exogenous growth factors may permit effective clonal expansion in vivo. The latter feature is likely essential for effective in vivo suppression.

Among the genes that fail to be upregulated in Foxp3-expressing cells is the PTPN22 phosphatase that has a role in dephosphorylating p56^{lck} and Zap-70 [17]. Interestingly, a gain of function mutation of this gene has been postulated to affect several autoimmune diseases and it is presently not clear whether this mutant affects Tregs that control autoimmune disease or effector T cells that cause autoimmune disease [18].

Another important characteristic of Tregs is that they do express an αβTCR that confers antigen specificity. This is worthwhile pointing out since many studies on Tregs ignore this fact. It is our belief that antigen specificity of Tregs is absolutely crucial for antigen-specific suppression of immune responses and hence considerable attention has to be paid to the role of TCR specificity in the generation, homing and effector function of Tregs [19]. As all T cells with αβTCRs, Tregs also undergo stringent TCR-dependent selection in primary and secondary lymphoid organs [20] which eventually may be exploited to generate Tregs of any desired specificity and to interfere specifically with unwanted immune responses in the clinic.

Intra- and Extrathymic Generation of Tregs

Experiments in TCR transgenic mice in which the transgenic TCR was the only TCR expressed by

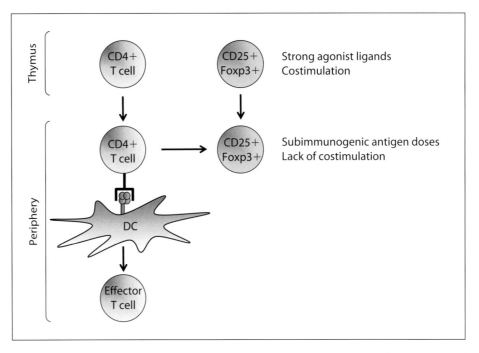

Fig. 1. Pathways of Treg generation in vivo. In addition to the thymus, Treg can also be generated outside the thymus when initially naive CD4+CD25– T cells are stimulated with peptide agonist ligands presented by DCs in peripheral lymphoid organs. Both pathways exhibit specific stimulation and cytokine requirements. The relative contribution of thymic and extrathymic generation to the peripheral Treg pool is currently not known.

developing T cells have clearly shown that ligation of the αβTCR by agonist ligands can play an essential role in the intrathymic generation of Tregs [21, 22]. These results are compatible with analysis of the Treg TCR repertoire in normal mice that were interpreted to indicate a focus on self antigens [23]. It became especially obvious that expression of TCR ligands by thymic epithelial cells represented a powerful means to commit developing CD4+ T cells to the Treg lineage [22]. In this context it is of considerable interest to note that thymic epithelial cells and especially thymic medullary epithelial cells can express 'ectopically' a variety of proteins that otherwise would be considered 'organ-specific' such as preproinsulin-2 that is expressed in pancreatic β cells but also in thymic medullary epithelial cells [24, 25]. Such ectopic expression can be regulated, at least in part, by the AIRE (autoimmune immune regulator) transcription factor [26] and it is thus conceivable that the ectopic expression of 'organ-specific' antigen by thymic epithelium plays a decisive role in the generation of Tregs specific for such antigens, even though experiments addressing that question have so far yielded negative results [27, 28]. However, negative results by no means rule out that AIRE-regulated antigens contribute to the generation of Tregs under more favorable experimental conditions.

The intrathymic generation of Tregs by strong agonist ligands appears to require costimulation of developing cells by B7-1 (CD80) [29] ligands that are expressed on thymic epithelial cells as well as on antigen-presenting cells of hemopoietic origin at least under certain experimental conditions. This is a somewhat astonishing observation in the light of findings that Treg generation in peripheral lymphoid tissue is most effective under conditions that avoid costimulation (see below). Conceivably this could be due to the different stages of development of thymic and extrathymic T cells which may require different signaling inputs for Treg commitment. From thymus transplantation experiments it is clear that Treg generated by ligands expressed on thymic epithelium only, can migrate into peripheral lymphoid tissue and patrol the body for long periods of time without being confronted with the same ligand that was involved in their generation [22, 30]. This does not exclude that lower affinity ligands in peripheral lymphoid tissue may contribute to survival much like they can contribute to survival of CD4 and CD8 conventional T cells [31].

Considering the intrathymic generation of Tregs, it is of interest to note that generation of Tregs from cells with one particular αβTCR is not mutually exclusive to deletion of some of these cells [22]. Thus both processes depend on recognition of agonist ligands by developing CD4+ T cells but under some conditions such recognition results in deletion and under other conditions in Treg generation even within the same thymus, perhaps because some of these cells encounter their TCR ligands on different cells, for instance either on cross-presenting dendritic cells or directly on thymic epithelial cells [32].

Whereas the intrathymic generation of Tregs would mostly depend on instruction of lineage commitment by self antigens, the peripheral generation of Tregs may also include instruction by foreign antigens. It is therefore of considerable interest to define conditions permissible for extrathymic Treg generation. To this end we have exploited protocols of subimmunogenic antigen presentation because circumstantial and historic evidence suggested that one might be able to induce 'dominant' tolerance in this way. Indeed it was found that either constant delivery of peptides by osmotic mini-pumps [33] or by targeting dendritic cells with peptide-containing fusion antibodies directed against the DEC205 endocytic receptor on dendritic cells [8] allowed the conversion of naive T cells into Foxp3 Tregs. The conversion process depended on an intact TGF-βRII receptor on naive T cells, i.e. was TGF-β-dependent, and conditions that avoided activation of dendritic cells as well as IL-2 production by naive T cells. It was clear that Tregs were generated by conversion rather than expansion of already committed Tregs since the experiments were performed in mice expressing only one particular transgenic TCR in the absence of coexpression of a TCR agonist ligand resulting in the unique constellation that none of the generated CD4+ T cells exhibited initially a Treg phenotype and only a certain percentage (~30%) assumed it after the artificial introduction of the respective TCR agonist ligand [8].

The generation of Treg by subimmunogenic antigen delivery and the negative impact of strong costimulation on conversion of naive T cells into Treg [8] correlates with the fact that costimulation results in the accumulation of Fos and Jun containing AP-1 that interacts with NFAT and thereby blocks the formation of a Foxp3-NFAT complex that is required for the generation of functional Treg [16]. The latter data are well in line with the observation that Foxp3 overexpression in T-cell hybridomas, that are not activated through their TCR results in weak binding of Foxp3 to target genes but very little regulation of target genes, while in contrast activation of such hybridomas results in activation as well as Foxp3-dependent down- and upregulation of genes [17]. Thus, TCR signals and Foxp3 need to synergize in the generation of functional Tregs [16, 17], but it is unclear at present whether a Foxp3-NFAT complex has an essential role in the generation of Treg.

Importantly, the peripherally generated Tregs exhibited a similar global gene expression pattern as intrathymically generated Tregs [32] and much like intrathymically generated Tregs exhibited a long lifespan that was independent on further supply of the TCR agonist ligand. Thus by these maneuvers a Treg 'memory' to external TCR ligands could be induced, resulting in the subsequent suppression of immune responses elicited by the same agonist ligand, i.e. this protocol succeeded in generating specific immunological tolerance. Hopefully this protocol can be extended to many other antigens and thus help the prevention of unwanted immune responses. Recently some of us [39] succeeded in inducing transplantation tolerance in wild-type female mice by infusing them with male peptide, resulting in the generation of male-specific Foxp3+ Tregs. Of note, this particular protocol only works with naive T cells and not with T cells that have been already activated in vivo. Thus, the induction of Treg can presumably not be used to suppress already established autoimmunity in which most antigen-specific T cells are already activated. In such cases the in vitro generation of Tregs by Foxp3 transduction would likely be more appropriate (see below) [32].

Recently it has been reported that retinoic acid generated in CD103+ DC in the gut helps the conversion of naive T cells into Foxp3+ Tregs thereby giving credibility to the disputed concept of oral tolerance [34–37]. Interestingly, retinoic acid appears to interfere with the negative effect of costimulation on TGF-β-dependent conversion of naive T cells into Tregs [37] providing a possible mechanism for its effect, since by itself in the absence of TGF-β retinoic acid does not affect conversion. Thus, there is an interesting difference between intra- and extrathymic Treg generation: while the former requires costimulation and takes place even in the absence of TGF-β, the latter is essentially dependent on TGF-β and takes place in the absence of costimulation. It is worthwhile pointing out that even in the presence of retinoic acid, the TGF-β-dependent conversion works effectively only with naive T cells

while preactivated T cells, perhaps because of their high AP-1 content, are relatively resistant to a TCR-induced conversion process.

At present one can only speculate why costimulation interferes with the upregulation of Foxp3 in naive T cells: it may be that AP-1 interferes with regulation of the Foxp3 locus by TCR and TGF-β-dependent signals that eventually results in stable Foxp3 expression. Whether it does so by interfering with the action of TGF-β-induced Foxp3 regulation or autoregulation by Foxp3 is unknown. It is also possible that AP-1 interferes somehow with demethylation of the Foxp3 locus. In this context it is of interest to note that the slow in vivo conversion process generates long-lived and stable Foxp3-expressing Tregs whereas the conversion process in vitro utilizing costimulation and TGF-β often results in cells with unstable Foxp3 expression, at least when these cells are analyzed during antigenic stimulation. The stability of Foxp3 expression was shown to correlate with the degree of demethylation of Foxp3.

Function of Tregs

One question to which the answer has remained rather elusive concerns the molecular mechanisms by which Tregs control other T cells. There are probably several not mutually exclusive mechanisms, some of which may dominate in certain situations [19]. In vitro data have emphasized the role of close cell-to-cell contact and dispensable cytokines such as IL-10 or TGF-β. All in vivo data published so far have emphasized the crucial role of the TGF-βRII on suppressed cells since a dominant negative form of that receptor is usually associated with ineffective Treg suppression and with generalized autoimmunity. It is still not clear whether this results from the fact that Tregs produce TGF-β (which they do but only in moderate amounts) or whether in general TGF-β-induced signaling 'conditions' effector cells for more stringent suppression by a mechanism that does not involve increased TGF-β production but depends on specific Treg activation [19]. A good example for such a scenario is the suppression of tumor-specific CD8 T cells by CD4 Tregs that crucially depends on an intact TGF-βRII receptor on the CD8 T cells. In this particular model the suppression affects the function of fully differentiated cytotoxic T lymphocytes (CTL), notably the secretion of cytolytic granules. However, in vitro experiments with fully differentiated CTL have shown that TGF-β does not have any negative impact on cytolysis when added during the effector phase. This is consistent with the hypothesis that TGF-β-dependent signaling 'conditions' the CD8 T cells for Treg suppression rather than representing the sole suppressor mechanism [38].

These experiments also make another important point, namely that it is apparently never too late to interfere with an immune response by Treg suppression since the experiments show that suppression can affect fully differentiated effector cells. This is good news in the sense that the obviously effective suppression late during an immune response can revert rather than prevent unwanted immunity, a concept that may become extremely useful in the clinic.

Different experiments attempting to reverse rather than prevent diabetes are fully consistent with that view: CD4 T cells specific for an islet-derived antigen of unknown nature could be activated in vitro and retrovirally transduced with Foxp3 such that within 24 h they assumed a phenotype of Tregs. When 10^5 of such converted cells were injected into NOD mice that had just become diabetic because of beginning destruction of their islet cells, these islet-specific Tregs cured the mice of diabetes and they remained diabetes-free for at least 3 months when the experiment was terminated. Again, this experiment suggests that Tregs can silence already fully developed effector cells [13].

Additional controls make important points with regard to the role of Treg antigen receptors in this process and hence the specificity of immunosuppression: while the injection of 10^5 cells with islet-antigen specificity was sufficient to abolish disease, the injection of 10^6 Tregs with specificity for a large variety of different antigens or the injection of Tregs with specificity for an antigen not present in the pancreatic lymph node did not have any effect and the animals died several days later from complete destruction of β cells and resulting diabetes that obviously at this point could be no longer reversed by Tregs [13]. Thus, antigen specificity of Tregs which permits specific activation and homing plays an important role in suppression of autoimmune disease. These results and similar results by others employing in vitro expanded Tregs [14, 15] are very encouraging since they suggest that by adoptive Treg therapy early-diagnosed diabetes may be cured, in spite of the fact that the generation of sufficient numbers of islet-antigen-specific Tregs still represents a staggering logistic problem.

In spite of our ignorance concerning molecular mechanisms of Treg-mediated suppression (even though a variety have been proposed [19]), we have promising evidence from murine models of disease that Tregs have the capacity to interfere with unwanted immunity early and/or late during the immune response in an antigen-specific way since they interfere with such immunity in a local milieu only while leaving the remainder of the immune system intact.

There is also no compelling reason why the findings made in the somewhat popular models of type 1 diabetes should not be extended to other autoimmune diseases such as rheumatic diseases provided that there are clues about relevant antigens that are presented in local lymphoid tissue.

Concluding Remarks

The described properties of Tregs, i.e. the possibility to generate them extrathymically in vivo or in vitro with any desired antigen specificity, their ability to co-home with T-effector cells into antigen-draining lymph nodes and/or sites of inflammation, their potential to suppress effector cells at early and late stages of differentiation and last but not least to suppress neighboring T-effector cells of any antigenic specificity, make these cells an ideal tool to intervene with unwanted immunity in an antigen-specific way. Thus one would eventually hope that the exploitation of evolutionarily selected mechanisms to deal with unwanted immune responses against self will replace indiscriminatory immunosuppression by drugs with potentially deadly side effects. This is not to say that such drugs may be completely useless: their transient application may help to set the immune system to a stage where Tregs can be more effective in dealing specifically with unwanted immunity. What should be avoided, however, is the long-term indiscriminatory use of the drugs that eventually will ruin the protection against infections and malignant disease afforded by the immune system.

References

1   Itoh M, Takahashi T, Sakaguchi N, Kuniyasu Y, Shimizu J, Otsuka F, Sakaguchi S: Thymus and autoimmunity: production of CD25+CD4+ naturally anergic and suppressive T cells as a key function of the thymus in maintaining immunologic self-tolerance. J Immunol 1999;162:5317–5326.

2   Bruder D, Probst-Kepper M, Westendorf AM, Geffers R, Beissert S, Loser K, von Boehmer H, Buer J, Hansen W: Neuropilin-1: a surface marker of regulatory T cells. Eur J Immunol 2004;34:623–630.

3   Huehn J, Siegmund K, Lehmann JC, Siewert C, Haubold U, Feuerer M, Debes GF, Lauber J, Frey O, Przybylski GK, Niesner U, de la Rosa M, Schmidt CA, Brauer R, Buer J, Scheffold A, Hamann A: Developmental stage, phenotype, and migration distinguish naive- and effector/memory-like CD4+ regulatory T cells. J Exp Med 2004;199:303–313.

4   Hansen W, Loser K, Westendorf AM, Bruder D, Pfoertner S, Siewert C, Huehn J, Beissert S, Buer J: G-protein-coupled receptor 83 overexpression in naive CD4+CD25– T cells leads to the induction of Foxp3+ regulatory T cells in vivo. J Immunol 2006;177:209–215.

5   Shimizu J, Yamazaki S, Takahashi T, Ishida Y, Sakaguchi S: Stimulation of CD25+CD4+ regulatory T cells through GITR breaks immunological self-tolerance. Nat Immunol 2002;3:135–142.

6   Bachmann MF, Kohler G, Ecabert B, Mak TW, Kopf M: Cutting edge: lymphoproliferative disease in the absence of CTLA-4 is not T cell autonomous. J Immunol 1999;163:1128–1131.

7   Liu W, Putnam AL, Xu-Yu Z, Szot GL, Lee MR, Zhu S, Gottlieb PA, Kapranov P, Gingeras TR, de St Groth BF, Clayberger C, Soper DM, Ziegler SF, Bluestone JA: CD127 expression inversely correlates with FoxP3 and suppressive function of human CD4+ Treg cells. J Exp Med 2006;203:1701–1711.

8   Kretschmer K, Apostolou I, Hawiger D, Khazaie K, Nussenzweig MC, von Boehmer H: Inducing and expanding regulatory T cell populations by foreign antigen. Nat Immunol 2005;6:1219–1227.

9   Fontenot JD, Rasmussen JP, Williams LM, Dooley JL, Farr AG, Rudensky AY: Regulatory T cell lineage specification by the forkhead transcription factor Foxp3. Immunity 2005;22:329–341.

10 Wan YY, Flavell RA: Identifying Foxp3-expressing suppressor T cells with a bicistronic reporter. Proc Natl Acad Sci USA 2005;102:5126–5131.

11 Hori S, Nomura T, Sakaguchi S: Control of regulatory T cell development by the transcription factor Foxp3. Science 2003;299:1057–1061.

12 Fontenot JD, Gavin MA, Rudensky AY: Foxp3 programs the development and function of CD4+CD25+ regulatory T cells. Nat Immunol 2003;4:330–336.

13 Jaeckel E, von Boehmer H, Manns MP: Antigen-specific Foxp3-transduced T-cells can control established type 1 diabetes. Diabetes 2005;54:306–310.

14 Tang Q, Henriksen KJ, Bi M, Finger EB, Szot G, Ye J, Masteller EL, McDevitt H, Bonyhadi M, Bluestone JA: In vitro-expanded antigen-specific regulatory T cells suppress autoimmune diabetes. J Exp Med 2004;199:1455–1465.

15 Tarbell KV, Yamazaki S, Olson K, Toy P, Steinman RM: CD25+CD4+ T cells, expanded with dendritic cells presenting a single autoantigenic peptide, suppress autoimmune diabetes. J Exp Med 2004;199:1467–1477.

16 Wu Y, Borde M, Heissmeyer V, Feuerer M, Lapan AD, Stroud JC, Bates DL, Guo L, Han A, Ziegler SF, Mathis D, Benoist C, Chen L, Rao A: Foxp3 controls regulatory T cell function through cooperation with NFAT. Cell 2006;126:375–387.

17 Marson A, Kretschmer K, Frampton GM, Jacobsen ES, Polansky JK, MacIsaac KD, Levine SS, Fraenkel E, von Boehmer H, Young RA: Foxp3 occupancy and regulation of key target genes during T-cell stimulation. Nature 2007;445:931–935.

18 Bottini N, Vang T, Cucca F, Mustelin T: Role of PTPN22 in type 1 diabetes and other autoimmune diseases. Semin Immunol 2006;18:207–213.

19 Von Boehmer H: Mechanisms of suppression by suppressor T cells. Nat Immunol 2005;6:338–344.

20 Von Boehmer H: Selection of the T-cell repertoire: receptor-controlled checkpoints in T-cell development. Adv Immunol 2004;84:201–238.

21 Jordan MS, Boesteanu A, Reed AJ, Petrone AL, Holenbeck AE, Lerman MA, Naji A, Caton AJ: Thymic selection of CD4+CD25+ regulatory T cells induced by an agonist self peptide. Nat Immunol 2001;2:301–306.

22 Apostolou I, Sarukhan A, Klein L, von Boehmer H: Origin of regulatory T cells with known specificity for antigen. Nat Immunol 2002;3:756–763.

23 Hsieh CS, Liang Y, Tyznik AJ, Self SG, Liggitt D, Rudensky AY: Recognition of the peripheral self by naturally arising CD25+CD4+ T cell receptors. Immunity 2004;21:267–277.

24 Derbinski J, Schulte A, Kyewski B, Klein L: Promiscuous gene expression in medullary thymic epithelial cells mirrors the peripheral self. Nat Immunol 2001;2:1032–1039.

25 Vafiadis P, Bennett ST, Todd JA, Nadeau J, Grabs R, Goodyer CG, Wickramasinghe S, Colle E, Polychronakos C: Insulin expression in human thymus is modulated by INS VNTR alleles at the IDDM2 locus. Nat Genet 1997;15:289–292.

26 Anderson MS, Venanzi ES, Klein L, Chen Z, Berzins SP, Turley SJ, von Boehmer H, Bronson R, Dierich A, Benoist C, Mathis D: Projection of an immunological self shadow within the thymus by the AIRE protein. Science 2002;298:1395–1401.

27 Liston A, Gray DH, Lesage S, Fletcher AL, Wilson J, Webster KE, Scott HS, Boyd RL, Peltonen L, Goodnow CC: Gene dosage-limiting role of AIRE in thymic expression, clonal deletion, and organ-specific autoimmunity. J Exp Med 2004;200:1015–1026.

28 Anderson MS, Venanzi ES, Chen Z, Berzins SP, Benoist C, Mathis D: The cellular mechanism of AIRE control of T cell tolerance. Immunity 2005;23:227–239.

29 Tai X, Cowan M, Feigenbaum L, Singer A: CD28 costimulation of developing thymocytes induces Foxp3 expression and regulatory T cell differentiation independently of interleukin-2. Nat Immunol 2005;6:152–162.

30 Klein L, Khazaie K, von Boehmer H: In vivo dynamics of antigen-specific regulatory T cells not predicted from behavior in vitro. Proc Natl Acad Sci USA 2003;100:8886–8891.

31 Hao Y, Legrand N, Freitas AA: The clone size of peripheral CD8 T cells is regulated by TCR promiscuity. J Exp Med 2006;203:1643–1649.

32 Kretschmer K, Apostolou I, Jaeckel E, Khazaie K, von Boehmer H: Making regulatory T cells with defined antigen specificity: role in autoimmunity and cancer. Immunol Rev 2006;212:163–169.

33 Apostolou I, Von Boehmer H: In vivo instruction of suppressor commitment in naive T cells. J Exp Med 2004;199:1401–1408.

34 Coombes JL, Siddiqui KR, Arancibia-Carcamo CV, Hall J, Sun CM, Belkaid Y, Powrie F: A functionally specialized population of mucosal CD103+ DCs induces Foxp3+ regulatory T cells via a TGF-β and retinoic acid-dependent mechanism. J Exp Med 2007;204:1757–1764.

35 Sun CM, Hall JA, Blank RB, Bouladoux N, Oukka M, Mora JR, Belkaid Y: Small intestine lamina propria dendritic cells promote de novo generation of Foxp3 Treg cells via retinoic acid. J Exp Med 2007;204:1775–1785.

36 Benson MJ, Pino-Lagos K, Rosemblatt M, Noelle RJ: All-trans retinoic acid mediates enhanced Treg cell growth, differentiation, and gut homing in the face of high levels of co-stimulation. J Exp Med 2007;204:1765–1774.

37 Von Boehmer H: Oral tolerance: is it all retinoic acid? J Exp Med 2007;204:1737–1739.

38 Mempel TR, Pittet MJ, Khazaie K, Weninger W, Weissleder R, von Boehmer H, von Andrian UH: Regulatory T cells reversibly suppress cytotoxic T cell function independent of effector differentiation. Immunity 2006;25:129–141.

39 Verginis P, McLaughlin KA, Wucherpfennig KW, von Boehmer H, Apostolou I: Induction of antigen-specific regulatory T cells in wild-type mice: visualization and targets of suppression. Proc Natl Acad Sci USA 2008;105:3479–3484.

Harald von Boehmer
Harvard Medical School, Dana-Farber Cancer Institute
44 Binney Street, Boston, MA 02115 (USA)
Tel. +1 617 632 6880, Fax +1 617 632 6881
E-Mail Harald_von_Boehmer@dfci.harvard.edu

Blaser K (ed): T Cell Regulation in Allergy, Asthma and Atopic Skin Diseases.
Chem Immunol Allergy. Basel, Karger, 2008, vol 94, pp 16–28

Molecular Mechanisms of Regulatory T-Cell Development

Talal A. Chatila

Division of Immunology, Allergy and Rheumatology, Department of Pediatrics,
The David Geffen School of Medicine at the University of California at Los Angeles,
Los Angeles, Calif., USA

Abstract

CD4+CD25+ natural regulatory T (nT_R) lymphocytes represent a separate, thymus-derived T-cell lineage that is essential to the maintenance of immunological tolerance in the host. Their deficiency or dysfunction has been implicated in the pathogenesis of allergic and autoimmune diseases. The discovery of Foxp3 as a transcription factor essential to the differentiation of CD4+CD25+ T_R cells ushered detailed studies into the molecular mechanisms of T_R cell development, peripheral homeostasis and effector functions. A second group of induced T_R (iT_R) cells can be derived de novo from conventional CD4+ T cells upon antigenic stimulation in the presence of TGF-β and IL-2. This process is especially active at the mucosal interface in the gut, and plays a critical role in the induction of oral tolerance to allergens and other antigens. Augmentation of T_R cells by immunotherapy and pharmacologic agents is a promising strategy in the treatment of allergic and autoimmune diseases.

Regulatory T (T_R) cells represent a distinct T-cell lineage that plays a key role in tolerance to self antigen and prevention of autoimmune diseases, as well as in inappropriate immune responses involved in allergic diseases [1–3]. T_R cells are characterized by a set of phenotypic and functional attributes that distinguish them from conventional T (T_{conv}) cells: they are predominantly CD4+ CD25+, T-cell receptor (TCR) $\alpha\beta$+. T_R cells are anergic and do not produce IL-2 [reviewed in 4]. When activated, they suppress the proliferation and cytokine production of conventional CD4+ CD25− T cells as well as that of CD8+ T cells and established Th1 and Th2 cells [5–8]. CD4+ CD25+T_R cells produce TGF-β and IL-10, two cytokines endowed with immunosuppressive functions and which play critical functions in T_R cell biology. The majority of peripheral T_R cells are programmed in the thymus and are known as natural T_R (nT_R) cells [3]. Other T_R cells known as induced or adaptive (iT_R) cells are derived de novo from a naive CD4+ precursor pool in peripheral lymphoid tissues after encountering exogenous antigen under the influence of TGF-β. Intense effort has gone into defining the molecular events that guide T_R cells through development and lineage commitment, and those that enable the acquisition and maintenance of T_R cell phenotypic and functional attributes. The recent advances made in elucidating those pathways are reviewed below.

Role of Foxp3 in T_R Cell Function

While T_R cells are characterized by the expression of a distinctive combination of surface antigens including CD25, CTLA-4 and GITR, the cardinal hallmark of a T_R cell is the forkhead-family transcription factor forkhead box p3 (Foxp3), which is indispensable to their suppressive activity, phenotype stability and survival in the periphery [3]. Loss of function mutations in the Foxp3 gene underlie the lymphoproliferative disease of the scurfy mouse and the homologous autoimmune lymphoproliferative disorder in man, termed immune dysregulation polyendocrinopathy enteropathy X-linked syndrome (IPEX). In both mice and humans, female carriers are asymptomatic, consistent with X-linked recessive inheritance. The immunopathology of Foxp3 deficiency results from unchecked T-cell activation due to the lack of regulatory restraint by CD4+CD25+ T_R cells [9, 10]. That Foxp3 is essential for T_R cell function is supported by the observation that forced expression of Foxp3 in effector T cells endows them with regulatory properties and some, but not all, of the phenotypic markers of T_R cells [11, 12]. Also, adoptive transfer of CD4+CD25+ T_R cells rescues scurfy mice from disease, and Foxp3-transduced CD4+CD25− T cells suppressed wasting and colitis induced by the transfer of CD4+CD25− T cells into RAG−/− mice [11, 13]. While there are reports of Foxp3 expression in non-lymphoid tissues such as mammary epithelial cells, the function of Foxp3 in immune regulation could be specifically attributed to its expression in T cells, as T-cell-specific disruption of *Foxp3* reproduces the full manifestation of global Foxp3 deficiency [14]. These results established an essential function for Foxp3 in CD4+CD25+ T_R development.

Foxp3 deficiency is permissive to the development in the thymus of T_R cell precursors that share many of the phenotypic and genetic attributes of T_R cells. However, unlike Foxp3-sufficient T_R cells, Foxp3-deficient T_R cell precursors fail to mediate suppression [15, 16]. Once in the periphery, they acquire attributes of an activated cytotoxic cell phenotype. They express high levels of mRNA encoding granzymes, some killer cell markers and a mixed Th1 and Th2 cytokine profile. In particular, they secrete large amounts of IL-4 and other Th2 cytokines, which accounts for much of the allergic dysregulation associated with Foxp3 deficiency [15–17]. Circulating Foxp3-deficient T_R cell precursors also exhibit a high rate of apoptotic death, possibly due to suboptimal response to growth factors such as IL-2. The continued requirement for Foxp3 expression to maintain the phenotype of mature T_R cell in the periphery was demonstrated in experiments in which the acute inactivation of the Foxp3 locus rapidly led to the loss of T_R cell regulatory function. Acute Foxp3 deficiency also alters the transcriptional program of T_R cells in a manner reminiscent of that of Foxp3-deficient T_R cell precursors [18].

Molecular Mechanisms of nT_R Cell Development in the Thymus

nTR cells develop in the thymus and are almost exclusively TCR $\alpha\beta$+. Several studies have sought to establish the nature of the TCR ligands and the signaling pathways that induce the development of the CD4+CD25+ nT_R cells in the thymus. These studies, which relied upon TCR transgenic mice that also expressed the cognate antigen, suggested an 'instructive' model of nT_R cell development, whereby the development of CD4+CD25+ nT_R in the thymus was driven by 'higher' avidity interactions between the developing T cell and the thymic epithelium [19–24]. In this model, the avidity window for T_R cell selection is narrow and shifted, residing between that required for the positive and negative selection of CD4+CD25− T cells. This would limit the number of nT_R cells that develop, and would favor a regulatory function for those peripheral T cells expressing TCRs with the greatest affinity for self peptide/MHC complexes, thereby avoiding auto-immunity [25]. More recently, a refinement of the instructive model was proposed whereby TCR signaling primes a CD25+ Foxp3− CD4-SP population to become responsive to the γc cytokines IL-2 and IL-15, which in turn upregulate Foxp3 expression [26, 27].

A TCR-based instructive model would suggest that the repertoires of T_R cell and CD4+ T_{conv} cells may be different. Several studies using transgenic approaches in mice that limit rearrangement diversity have supported such a conclusion, finding the T_R cell and T_{conv} cell TCR repertoires to be equally diverse yet substantially different, with most studies finding only a modest overlap in CDR3 amino acid sequences [28–31]. However, an alternative stochastic-selective model of nT_R cell lineage commitment has been proposed whereby the decision to become an nT_R cell occurs early in thymocyte development prior to negative selection. In this model, the promotion of CD4+CD25+ T_R cell development by agonistic ligands reflects their relative resistance to negative selection as compared to CD4+CD25− T cells [32]. Studies demonstrating that the antigen specificity of nT_R cells is no more skewed towards self antigens than T_{conv} cells were also interpreted to argue against an instructive model of nT_R cell development driven by high avidity to self antigens [33]. A non-instructive model of nT_R cell development has been proposed that invokes transacting factors that act on CD4−CD8− developing thymocytes [34]. It is quite possible that nT_R cells development may involve a combination of early stochastic-selective events that endow a developing thymocyte with the potential to develop into an nT_R cell, followed by TCR-dependent instructive events that allows the realization of that potential.

Function of Foxp3 in nT_R Cell Development

The function of Foxp3 in nT_R cell development was recently examined in mice harboring locus-tagged wild-type or mutant Foxp3 allele, which allowed comparative analysis of nT_R cell development in the presence or absence or a functional Foxp3 protein. In our own studies, a cassette encoding a mutant, non-functional Foxp3-enhanced green fluorescent protein (EGFP) was engineered within the Foxp3 locus ($Foxp3^{\Delta EGFP}$). The development of EGFP+ thymocyte precursors in $Foxp3^{\Delta EGFP}$ mice was compared to that in mice harboring an EGFP-tagged Foxp3 allele that expresses the wild-type Foxp3 protein ($Foxp3^{EGFP}$) [16]. The total number of EGFP+ cells in CD4 single positive (SP) compartment of $Foxp3^{EGFP}$ (wild-type) or the $Foxp3^{\Delta EGFP}$ (mutant) mice was found to be similar. The cell surface phenotype of the EGFP+ CD4-SP wild-type and mutant populations was also similar. However, the mutant cells were totally lacking in suppressor function. Using a slightly different approach to generate T_R precursor cells that lacked Foxp3 but expressed EGFP, another group arrived at a similar conclusion [15]. These results indicated that nT_R cell lineage commitment occurs prior to, and independent of Foxp3 expression, but that Foxp3 expression is essential for the mature, differentiated functions of nT_R cells.

Transcriptional Regulation by Foxp3

Foxp3 was initially thought to function as a transcriptional repressor [35]. However, it has become clear that Foxp3 may function as either a transcriptional activator or repressor depending on the context [36, 37]. The transcriptional functions of Foxp3 are enabled by the capacity of its different domains to interact with distinct sets of regulatory proteins to form large macromolecular transcriptional complexes. An N-terminal domain that mediates transcriptional activation and repression associates with the histone acetyltransferase TIP60 (Tat-interactive protein, 60 kDa) and class II histone deacetylases HDAC7 and HDAC9 [38]. A zinc finger and leucine zipper

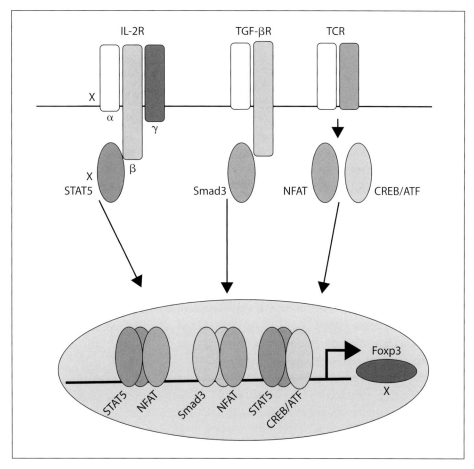

Fig. 1. Transcriptional circuitries in T_R cells. Activation of the Foxp3 promoter/enhancer. Signaling by the TCR/NFAT, IL-2/STAT5 and TGF-β/Smad3 pathways converge on the Foxp3 promoter/enhancer to efficiently activate Foxp3 gene expression. X denotes genetic defects associated with IPEX (Foxp3) and IPEX-like syndromes (IL-2Rα chain and STAT5b).

domains mediate a second set of interactions, with the leucine zipper domain being especially important for homo- and heteroligmerization of Foxp3 with related members of the Foxp family [39]. The distal part of the protein includes a carboxyl-terminal forkhead domain that mediates binding to specific DNA response elements. It also includes residues that contribute to the physical association of Foxp3 with other transcription factors including the nuclear factor of activated T cells (NFAT) and Runx1/AMl1, both of which contribute to the transcriptional program and suppressive functions of T_R cells [40, 41] (fig. 1). An isoform of Foxp3 is expressed that lacks an N-terminal domain 33-amino-acid peptide encoded by exon 2. This isoform is ineffective in conferring regulatory function upon its expression in T_{conv} cells [42].

The Foxp3 Transcriptional Program and the T_R Cell Transcriptosome

T_R cells isolated from lymphoid organs are endowed with a distinct genetic signature, characterized by a reproducible set of canonical transcripts that together distinguish T_R from T_{conv} cells [43]. These transcripts include *Il2ra, Ctla4, Itgae, CD83, gpr83, Gzmb, Helios, Icos, Il1r2, Il1rl1, Klrg1, S100a4, S100a6, Tiam1, Tnfrsf4, Tnfrsf9* and *Tnfrsf18* [43–46]. The role of Foxp3 in the formation of the T_R cell transcriptosome was analyzed by comparing the expression profiles of CD4+EGFP+ cells of *Foxp3*^{EGFP} mice, whose T_R cells co-express a normal Foxp3 protein and EGFP, and those of *Foxp3*$^{\Delta EGFP}$ mice, which express an inactive Foxp3-EGFP fusion protein. The transcriptosome of the respective cell type was compared to that CD4+EGFP$^-$ T_{conv} cells of *Foxp3*^{EGFP} mice. Strikingly, the analysis revealed that the majority of genes previously identified to constitute a T_R cell genetic signature were shared among the two populations. These results lead to the surprising conclusion that acquisition of the nT_R cell genetic signature is largely independent of Foxp3 activity.

Insight into the Foxp3-dependent component of the T_R cell genetic signature was gained by directly comparing the gene expression profiles of CD4+EGFP+ T cells from *Foxp3*^{EGFP} and *Foxp3*$^{\Delta EGFP}$ mice. Surprisingly, few transcripts characteristic of the T_R cell genetic signature were overexpressed at ≥2-fold in CD4+EGFP+ T cells of *Foxp3*^{EGFP} as compared to *Foxp3*$^{\Delta EGFP}$ mice. The most prominent member of this group was *Itgae* (about 3-fold enrichment). *Il2ra, Ctla4, Gpr83* and *Npl1* were also enriched but at more modest levels (<2-fold), consistent with the potentiation by Foxp3 of their transcription. In contrast, CD4+EGFP+ T cells of *Foxp3*$^{\Delta EGFP}$ mice overexpressed genes encoding numerous cell cycle regulators, consistent with their intense proliferation. Of particular interest was the marked overexpression in CD4+EGFP+ T cells

from *Foxp3*$^{\Delta EGFP}$ mice of genes associated with a cytotoxic effector program including those encoding granzymes the inhibitory receptor gp49b *Lilrb4, Slamf7* (Cracc), *Nkg7, Lgals3* (galectin 3), *Fasl* (Fas ligand) *Cd160* and the transcription factor *Tbx21*, a key regulator of Th1 differentiation in CD4+ T cells and the cytotoxic effector programs of CD8+, natural killer and natural killer T cells [47]. CD4+EGFP+ T cells from *Foxp3*$^{\Delta EGFP}$ mice also overexpressed a number of cytokine genes, most notably *Il4, Ifng* and *Il21*, and in lower amounts *Ebi3* (encodes IL-27) and *Tnfsf14* (encodes LIGHT). They also exhibited a profile of chemokine and chemokine receptor gene expression associated with tissue-infiltrating inflammatory T cells, including *Cxcr6, Ccl1, Ccl3, Ccl4,* and *Ccl5* [48]. Together, these data indicated that while Foxp3 does not direct the acquisition of nT_R cell genetic signature, it reinforces it and accordingly acts to 'fix' the phenotype of nT_R cells [15, 16, 36, 37].

Analysis of the genes directly bound by Foxp3 revealed that they constitute only a subset of the T_R cell transcriptosome, indicating that much of the effect of Foxp3 on the T-cell transcriptosome occurs indirectly through its modulation of the expression of other transcriptional factors [36, 37]. Thus a critical mechanism by which Foxp3 stabilizes the phenotype of T_R cells in the periphery is by coordinating and reinforcing transcriptional circuitries activated by key T_R cell signaling pathways, including the TCR and the cytokines IL-2 and TGF-β [49, 50]. Foxp3 upregulates the expression of components of the IL-2 signaling pathway, most notably the IL-2 receptor α-chain (CD25). It similarly upregulates expression of TGF-β signaling components, including TGF-β receptor II. Foxp3 also potentiates TGF-β signaling by promoting the retention in the nucleus of TGF-β-responsive Smad transcription factors (fig. 1) [49, 50]. In turn, those pathways upregulate Foxp3 expression and maintain T_R cells in a fit condition. A target of Foxp3 is the Foxp3 gene itself, which is endowed with a number of forkhead factor response elements [15]. Foxp3 deficiency is associated with decreased Foxp3 expression in the T_R cell precursors that do develop, consistent with autoinduction of Foxp3 by a positive feedback loop.

One of the persisting enigmas not clarified by the gene expression studies is the nature of the suppressor mechanism(s) endowed on T_R cells by Foxp3. Functional studies have revealed several candidate mechanisms including cell contact and cytoxicity-dependent suppression, cytokine (IL-10, TGF-β) dependent regulation, cell surface marker dependent suppression (CTLA-4), and an IL-2 'sink' effect that deprives T_{conv} cells of IL-2 [51, 52]. However, gene array studies have failed to satisfactory correlate T_R cell suppressor mechanisms with Foxp3 expression. Specifically, the expression of components of these pathways such as the granzymes and IL-10 persists in the absence of a functional Foxp3, suggesting the presence of additional components or alternative pathways through which Foxp3 enables suppression [16].

Transcriptional Regulation of *Foxp3*

Details of the mechanisms governing the induction of Foxp3 expression in nT_R cells in the thymus and iT_R cells in the periphery remain sketchy. The Foxp3 promoter contains binding sites for several transcription factors that have been linked to signaling pathways involved in inducible Foxp3 expression, including NFAT, Sp1, AP-1 CREB/ATF and STAT5 (fig. 2) [53–55]. An evolutionary conserved Foxp3 enhancer that binds NFAT and Smad3, allowing responsiveness to TCR and TGF-β signaling, respectively [56]. Concerted action of NFAT and Smad3 is required for histone H4 acetylation of the enhancer region and for Foxp3 induction. TGF-β is important for induction of iT_R cells and for the maintenance of T_R cells in the periphery, but is dispensable for the induction of nT_R cells in the thymus [57].

Whether alternative pathways of Smad3 activation occur in developing nT_R cells the thymus (through the agency of activins or bone morphogenic proteins), or whether Smad3-independent pathways of Foxp3 induction are operative the thymus remains to be established.

nT_R versus iT_R Cells

T_R cells are unique among the effector T-cell subsets in being comprised of two developmentally distinct populations: nT_R cells, which develop in the thymus and adaptive or induced iT_R cells that are induced de novo in the periphery from T_{conv} cells. The two populations display a close affinity in their regulatory function and phenotype, but are not identical. The phenotypic and genetic attributes of nT_R cells are 'hard-wired', with most them persisting even in the absence of Foxp3. This is reflection of an irreversible commitment to the T_R cell lineage that occurs in the course of thymic selection and maturation of nT_R cells. In contrast, iT_R cells are 'plastic', developing upon antigenic stimulation of T_{conv} cells in the presence of TGF-β and IL-2 (fig. 2) [58–61]. Foxp3, whose expression in iT_R cells is induced by the action of TGF-β and TCR signaling, is absolutely required for the suppressive functions of iT_R cells, similar to the situation of their iT_R cells counterparts [D. Haribhai, T.A. Chatila and C.B. Williams, unpubl. observations]. iT_R cells have been demonstrated to develop during induction of oral tolerance, to an allergen and may play an important role in tolerance induction in immunotherapy [62, 63]. Their phenotype, however, is less stable than that of nT_R cells. Whereas the Foxp3 locus is stably hypomethylated in nT_R cells, it is weakly so in adaptive T_R cells [64]. The suppressive function and Foxp3 expression levels of the latter may accordingly decline over time.

One of the important recent developments in understanding the development of iT_R cells is the emergence of an important role for retinoic acid

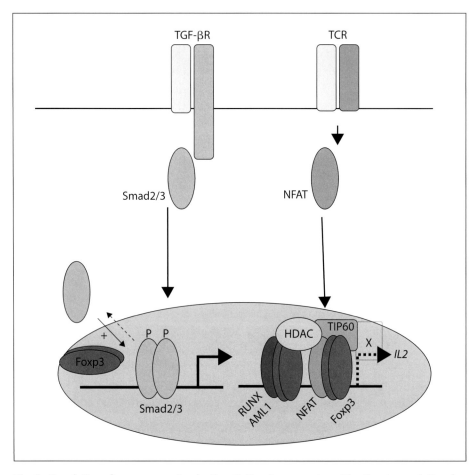

Fig. 2. Regulation of gene expression by Foxp3. Foxp3 cooperates with other transcription factors, including NFAT and RUNX1/AML1, to suppress transcription of a number of genes (e.g. *IL2*) and activate others. It also potentiates transcriptional activation by the TGF-βR pathway, in part by promoting the retention of phosphorylated Smad2/3 proteins in the nucleus [49, 50].

in this process. It is well established that the induction of oral tolerance is associated with the in situ production of Foxp3+ iT_R cells. The in situ conversion of naive T cells into iT_R cells, which takes place upon antigen presentation by CD103+ dendritic cells in gut-associated lymphoid tissue and is strictly TGF-β-dependent, is greatly augmented by retinoic acid, and reciprocally antagonized by inhibitors of retinal dehydrogenase (fig. 3) [65–69]. Importantly, retinoic acid inhibits the IL-6-driven programming of

TGF-β-treated T cells into pro-inflammatory Th17 cells in favor of iT_R cells differentiation [67, 70]. The use of retinoic acid congeners as therapeutic agents in boosting oral tolerance is thus of intense current interest.

Heritable Disorders of T_R Cells

In humans, loss of function Foxp3 mutations result in the IPEX syndrome [1, 71]. The hallmark of

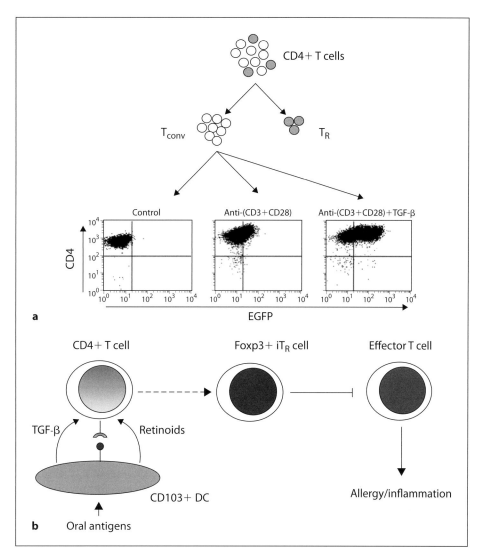

Fig. 3. Induction of iT_R cells in vitro and in vivo. **a** CD4+ T cells from mice whose *Foxp3* locus expresses both Foxp3 and an enhanced green fluorescent protein (EGFP) were sorted into CD4+EGFP+ (Foxp3+ T_R cells; schematically represented as green cells) and CD4+EGFP– (T_{conv} cells). The T_{conv} cells were either left unstimulated or stimulated with anti-CD3+ anti-CD28 antibodies without and with TGF-β. The different cell populations were analyzed for CD4 and EGFP expression, the latter as a measure of Foxp3 expression. Only the combination of anti-CD3+ anti-CD28 antibodies (which provides TCR activation and Il-2 production) together with TGF-β resulted in high level expression of Foxp3, characteristic of T_R cells. **b** Schematic representation of the induction of iT_R cells in vivo in the gut. Antigen presentation by specialized CD103+ dendritic cells in the presence of TGF-β and retinoic acid results in the conversion of CD4+ T_{conv} cells in iT_R cells, which then suppress T-effector cells reactive to foods or to the microbial flora.

IPEX is immune dysregulation due to the lack of functional T_R cells. It typically presents during infancy with enteropathy, autoimmune endocrinopathy, immune-mediated cytopenias, dermatitis. There is a striking allergic dysregulation that manifests in particular as food allergy, eosinophilia and very elevated IgE levels [72, 73]. Foxp3 deficiency in mice, whether due to natural or induced mutations, gives rise to a fatal autoimmune and inflammatory disorder called *scurfy* that has many of the features of IPEX including the allergic dysregulation and hyper-IgE phenotype [74]. Some of the allergic dysregulation in IPEX results from the presence in circulation of T_R cell precursors that secrete large amounts of Th2 cytokines especially IL-4, and it is tempting to speculate that the food allergy is a manifestation of iT_R cell deficiency [15, 16, 75]. IPEX-like syndromes in humans and in mice also arise from mutations along the IL-2 signaling pathway, including loss of function mutations in IL-2 receptor α-chain (CD25) and the IL-2-responsive transcription factor STAT5b, the latter also presenting with an associated phenotype of resistance to growth hormone [76–78].

T_R Cell-Directed Therapeutic Interventions in Allergy and Autoimmunity

Manipulation of T_R cells is an attractive strategy for immunotherapy, as suggested by adoptive transfer of T_R cells to treat experimental autoimmune diseases [79, 80]. Similar treatment strategies are now being developed in humans in whom it is envisaged that the cellular therapy with antigen-specific T_R cells may allow the development of long-term immune modulation strategies without the problem of general immunosuppression and systemic toxicity [81, 82]. Other approaches include the derivation for therapeutic use of human cell lines that stably express ectopic Foxp3, which converts both naive and antigen-specific memory CD4+ T cells into cells with T_R cell-like properties [83]. T_R cell therapy may also be rendered more effective by

combining it with immunomodulatory drugs that spare T_R cells while targeting T_{conv} cells. One such drug is rapamycin, an inhibitor of the mTor pathway, which plays an important role in T-cell proliferation and survival. The mTor pathway is relatively inactive in T_R cells, which employ an alternative IL-2 receptor-coupled STAT5 pathway to mediate cell growth and proliferation [84, 85]. A second approach is to use histone deacetylase inhibitors, which promote the development of Foxp3+ iT_R cells [86].

A pharmacological approach of particular therapeutic relevance to allergic diseases is to bolster iT_R cell-dependent oral tolerance by manipulating the retinoic acid pathway. It is well established that the induction of oral tolerance is associated with the in situ production of Foxp3+ iT_R cells [62, 87]. The in situ conversion of naive CD4+ T cells into iT_R cells, which takes place upon antigen presentation by CD103+ dendritic cells in gut-associated lymphoid tissue and is strictly TGF-β-dependent, is greatly augmented by retinoic acid, and reciprocally antagonized by inhibitors of retinal dehydrogenase [65–69]. Importantly, retinoic acid inhibits the IL-6-driven programming of TGF-β-treated T cells into pro-inflammatory Th17 cells in favor of iT_R cell differentiation [67, 70]. These findings, if proven applicable to the human mucosal immune system, open up the possibility of pharmacologically enhancing oral tolerogenic therapies such as sublingual immunotherapy with retinoic acid analogues or concurrent vitamin A supplementation [88, 89]. They also usher the potential to shift effector T-cell differentiation in inflammatory diseases away from Th17 and in favor of the T_R cell lineage.

Concluding Remarks

Impressive progress has been made in elucidating molecular mechanisms underlying T_R cell development and differentiated functions. The stage is now set to tackle some important outstanding issues in the field. These include the nature of the molecular circuitry governing the early development of nT_R cells in the thymus, the mechanisms underlying suppressive function of T_R cells, the respective roles of nT_R and iT_R cells in dominant tolerance, and the nature of the molecular pathways mediating their non-redundant functions. The striking allergic dysregulation and food allergy associated with the IPEX syndrome indicates a fundamental role for T_R cells in tolerance to allergens especially foods. Pharmacological interventions that aim to bolster T_R cell development and function, alone or together with immunotherapy, offer the potential for novel therapeutic strategies in the treatment of allergic and autoimmune diseases.

References

1 Chatila TA: Role of regulatory T cells in human diseases. J Allergy Clin Immunol 2005;116:949–960.

2 Bacchetta R, Gambineri E, Roncarolo MG: Role of regulatory T cells and FOXP3 in human diseases. J Allergy Clin Immunol 2007;120:227–237.

3 Zheng Y, Rudensky AY: Foxp3 in control of the regulatory T cell lineage. Nat Immunol 2007;8:457–462.

4 Shevach EM: CD4+CD25+ suppressor T cells: more questions than answers. Nat Rev Immunol 2002;2:389–400.

5 Thornton AM, Shevach EM: CD4+CD25+ immunoregulatory T cells suppress polyclonal T cell activation in vitro by inhibiting interleukin-2 production. J Exp Med 1998;188:287–296.

6 Xu D, Liu H, Komai-Koma M, Campbell C, McSharry C, Alexander J, Liew FY: CD4+CD25+ regulatory T cells suppress differentiation and functions of Th1 and Th2 cells, *Leishmania major* infection, and colitis in mice. J Immunol 2003;170:394–399.

7 Stassen M, Jonuleit H, Muller C, Klein M, Richter C, Bopp T, Schmitt S, Schmitt E: Differential regulatory capacity of CD25+ T regulatory cells and preactivated CD25+ T regulatory cells on development, functional activation, and proliferation of Th2 cells. J Immunol 2004;173:267–274.

8 Suvas S, Kumaraguru U, Pack CD, Lee S, Rouse BT: CD4+CD25+ T cells regulate virus-specific primary and memory CD8+ T cell responses. J Exp Med 2003;198:889–901.

9 Clark LB, Appleby MW, Brunkow ME, Wilkinson JE, Ziegler SF, Ramsdell F: Cellular and molecular characterization of the scurfy mouse mutant. J Immunol 1999;162:2546–2554.

10 Blair PJ, Bultman SJ, Haas JC, Rouse BT, Wilkinson JE, Godfrey VL: CD4+CD8– T cells are the effector cells in disease pathogenesis in the scurfy (sf) mouse. J Immunol 1994;153:3764–3774.

11 Fontenot JD, Gavin MA, Rudensky AY: Foxp3 programs the development and function of CD4+CD25+ regulatory T cells. Nat Immunol 2003;4:330–336.

12 Hori S, Nomura T, Sakaguchi S: Control of regulatory T cell development by the transcription factor Foxp3. Science 2003;299:1057–1061.

13 Khattri R, Cox T, Yasayko SA, Ramsdell F: An essential role for Scurfin in CD4+CD25+ T regulatory cells. Nat Immunol 2003;4:337–342.

14 Liston A, Farr AG, Chen Z, Benoist C, Mathis D, Manley NR, Rudensky AY: Lack of Foxp3 function and expression in the thymic epithelium. J Exp Med 2007;204:475–480.

15 Gavin MA, Rasmussen JP, Fontenot JD, Vasta V, Manganiello VC, Beavo JA, Rudensky AY: Foxp3-dependent programme of regulatory T-cell differentiation. Nature 2007;445:771–775.

16 Lin W, Haribhai D, Relland LM, Truong N, Carlson MR, Williams CB, Chatila TA: Regulatory T cell development in the absence of functional Foxp3. Nat Immunol 2007;8:359–368.

17 Chatila TA, Blaeser F, Ho N, Lederman HM, Voulgaropoulos C, Helms C, Bowcock AM: JM2, encoding a forkhead-related protein, is mutated in X-linked autoimmunity-allergic dysregulation syndrome. J Clin Invest 2001;106:R75–R81.

18 Williams LM, Rudensky AY: Maintenance of the Foxp3-dependent developmental program in mature regulatory T cells requires continued expression of Foxp3. Nat Immunol 2007;8:277–284.

19 Jordan MS, Boesteanu A, Reed AJ, Petrone AL, Holenbeck AE, Lerman MA, Naji A, Caton AJ: Thymic selection of CD4+CD25+ regulatory T cells induced by an agonist self-peptide. Nat Immunol 2001;2:301–306.

20 Shevach EM: Certified professionals: CD4+CD25+ suppressor T cells. J Exp Med 2001;193:F41–F46.

21 Jordan MS, Riley MP, von Boehmer H, Caton AJ: Anergy and suppression regulate CD4+ T cell responses to a self peptide. Eur J Immunol 2000;30:136–144.

22 Kawahata K, Misaki Y, Yamauchi M, Tsunekawa S, Setoguchi K, Miyazaki J, Yamamoto K: Generation of CD4+CD25+ regulatory T cells from autoreactive T cells simultaneously with their negative selection in the thymus and from nonautoreactive T cells by endogenous TCR expression. J Immunol 2002;168:4399–4405.

23 Fontenot JD, Gavin MA, Rudensky AY: Foxp3 programs the development and function of CD4+CD25+ regulatory T cells. Nat Immunol 2003;4:330–336.

24 Walker LS, Chodos A, Eggena M, Dooms H, Abbas AK: Antigen-dependent proliferation of CD4+CD25+ regulatory T cells in vivo. J Exp Med 2003;198:249–258.

25 Maloy KJ, Powrie F: Regulatory T cells in the control of immune pathology. Nat Immunol 2001;2:816–822.

26 Burchill MA, Yang J, Vang KB, Moon JJ, Chu HH, Lio CW, Vegoe AL, Hsieh CS, Jenkins MK, Farrar MA: Linked T cell receptor and cytokine signaling govern the development of the regulatory T cell repertoire. Immunity 2008;28: 112–121.

27 Lio CW, Hsieh CS: A two-step process for thymic regulatory T cell development. Immunity 2008;28:100–111.

28 Hsieh CS, Liang Y, Tyznik AJ, Self SG, Liggitt D, Rudensky AY: Recognition of the peripheral self by naturally arising CD25+CD4+ T cell receptors. Immunity 2004;21:267–277.

29 Hsieh CS, Zheng Y, Liang Y, Fontenot JD, Rudensky AY: An intersection between the self-reactive regulatory and nonregulatory T cell receptor repertoires. Nat Immunol 2006;7:401–410.

30 Pacholczyk R, Ignatowicz H, Kraj P, Ignatowicz L: Origin and T cell receptor diversity of Foxp3+CD4+CD25+ T cells. Immunity 2006;25:249–259.

31 Wong J, Mathis D, Benoist C: TCR-based lineage tracing: no evidence for conversion of conventional into regulatory T cells in response to a natural self-antigen in pancreatic islets. J Exp Med 2007;204:2039–2045.

32 Van Santen HM, Benoist C, Mathis D: Number of Treg cells that differentiate does not increase upon encounter of agonist ligand on thymic epithelial cells. J Exp Med 2004;200:1221–1230.

33 Pacholczyk R, Kern J, Singh N, Iwashima M, Kraj P, Ignatowicz L: Nonself-antigens are the cognate specificities of Foxp3+ regulatory T cells. Immunity 2007;27:493–504.

34 Pennington DJ, Silva-Santos B, Silberzahn T, Escorcio-Correia M, Woodward MJ, Roberts SJ, Smith AL, Dyson PJ, Hayday AC: Early events in the thymus affect the balance of effector and regulatory T cells. Nature 2006; 444:1073–1077.

35 Schubert LA, Jeffery E, Zhang Y, Ramsdell F, Ziegler SF: Scurfin (FOXP3) acts as a repressor of transcription and regulates T cell activation. J Biol Chem 2001;276:37672–37679.

36 Marson A, Kretschmer K, Frampton GM, Jacobsen ES, Polansky JK, MacIsaac KD, Levine SS, Fraenkel E, von Boehmer H, Young RA: Foxp3 occupancy and regulation of key target genes during T-cell stimulation. Nature 2007;445:931–935.

37 Zheng Y, Josefowicz SZ, Kas A, Chu TT, Gavin MA, Rudensky AY: Genome-wide analysis of Foxp3 target genes in developing and mature regulatory T cells. Nature 2007;445:936–940.

38 Li B, Samanta A, Song X, Iacono KT, Bembas K, Tao R, Basu S, Riley JL, Hancock WW, Shen Y, Saouaf SJ, Greene MI: FOXP3 interactions with histone acetyltransferase and class II histone deacetylases are required for repression. Proc Natl Acad Sci USA 2007;104:4571–4576.

39 Li B, Samanta A, Song X, Iacono KT, Brennan P, Chatila TA, Roncador G, Banham AH, Riley JL, Wang Q, Shen Y, Saouaf SJ, Greene MI: FOXP3 is a homo-oligomer and a component of a supramolecular regulatory complex disabled in the human XLAAD/ IPEX autoimmune disease. Int Immunol 2007; 19:825–835.

40 Ono M, Yaguchi H, Ohkura N, Kitabayashi I, Nagamura Y, Nomura T, Miyachi Y, Tsukada T, Sakaguchi S: Foxp3 controls regulatory T-cell function by interacting with AML1/Runx1. Nature 2007;446:685–689.

41 Wu Y, Borde M, Heissmeyer V, Feuerer M, Lapan AD, Stroud JC, Bates L, Guo L, Han A, Ziegler SF, Mathis D, Benoist C, Chen L, Rao A: FOXP3 controls regulatory T cell function through cooperation with NFAT. Cell 2006;126:375–387.

42 Allan SE, Passerini L, Bacchetta R, Crellin N, Dai M, Orban PC, Ziegler SF, Roncarolo MG, Levings MK: The role of 2 FOXP3 isoforms in the generation of human CD4+ Tregs. J Clin Invest 2005;115:3276–3284.

43 Fontenot JD, Rasmussen JP, Williams LM, Dooley JL, Farr AG, Rudensky AY: Regulatory T cell lineage specification by the forkhead transcription factor Foxp3. Immunity 2005;22:329–341.

44 Gavin MA, Clarke SR, Negrou E, Gallegos A, Rudensky A: Homeostasis and anergy of CD4+CD25+ suppressor T cells in vivo. Nat Immunol 2002;3: 33–41.

45 Chen Z, Herman AE, Matos M, Mathis D, Benoist C: Where CD4+CD25+ Treg cells impinge on autoimmune diabetes. J Exp Med 2005;202: 1387–1397.

46 Sugimoto N, Oida T, Hirota K, Nakamura K, Nomura T, Uchiyama T, Sakaguchi S: Foxp3-dependent and -independent molecules specific for CD25+CD4+ natural regulatory T cells revealed by DNA microarray analysis. Int Immunol 2006;18:1197–1209.

47 Glimcher LH, Townsend MJ, Sullivan BM, Lord GM: Recent developments in the transcriptional regulation of cytolytic effector cells. Nat Rev Immunol 2004;4:900–911.

48 Kim CH, Kunkel EJ, Boisvert J, Johnston B, Campbell JJ, Genovese MC, Greenberg HB, Butcher EC: Bonzo/CXCR6 expression defines type 1-polarized T-cell subsets with extra-lymphoid tissue homing potential. J Clin Invest 2001;107:595–601.

49 Hill JA, Feuerer M, Tash K, Haxhinasto S, Perez J, Melamed R, Mathis D, Benoist C: Foxp3 transcription-factor-dependent and -independent regulation of the regulatory T cell transcriptional signature. Immunity 2007;27:786–800.

50 Chatila T: The regulatory T cell transcriptosome: e pluribus unum. Immunity 2007;27:693–695.

51 Miyara M, Sakaguchi S: Natural regulatory T cells: mechanisms of suppression. Trends Mol Med 2007;13:108–116.

52 Pandiyan P, Zheng L, Ishihara S, Reed J, Lenardo MJ: CD4+CD25+Foxp3+ regulatory T cells induce cytokine deprivation-mediated apoptosis of effector CD4+ T cells. Nat Immunol 2007;8:1353–1362.

53 Mantel PY, Ouaked N, Ruckert B, Karagiannidis C, Welz R, Blaser K, Schmidt-Weber CB: Molecular mechanisms underlying FOXP3 induction in human T cells. J Immunol 2006;176: 3593–3602.

54 Burchill MA, Yang J, Vogtenhuber C, Blazar BR, Farrar MA: IL-2 receptor β-dependent STAT5 activation is required for the development of Foxp3+ regulatory T cells. J Immunol 2007;178:280–290.

55 Kim HP, Leonard WJ: CREB/ATF-dependent T cell receptor-induced FoxP3 gene expression: a role for DNA methylation. J Exp Med 2007;204: 1543–1551.

56 Tone Y, Furuuchi K, Kojima Y, Tykocinski ML, Greene MI, Tone M: Smad3 and NFAT cooperate to induce Foxp3 expression through its enhancer. Nat Immunol 2008;9:194–202.

57 Marie JC, Letterio JJ, Gavin M, Rudensky AY: TGF-β$_1$ maintains suppressor function and Foxp3 expression in CD4+CD25+ regulatory T cells. J Exp Med 2005;201:1061–1067.

58 Chen W, Jin W, Hardegen N, Lei KJ, Li L, Marinos N, McGrady G, Wahl SM: Conversion of peripheral CD4+CD25− naive T cells to CD4+CD25+ regulatory T cells by TGF-β induction of transcription factor Foxp3. J Exp Med 2003;198:1875–1886.

59 Fantini MC, Becker C, Monteleone G, Pallone F, Galle PR, Neurath MF: Cutting edge: TGF-β induces a regulatory phenotype in CD4+CD25− T cells through Foxp3 induction and down-regulation of Smad7. J Immunol 2004;172:5149–5153.

60 Zheng SG, Wang J, Wang P, Gray JD, Horwitz DA: IL-2 is essential for TGF-β to convert naive CD4+CD25− cells to CD25+Foxp3+ regulatory T cells and for expansion of these cells. J Immunol 2007;178:2018–2027.

61 Davidson TS, DiPaolo RJ, Andersson J, Shevach EM: Cutting Edge: IL-2 is essential for TGF-β-mediated induction of Foxp3+ T regulatory cells. J Immunol 2007;178:4022–4026.

62 Mucida D, Kutchukhidze N, Erazo A, Russo M, Lafaille JJ, Curotto de Lafaille MA: Oral tolerance in the absence of naturally occurring Tregs. J Clin Invest 2005;115:1923–1933.

63 Apostolou I, von Boehmer H: In vivo instruction of suppressor commitment in naive T cells. J Exp Med 2004;199: 1401–1408.

64 Floess S, Freyer J, Siewert C, Baron U, Olek S, Polansky J, Schlawe K, Chang HJ, Bopp T, Schmitt E, Klein-Hessling S, Serfling E, Hamann A, Huehn J: Epigenetic control of the Foxp3 locus in regulatory T cells. PLoS Biol 2007;5:e38.

65 Benson MJ, Pino-Lagos K, Rosemblatt M, Noelle RJ: All-trans retinoic acid mediates enhanced T reg cell growth, differentiation, and gut homing in the face of high levels of co-stimulation. J Exp Med 2007;204:1765–1774.

66 Coombes JL, Siddiqui KR, Arancibia-Carcamo CV, Hall J, Sun CM, Belkaid Y, Powrie F: A functionally specialized population of mucosal CD103+ DCs induces Foxp3+ regulatory T cells via a TGF-β and retinoic acid-dependent mechanism. J Exp Med 2007;204: 1757–1764.

67 Mucida D, Park Y, Kim G, Turovskaya O, Scott I, Kronenberg M, Cheroutre H: Reciprocal TH17 and regulatory T cell differentiation mediated by retinoic acid. Science 2007;317:256–260.

68 Sun CM, Hall JA, Blank RB, Bouladoux N, Oukka M, Mora JR, Belkaid Y: Small intestine lamina propria dendritic cells promote de novo generation of Foxp3 Treg cells via retinoic acid. J Exp Med 2007;204:1775–1785.

69 Kang SG, Lim HW, Andrisani OM, Broxmeyer HE, Kim CH: Vitamin A metabolites induce gut-homing FoxP3+ regulatory T cells. J Immunol 2007;179:3724–3733.

70 Elias KM, Laurence A, Davidson TS, Stephens G, Kanno Y, Shevach EM, O'Shea JJ: Retinoic acid inhibits Th17 polarization and enhances FoxP3 expression through a Stat-3/Stat-5 independent signaling pathway. Blood 2008;111:1013–1020.

71 Torgerson TR, Ochs HD: Immune dysregulation, polyendocrinopathy, enteropathy, X-linked: forkhead box protein 3 mutations and lack of regulatory T cells. J Allergy Clin Immunol 2007;120:744–751.

72 Chatila TA, Blaeser F, Ho N, Lederman HM, Voulgaropoulos C, Helms C, Bowcock AM: JM2, encoding a forkhead-related protein, is mutated in X-linked autoimmunity-allergic dysregulation syndrome. J Clin Invest 2000;106:R75–R81.

73 Torgerson TR, Linane A, Moes N, Anover S, Mateo V, Rieux-Laucat F, Hermine O, Vijay S, Gambineri E, Cerf-Bensussan N, Fischer A, Ochs HD, Goulet O, Ruemmele FM: Severe food allergy as a variant of IPEX syndrome caused by a deletion in a non-coding region of the FOXP3 gene. Gastroenterology 2007;132:1705–1717.

74 Lin W, Truong N, Grossman WJ, Haribhai D, Williams CB, Wang J, Martin MG, Chatila TA: Allergic dysregulation and hyperimmunoglobulinemia E in Foxp3 mutant mice. J Allergy Clin Immunol 2005;116: 1106–1115.

75 Gavin MA, Torgerson TR, Houston E, DeRoos P, Ho WY, Stray-Pedersen A, Ocheltree EL, Greenberg PD, Ochs HD, Rudensky AY: Single-cell analysis of normal and FOXP3-mutant human T cells: FOXP3 expression without regulatory T cell development. Proc Natl Acad Sci USA 2006;103:6659–6664.

76 Caudy AA, Reddy ST, Chatila T, Atkinson JP, Verbsky JW: CD25 deficiency causes an immune dysregulation, polyendocrinopathy, enteropathy, X-linked-like syndrome, and defective IL-10 expression from CD4 lymphocytes. J Allergy Clin Immunol 2007;119:482–487.

77 Cohen AC, Nadeau KC, Tu W, Hwa V, Dionis K, Bezrodnik L, Teper A, Gaillard M, Heinrich J, Krensky AM, Rosenfeld RG, Lewis DB: Cutting edge: decreased accumulation and regulatory function of CD4+CD25^{high} T cells in human STAT5b deficiency. J Immunol 2006;177:2770–2774.

78 Malek TR: The biology of interleukin-2. Annu Rev Immunol 2008;26:453–479.

79 Wing K, Fehervari Z, Sakaguchi S: Emerging possibilities in the development and function of regulatory T cells. Int Immunol 2006;18:991–1000.

80 Verbsky JW: Therapeutic use of T regulatory cells. Curr Opin Rheumatol 2007;19:252–258.

81 Roncarolo MG, Battaglia M: Regulatory T-cell immunotherapy for tolerance to self antigens and alloantigens in humans. Nat Rev Immunol 2007;7:585–598.

82 Tang Q, Bluestone JA: Regulatory T-cell physiology and application to treat autoimmunity. Immunol Rev 2006;212:217–237.

83 Allan SE, Alstad AN, Merindol N, Crellin NK, Amendola M, Bacchetta R, Naldini L, Roncarolo MG, Soudeyns H, Levings MK: Generation of potent and stable human CD4+ T regulatory cells by activation-independent expression of FOXP3. Mol Ther 2008;16:194–202.

84 Battaglia M, Stabilini A, Roncarolo MG: Rapamycin selectively expands CD4+CD25+FoxP3+ regulatory T cells. Blood 2005;105:4743–4748.

85 Zeiser R, Leveson-Gower DB, Zambricki EA, Kambham N, Beilhack A, Loh J, Hou JZ, Negrin RS: Differential impact of mTOR inhibition on CD4+CD25+Foxp3+ regulatory T cells as compared to conventional CD4+ T cells. Blood 2008;111:453–462.

86 Tao R, de Zoeten EF, Ozkaynak E, Chen C, Wang L, Porrett PM, Li B, Turka LA, Olson EN, Greene MI, Wells AD, Hancock WW: Deacetylase inhibition promotes the generation and function of regulatory T cells. Nat Med 2007;13:1299–1307.

87 Akdis M, Akdis CA: Mechanisms of allergen-specific immunotherapy. J Allergy Clin Immunol 2007;119: 780–791.

88 Von Boehmer H: Oral tolerance: is it all retinoic acid? J Exp Med 2007;204: 1737–1739.

89 Chatila TA: Extraintestinal manifestations of gastrointestinal allergy: effector and regulatory T cells in the balance. Clin Exp Allergy 2007;37:1417–1418.

Talal A. Chatila
Division of Immunology, Allergy and Rheumatology, Department of Pediatrics
The David Geffen School of Medicine at the University of California at Los Angeles, MDCC 12-430
10833 Le Conte Ave, Los Angeles, CA 90095-1752 (USA)
Tel. +1 310 825 6481, Fax +1 310 825 9832, E-Mail tchatila@mednet.ucla.edu

Blaser K (ed): T Cell Regulation in Allergy, Asthma and Atopic Skin Diseases.
Chem Immunol Allergy. Basel, Karger, 2008, vol 94, pp 29–39

Interaction of Regulatory T Cells with Antigen-Presenting Cells in Health and Disease

Karsten Mahnke · Sabine Ring · Tanja Bedke ·
Svetlana Karakhanova · Alexander H. Enk

Department of Dermatology, University Hospital Heidelberg, Heidelberg, Germany

Abstract

Among antigen-presenting cells (APCs), dendritic cells as well as monocytes acquire immunostimulatory capacity only after appropriate maturation. Therefore, blockade of the maturation/activation results in a steady state or alternatively activated phenotype, which induces tolerance rather than immunity. Functional analyses revealed recently that steady-state dendritic cells and alternatively activated macrophages, respectively, actively induce regulatory T cells (Tregs) in the periphery of the body. Thus, production of Tregs does not rely exclusively on thymic development. Vice versa, Tregs respond to APCs by several means. Recent lines of evidence indicate that Tregs prevent terminal differentiation of subpopulations of APCs or lead to upregulation of surface expression of immunosuppressive molecules. Thus, Tregs foster an environment that further promotes their development. In conclusion, the mutual interaction of Tregs and APCs enables Tregs to sustain their immunosuppressive function(s), which in healthy individuals may be crucial for the maintenance of peripheral tolerance. Since macrophages bridge the innate and the acquired immune system, Tregs are able to gain influence on the innate immune system by interacting with macrophages beyond the mere interaction with effector T cells.

Dendritic Cells and Regulatory T Cells

Maturation Status of Dendritic Cells Is Critical for Induction of Regulatory T Cells

Dendritic cells (DCs) have long been regarded as key cells for the induction of immunity and are defined as nature's adjuvants [1]. However, these function(s) are only assigned to DCs after proper maturation. Fully matured DCs express a multitude of MHC and other T-cell costimulatory molecules, which enable them to induce immune reactions. In contrast, non-activated tissue resident DCs have been shown not to possess these T-cell-stimulating capacities [1]. For this reason they were regarded as immature precursors that later become a 'real' and fully developed DC after activation.

Recently it has been shown that instead of being bystanders [2], immature DCs actively exert tolerogenic function(s). Among the first reports in this regard was the observation that repeated coculture of ex vivo prepared immature DCs with allogenic CD4+ T cells leads to the enhanced expression of the IL-2 receptor α-chain (CD25) on the surface of the T cells and to the acquisition of suppressive capacity. These changes in phenotype are indicative for so-called naturally occurring regulatory T cells (Tregs). These T cells do not proliferate and are able to suppress proliferation of CD4+ and CD8+ effector T cells [3]. Beyond the mere in vitro characterization of these suppressive T cells, their in vivo relevance has been proven repeatedly. First, a subset of CD4+CD25+ naturally occurring Tregs was purified from blood and lymphatic organs, verifying their presence in vivo [4]; second, deletion of these Tregs by antibody depletion (in animal models) or by mutation (IPEX syndrome in humans), leads to vigorously enhanced autoimmunity in the affected animals and humans, respectively [5]. Thus, an in vivo homologue of the in vitro induced CD4+CD25+ Tregs not only exists, but these cells are also critically involved in the inhibition of potentially autoreactive T cells for the maintenance of peripheral tolerance.

The final proof for Treg induction by immature DCs in vivo was hampered by the fact DCs had to be isolated and loaded with antigens in vitro prior to analyzing the subsequent events of antigen presentation in vivo. This procedure however provides enough stimulation to render the DCs mature.

This problem was overcome when in vivo antigen targeting was applied to load DCs in situ without inducing maturation. This approach took advantage of the antigen receptor DEC-205, which is exclusively expressed by DCs [6] in comparison to the macrophage mannose receptor and Fc receptors that are also expressed on macrophages or B cells. Therefore, the DC-specific expression of DEC-205 provided the possibility to selectively target and load DCs in situ by means of antibody targeting.

To test DC-specific targeting, model antigens such as hen egg lysozyme (HEL) and ovalbumin (OVA) were covalently linked to anti-DEC-205 antibodies and injected into mice. This resulted in antigen loading of the lymph node DCs, followed by presentation of the antigens to T cells. Further analysis of immune responses induced by anti-DEC targeting revealed that tolerance against the respective antigens was obtained. Additionally, increased numbers of CD4+CD25+ Tregs could be recorded in anti-DEC antigen-conjugate-treated animals. These cells were also able to suppress proliferation of effector T cells and thus possess all qualities attributed to genuine Tregs [7, 8].

Beyond the proof of Treg induction with model antigens, such as OVA and HEL, several attempts have recently been made to exploit the therapeutic role of antigen targeting for the treatment of autoimmunity. Indeed, in animal models for contact hypersensitivity (CHS), diabetes and multiple sclerosis, treatment with the respective anti-DEC-antigen conjugates resulted in significant improvement of these diseases [9, 10]. Thus, antibody-mediated targeting of autoantigen(s) to steady-state DCs may provide a novel tool to specifically induce tolerance in various autoimmune diseases (fig. 1).

Regulatory T Cells Suppress DC Maturation
As outlined above, several lines of evidence indicate that DCs are crucially involved in the induction of Tregs. However, this interaction is not restricted to a DC-to-Treg one-way street, since several recent data revealed that Tregs in turn have an impact on DC development [11].

Recent in vitro coculture experiments made clear that Tregs influence the maturation and thus the function of DCs profoundly. Several means by which DCs are rendered immunosuppressive by the Tregs are currently discussed. For instance, the coculture of DCs and activated Tregs results in diminished expression of T-cell costimulatory ligands, leading to a reduced T-cell stimulatory capacity by DCs, indicating a Treg-driven block in DC maturation [12–14].

Moreover, we and others have shown that in addition to the mere blockade of DC maturation, the immunosuppressive molecules B7-H3 and

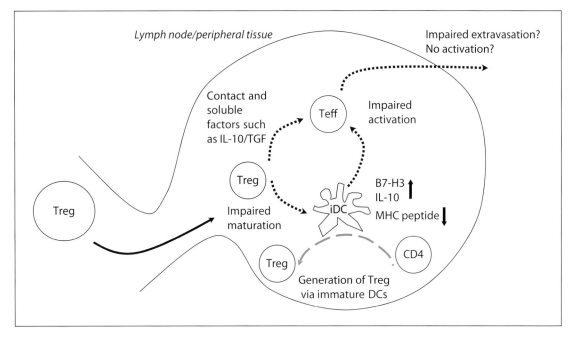

Fig. 1. Possible interactions between DCs and Tregs in peripheral lymphoid organs. In lymph nodes or in the peripheral tissues, Tregs encounter effector T cells (Teff) as well as dendritic cells (DCs). Here they can interact with Teff directly via cell-cell contact or secretion of IL-10 and TGF-β. In addition, Tregs are able to prevent DC maturation as indicated by reduced MHC class II complexes, or to convert DCs into a suppressive phenotype, that upregulates IL-10 and immunosuppressive B7-H molecules. Nevertheless, these actions augment the suppressive activity of Tregs, as immature DCs are prone to generate Tregs from a CD4+CD25– T-cell pool and these cells also convey suppressive signals to adjacent effector T cells.

B7-H4 are upregulated on the surface of DCs upon contact with Tregs [15, 16]. Although for both molecules the counter-receptor is not known, it is most likely that immunosuppressive signals will be conveyed. Functional data concerning B7-H3 and B7-H4 are still limited, since they have been described rather recently. Nevertheless, similar to other members of the B7-H family, B7-H3 has clear immunosuppressive functions, as this molecule has been shown to mediate the reduction of autoimmune EAE and addition of recombinant B7-H3 molecules to mixed leukocyte reactions suppresses T-cell proliferation in vitro [17–20].

Likewise, B7-H4 has been shown to be expressed by a suppressive subset of macrophages and is associated with an unfavorable prognosis in some cancers [21]. Thus, taken together, these data indicate that B7-H3 and B7-H4 respectively serve as negative regulators of T cells and are involved in conveying suppressive activity of Treg-exposed DCs to other T cells.

In addition to surface molecules, the presence and/or absence of cytokine production by DCs is influenced by Tregs in a way that tolerance rather than immunity is induced. For example, in mixed lymphocyte reactions with CD25–CD4+ T-cell DCs produce large amounts of the proinflammatory cytokine IL-6. However, the presence of Tregs in these cultures leads to abrogation of IL-6 expression and to production of the immunosuppressive cytokine IL-10. This effect is quite robust and neither the presence of CD8+ T cells nor of memory CD4+ T cells compensate this suppressive effect of Tregs [22].

The whole scenario changes when a potent inflammatory stimulus like LPS is present in the cultures. Under these circumstances, high amounts of IL-6 are continuously expressed and the secretion of the immunosuppressive cytokine IL-10 is abrogated.

In summary, the recent data show that Tregs are able to force DCs to acquire tolerogenic phenotype and function. This change in phenotype is indicated by downregulation of T-cell costimulatory molecules and upregulation of suppressive molecules such as B7-H3 and soluble factors like IL-10. One can thus speculate that Tregs multiply their suppressive activity in a closed loop, since (i) Tregs suppress proliferation of effector T cells directly and (ii) Tregs suppress activation of effector T cells via keeping the main stimulatory cells, namely DCs, in an immature state.

According to these recent data, Tregs may create their own suppressive environment by favoring the generation of additional Tregs by keeping DCs immature and thus further augmenting their immunosuppressive capacity in peripheral tissues (fig. 1).

This self-sustained cycle of T-cell regulation may play an important role for maintenance of peripheral tolerance. Here, steady-state DCs from the periphery of the body, entering secondary lymphoid organs, come in contact with Tregs. This interaction ensures that the DCs remain inactivated and those self antigens picked up in the periphery of the body are presented to T cells in a way that tolerance ensues. However, in the presence of proinflammatory, pathogen-derived stimuli (like LPS, CpG), the DCs mature regardless of the presence of Tregs and an immune response gets started [11].

Monocytes/Macrophages and Regulatory T Cells

Although closely related, monocytes/macrophages (MO) possess features that are distinct from DCs. Due to their limited expression of T-cell costimulatory molecules, MO are not able to prime T cells de novo, but rather stimulate effector/memory T cells by the secretion of cytokines, which support T-cell proliferation. As DCs, MO differentiate from myeloid precursors and form a heterogeneous population of antigen-presenting cells (APCs) that link the innate and adaptive immune systems. However, their ability to interact with T cells via MHC class II TCR interaction(s) as well as engagement of T-cell costimulatory receptors on their surface, makes close contact between MO and Tregs likely to occur in vivo.

Different types of activated MO have been characterized, which perform distinct immunological functions. Upon priming through the 'classical pathway' with IFN-γ and exposure to bacterially induced TNF-α, the MO acquire the ability to kill and degrade intracellular microorganisms and to support antigen-specific T-cell responses by antigen presentation and release of IL-12. Thus, these MO play a proinflammatory role. In contrast, the alternatively activated MO have rather immunomodulatory (i.e. suppressive) functions and are generated by MO activation in the presence of IL-4 or IgG immune complexes (type II MO). These alternatively activated MO are not efficient in Ag presentation, secret rather IL-10 and are able to suppress the proliferation of activated T cells. This suppression is not just mediated by the IL-10 secretion of the MO. Instead, recent findings indicate that these MO are also able to induce CD4+CD25+ Tregs, which additionally account for the drastically reduced T-cell proliferation induced by the MO [23] (fig. 2). Vice versa, Tregs 'respond' to MO since they are able to block MO maturation. This has been demonstrated by in vitro experiments, showing that MO that have been cultured in the presence of Tregs, exhibit

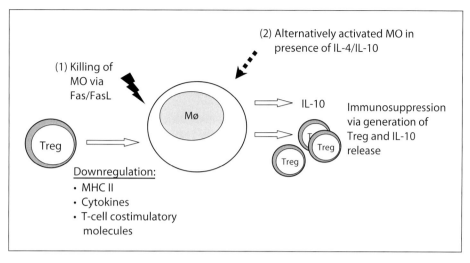

Fig. 2. Interaction of monocytes/macrophages (MO) with regulatory T cells (Treg). (1) Tregs are capable of preventing the full maturation of MO, resulting in reduced cytokine secretion and diminished expression of T-cell costimulatory molecules. Also, some investigations report that Tregs may be able to induce killing of MO via the Fas/FasL pathway. (2) When MO are activated in the presence of e.g. IL-4/IL-10, the activation is incomplete (alternatively activated MO). These MO secrete substantial amounts of IL-10 and are able to induce Treg.

minimal cytokine production and only reduced expression of the surface molecules CD80, CD86 and MHC class II [24].

Thus, these data indicate that similar to immature DCs, alternatively activated MO can induce immunosuppressive Tregs and that in return these Tregs are potent suppressors of MO maturation (fig. 2). Since MO bridge the innate and the acquired immune system, Tregs are able to gain influence on the innate immune system by interactions with MO.

This self-sustained balance of reciprocal activation and suppression of Tregs and MO may be important for maintenance of peripheral tolerance in healthy individuals. However, this balance can be impaired during infection and inflammation. Under septic shock conditions, increased Treg numbers can be seen in patients, which interfere with MO survival that ultimately leads to aggravation of the septic shock.

Normally, during bacterial infection LPS is present in large quantities in the body, which binds and activates CD14+ MO for the initiation of an adaptive T-cell response. Under septic shock conditions, however, MO subsequently stop antigen presentation and undergo augmented apoptosis. Recent data suggest that these effects are indeed mediated by Tregs [25]. The Tregs prevent the LPS-induced survival of MO by driving MO into apoptosis. This mechanism is Fas/FasL-dependent and involves a so far unknown soluble factor, released by Tregs. Thus, under septic shock conditions the increased Treg numbers may have fatal consequences, as MO-driven immune responses are downregulated during an ongoing infection.

As to how Tregs convey their suppressive capacity to MO is not entirely clear yet. At least in several in vitro culture systems, cell-to-cell contact is mandatory, which may indicate a surface molecule-receptor-based mechanism. A possible candidate molecule, which is involved in MO-driven Treg induction, is the F4/80 antigen. This molecule is a prototypic member of the EGF transmembrane receptor family, which is likely involved in cellular adhesion and the determination of cell fate. F4/80 is expressed by most tissue resident macrophages and even Langerhans' cells in the skin and is downregulated in response to activation stimuli. Evidence for molecular involvement of the molecule in the generation of Tregs derives from experiments using an anterior chamber-associated immune deviation (ACAID) model [26]. The ACAID model takes advantage of the fact that the visual axis has to be protected from devastating inflammation. Thus, foreign antigens that enter the eye are taken up by MO and are transported to the spleen, where CD8+ Tregs are induced in order to suppress immune responses in the eye. In their model, Lin et al. [26] show that upon transferal of antigens into the anterior chamber of F4/80-deficient mice, these mice were unable to generate Tregs in the spleen. However, this defect could be compensated by injection of F4/80+ MO, thus indicating that the presence of the F4/80 molecule is critically involved in the generation of Tregs by MO.

B Cells and Regulatory T Cells

As compared to DCs, B cells are very poor APCs and play a major role as source for antibodies. Upon stimulation by antigens and in the presence of T cells at the border of the T-cell–B-cell area, adjacent to follicles, B cells become antibody-secreting cells and eventually form a germinal center (GC) response. GCs are specialized follicles for B-cell expansion, somatic hypermutation, and class switch recombination, processes that are regulated by T cells, follicular DCs, and other cells. In this process of B-cell maturation, Tregs seem to play a critical role, as in several immune diseases, which are characterized by aberrant antibody production, the numbers of Tregs are changed as compared to healthy individuals. For instance, in autoimmune myasthenia gravis, which is normally accompanied by extensive expansion of antiacetylcholine receptor antibody-producing B cells, Treg function is severely impaired [27]. Also, in patients with chronic hepatitis C virus infection, which often develop a B-cell proliferative disorder with polyclonal activation, autoantibody production and vasculitis, the quantity of Tregs in peripheral tissues is substantially reduced [28].

These data only give circumstantial evidence that Tregs and B cells functionally interfere with each other, however direct impact of Tregs on B-cell maturation could be detected in several murine models. When Tregs were injected into mice during the initial 'priming phase' of the antibody response, the ultimate antibody production of the B cells was blocked [29, 30]. These effects were dependent of the interaction, i.e. the presence, of Tregs at the interface of the T-cell–B-cell zones and were accompanied by the downregulation of ICOS molecules by the T-helper cells, thus indicating that Tregs indirectly interfere with B-cell maturation by blocking T-cell 'help' in the GC (fig. 3).

However, recent data obtained in humans also suggest direct actions of Tregs on B cells, as Lim et al. [31] have shown that isolated Tregs can suppress antibody production and the class switching recombination of B cells in the absence of T-helper cells.

In addition to the inhibition of antibody production, Tregs have even more distinct means to curb B-cell-driven immune responses: they are able to kill antigen-presenting B cells [32]. This lytic activity resembles effects which can also be observed in the Treg–MO interaction(s) [25], however the killing of the B cells, in contrast to that of MO, seems to be independent from Fas/FasL interaction. Here, Tregs destroy B cells via the release of perforin and granzymes and this process was selective for antigen-presenting B cells [33]. In aggregate, these means enable Tregs to directly govern B-cell-driven immune responses and dysfunction of

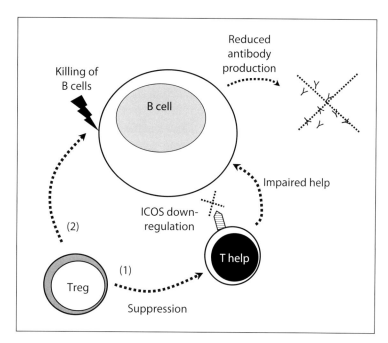

Fig. 3. Interaction of B cells with regulatory T cells (Treg). (1) Tregs exert their suppressive effects on B cells via T-helper cells (T help). Upon contact to Treg, T-helper cells downregulate expression of ICOS and abrogate helper functions for B-cell maturation, resulting in impaired antibody maturation and secretion by B cells. (2) Tregs can also directly interact with B cells, either preventing antibody responses or by killing B cells via an unknown mechanism.

Tregs during B-cell-mediated autoimmune diseases has to be taken into account (fig. 3).

Only limited data exist showing that B cells can directly influence Treg function(s), however several molecular interactions between these cells are possible. For instance, B and T cells can form a so-called immunological synapse, which involves a close contact and engagement of the TCR, costimulatory molecules as well as several adhesion molecules with their receptor counterparts [34]. Although at first described for DC–T-cell interactions, it is obvious that such a synapse can also be formed by B-cell–T-cell pairs. Here, the contact involves a different set of adhesion molecules and last up to several hours. More interestingly, when the synapse is formed between naive B cells and naive T cells, the T cells acquire a regulatory phenotype and can be regarded as Treg.

While these experiments were carried out in vitro, an in vivo correlate may be deduced from observations made in non-Hodgkin lymphoma-bearing mice [35]. Here it has been demonstrated

that the number of FoxP3+ Tregs are greatly enhanced within the tumor. This augmentation was critically dependent on the presence of CD70+ B cells. Moreover, removal of the B cells or blockade of the CD70 molecules, inhibited the intratumoral generation of Tregs, thus indicating that B cells, via interaction of the CD70–CD27 surface molecules, are able to induce Tregs in vivo.

Interaction between DCs and Regulatory T Cells during Allergic and Inflammatory Reactions

As a consequence of their immunosuppressive activity, Tregs may function as a cellular therapeutic agent that ameliorates allergies and autoimmune diseases. This has been proven in several disease models including asthma, inflammatory bowel disease, multiple sclerosis and CHS reactions. Others and we have studied the effects of in vivo applied Tregs as a possible therapeutical means to curb allergic and autoimmune disease, and thus it has clearly been shown in animal models of colitis, asthma and CHS reactions that injection of Tregs led to suppression of immune reactions [36–39].

Although the immunosuppressive effects of in vivo administered Tregs in various disease models are well documented, i.e. they always reduced inflammation/autoimmunity depending on the model used, the means by which Tregs act in vivo are not clear yet. Several in vitro data indicate that Tregs and effector T cells have to be in cell-to-cell contact in order to exert their suppressive functions. This has been indicated by Boyden-chamber experiments, which clearly demonstrated that separation of Tregs from effector T cells abrogated their suppressive activity, thus the mere transport of immunosuppressive mediators was not enough to convey the Treg-mediated suppression. However, these experiments were mainly done in vitro, whereas several in vivo studies suggest that other (soluble) factors may play essential roles [40, 41]. For example, in murine models of inflammatory bowel diseases, symptoms could only be prevented by transfer of IL-10-producing CD4+CD25+ T cells, as administration of antibodies against IL-10 or its receptor neutralized the suppressive effects of the Treg. Moreover, transfer of Tregs from IL-10-deficient mice failed to prevent colitis. In other colitis models, the injection of freshly isolated or activated Tregs halted the progression of the disease and reversed the symptoms. These effects were critically dependent on IL-10, TGF-β and CTLA-4, since injection of the mice with anti-IL-10 receptor, anti-CTLA-4 or anti-TGF-β abrogated the therapeutic effects of the transferred Tregs [39, 42, 43].

Our own experiments indicate that i.v. injection of Tregs is able to prevent CHS reactions, but the Tregs never entered the tissue site, i.e. the skin in which the allergic reaction takes place [36]. Rather, their suppressive action seems to be mediated by IL-10 and involves endothelial cells, as Ring et al. [36] have been shown that the adherence of effector T cells to inflamed vascular endothelium is blocked by Treg injections. Thus,

soluble factors as well as the spatial distributing of Tregs seem to be important for propagation of their suppressive actions in situ.

Consequently, the homing and the presence of Tregs in different organs during allergic and infections diseases further influences their suppressive capacity. The differential expression of tissue-specific homing receptors therefore allows a 'tailored' immunosuppression, by guiding Tregs to tissues where they are required [44]. For instance, a α4β7 integrin expressing subpopulation of Tregs has been described [45] which accumulates in the gastrointestinal mucosa where exposure to harmless but foreign antigen(s) may occur and thus an immunosuppressive environment is necessary to avoid overboarding immune responses.

Moreover, an even more detailed analysis of the effects that tissue-specific homing of Tregs exerts on immunosuppression can be performed in allergic reactions, as they can be dissected into a sensitization phase and into an elicitation phase. An example of a well-studied model is the hapten-induced CHS reaction. After the first application of a hapten onto the skin, it is picked up by tissue-residing DCs and transported to draining lymph nodes. Here the priming of CD8+ T cells against the respective antigen is accomplished resulting in a 'sensitized' individual. However, after a following application of the same allergen, a CD8-driven immune response is generated immediately by activation of CD8+ T cells in the locally affected tissues. Thus, sensitization and/or elicitation take places at different tissue sites. As a consequence, Tregs have to be present in the lymph node or at the tissue site, depending on whether sensitization or elicitation, respectively, should be blocked.

One of the prominent regulators of T-cell homing to lymph nodes in mice and humans is the CD62L molecule, and among naturally occurring Tregs approx. 85% express CD62L. When we separated CD62L+ and CD62L− Tregs and injected the subpopulations separately before sensitizing/challenging the mice, the CD62L+ subset was able to prevent the sensitization phase of CHS reactions, whereas the CD62L− cells failed to do so [pers. unpubl. observations]. Moreover, this effect was not dependent on IL-10.

As to how the expression of different homing molecules by Tregs is accomplished is not clear yet, but the differential homing of Tregs may be guided by DCs, whereby the DCs are able to program the homing of Tregs to specific tissues. This phenomenon has been described for UV-induced Tregs (UV-Tregs), which are generated by UV irradiation in the skin [46].

The UV-Tregs express the lymph node homing receptor CD62 ligand (CD62L) and upon i.v. injection they migrate into the lymph nodes. Therefore the UV-Tregs are able to prevent the sensitization against haptens (which takes place in the lymph node), but are unable to suppress the elicitation of a CHS reaction, as these events take place in the periphery, i.e. at the site of antigen challenge. However, the behavior of the UV-Tregs can be reprogrammed. It has been shown that UV-Tregs after coculture with skin-derived DCs (Langerhans' cells), but not with spleen or bone marrow-derived DCs, downregulate CD62L expression and upregulate PSGL-1, a molecule involved in skin homing. Consequently, after coculture with Langerhans' cells, the UV-Tregs were able to migrate to the skin sites and to suppress the challenging reaction in a CHS model. Thus these data indicate that DC are able to 'reprogram' Treg homing and therefore may govern immunosuppressive effects by inducing differential homing of Tregs.

These effects have to be taken into account when Tregs or subsets thereof (either isolated or generated ex vivo from precursors) are utilized for the treatment of autoimmune or inflammatory diseases.

Conclusion

Several studies have addressed different means of interaction between APCs and Treg. Functional data indicate that steady-state DCs as well as alternatively activated MO are prone to induce Tregs in vivo. Thus the activation status of the APCs seems to be a common denominator for the decision-making on whether effector T cells or Tregs are induced. As to how these effects are mediated is not clear but CTLA-4 as well as IL-10 and TGF-β seem to be involved. Vice versa, the Tregs can prevent terminal differentiation of subpopulations of APCs or lead to upregulation of surface expression of immunosuppressive molecules. Thus, Tregs foster an environment that further promotes their own development, by keeping APCs in a non-activated state.

In conclusion, the mutual interaction of Tregs and APCs enables Tregs to sustain their immunosuppressive function(s), which may be crucial for the maintenance of peripheral tolerance in healthy individuals. Since MO and DCs bridge the innate and the acquired immune system, this 'crosstalk' with MO and DCs permits Tregs to gain influence on the innate immune system. Furthermore, the impact on APCs offers Tregs to expand their suppression beyond the mere interaction with effector T cells.

References

1 Banchareau J, Steinman RM: Dendritic cells and the control of immunity. Nature 1998;392:245–252.
2 Mahnke K, Knop J, Enk AH: Induction of tolerogenic DCs: 'you are what you eat'. Trends Immunol 2003;24:646–651.
3 Jonuleit H, Schmitt E, Schuler G, Knop J, Enk AH: Induction of interleukin-10-producing, nonproliferating CD4+ T cells with regulatory properties by repetitive stimulation with allogeneic immature human dendritic cells. J Exp Med 2000;192:1213–1222.
4 Jonuleit H, Schmitt E, Stassen M, Tuettenberg A, Knop J, Enk AH: Identification and functional characterization of human CD4+CD25+ T cells with regulatory properties isolated from peripheral blood. J Exp Med 2001;193:1285–1294.

5 Sakaguchi S, Sakaguchi N: Regulatory T cells in immunologic self-tolerance and autoimmune disease. Int Rev Immunol 2005;24:211–226.

6 Mahnke K, Guo M, Lee S, Sepulveda H, Swain SL, Nussenzweig M, Steinman RM: The dendritic cell receptor for endocytosis, DEC-205, can recycle and enhance antigen presentation via major histocompatibility complex class II-positive lysosomal compartments. J Cell Biol 2000;151:673–684.

7 Bonifaz L, Bonnyay D, Mahnke K, Rivera M, Nussenzweig MC, Steinman RM: Efficient targeting of protein antigen to the dendritic cell receptor DEC-205 in the steady state leads to antigen presentation on major histocompatibility complex class I products and peripheral CD8+ T cell tolerance. J Exp Med 2002;196:1627–1638.

8 Mahnke K, Qian Y, Knop J, Enk AH: Induction of CD4+/CD25+ regulatory T cells by targeting of antigens to immature dendritic cells. Blood 2003; 101:4862–4869.

9 Bruder D, Westendorf AM, Hansen W, Prettin S, Gruber AD, Qian Y, von Böhmer H, Mahnke K, Buer J: On the edge of autoimmunity: T-cell stimulation by steady-state dendritic cells prevents autoimmune diabetes. Diabetes 2005;54:3395–3401.

10 Kretschmer K, Apostolou I, Hawiger D, Khazaie K, Nussenzweig MC, von Böhmer H: Inducing and expanding regulatory T cell populations by foreign antigen. Nat Immunol 2005;6:1219–1227.

11 Mahnke K, Johnson TS, Ring S, Enk AH: Tolerogenic dendritic cells and regulatory T cells: a two-way relationship. J Dermatol Sci 2007;46:159–167.

12 Min WP, Zhou D, Ichim TE, Strejan GH, Xia X, Yang J, Huang X, Garcia B, White D, Dutartre P, Jevnikar AM, Zhong R: Inhibitory feedback loop between tolerogenic dendritic cells and regulatory T cells in transplant tolerance. J Immunol 2003;170:1304–1312.

13 Misra N, Bayry J, Lacroix-Desmazes S, Kazatchkine MD, Kaveri SV: Cutting edge: human CD4+CD25+ T cells restrain the maturation and antigen-presenting function of dendritic cells. J Immunol 2004;172:4676–4680.

14 Cederbom L, Hall H, Ivars F: CD4+CD25+ regulatory T cells down-regulate co-stimulatory molecules on antigen-presenting cells. Eur J Immunol 2000;30:1538–1543.

15 Kryczek I, Wei S, Zou L, Zhu G, Mottram P, Xu H, Chen L, Zou W: Cutting edge: induction of B7-H4 on APCs through IL-10. Novel suppressive mode for regulatory T cells. J Immunol 2006;177:40–44.

16 Mahnke K, Ring S, Johnson TS, Schallenberg S, Schonfeld K, Storn V, Bedke T, Enk AH: Induction of immunosuppressive functions of dendritic cells in vivo by CD4+CD25+ regulatory T cells: role of B7-H3 expression and antigen presentation. Eur J Immunol 2007;37:2117–2126.

17 Suh WK, Gajewska BU, Okada H, Gronski MA, Bertram EM, Dawicki W, Duncan GS, Bukczynski J, Plyte S, Elia A, Wakeham A, Itie A, Chung S, Da CJ, Arya S, Horan T, Campbell P, Gaida K, Ohashi PS, Watts TH, Yoshinaga SK, Bray MR, Jordana M, Mak TW: The B7 family member B7-H3 preferentially down-regulates T-helper type 1-mediated immune responses. Nat Immunol 2003;4:899–906.

18 Schreiner B, Mitsdoerffer M, Kieseier BC, Chen L, Hartung HP, Weller M, Wiendl H: Interferon-β enhances monocyte and dendritic cell expression of B7-H1 (PD-L1), a strong inhibitor of autologous T-cell activation: relevance for the immune modulatory effect in multiple sclerosis. J Neuroimmunol 2004;155:172–182.

19 Selenko-Gebauer N, Majdic O, Szekeres A, Hofler G, Guthann E, Korthauer U, Zlabinger G, Steinberger P, Pickl WF, Stockinger H, Knapp W, Stockl J: B7-H1 (programmed death-1 ligand) on dendritic cells is involved in the induction and maintenance of T cell anergy. J Immunol 2003;170: 3637–3644.

20 Xu J, Huang B, Xiong P, Feng W, Xu Y, Fang M, Zheng F, Gong F: Soluble mouse B7-H3 down-regulates dendritic cell stimulatory capacity to allogenic T cell proliferation and production of IL-2 and IFN-γ. Cell Mol Immunol 2006;3:235–240.

21 Kryczek I, Zou L, Rodriguez P, Zhu G, Wei S, Mottram P, Brumlik M, Cheng P, Curiel T, Myers L, Lackner A, Alvarez X, Ochoa A, Chen L, Zou W: B7-H4 expression identifies a novel suppressive macrophage population in human ovarian carcinoma. J Exp Med 2006; 203:871–881.

22 Veldhoen M, Moncrieffe H, Hocking RJ, Atkins CJ, Stockinger B: Modulation of dendritic cell function by naive and regulatory CD4+ T cells. J Immunol 2006;176:6202–6210.

23 Hoves S, Krause SW, Schutz C, Halbritter D, Scholmerich J, Herfarth H, Fleck M: Monocyte-derived human macrophages mediate anergy in allogeneic T cells and induce regulatory t cells. J Immunol 2006;177:2691–2698.

24 Taams LS, van Amelsfort JM, Tiemessen MM, Jacobs KM, de Jong EC, Akbar AN, Bijlsma JW, Lafeber FP: Modulation of monocyte/macrophage function by human CD4+CD25+ regulatory T cells. Hum Immunol 2005;66: 222–230.

25 Venet F, Pachot A, Debard AL, Bohe J, Bienvenu J, Lepape A, Powell WS, Monneret G: Human CD4+CD25+ regulatory T lymphocytes inhibit lipopolysaccharide-induced monocyte survival through a Fas/Fas ligand-dependent mechanism. J Immunol 2006; 177:6540–6547.

26 Lin HH, Faunce DE, Stacey M, Terajewicz A, Nakamura T, Zhang-Hoover J, Kerley M, Mucenski ML, Gordon S, Stein-Streilein J: The macrophage F4/80 receptor is required for the induction of antigen-specific efferent regulatory T cells in peripheral tolerance. J Exp Med 2005;201:1615–1625.

27 Balandina A, Lecart S, Dartevelle P, Saoudi A, Berrih-Aknin S: Functional defect of regulatory CD4+CD25+ T cells in the thymus of patients with autoimmune myasthenia gravis. Blood 2005;105:735–741.

28 Boyer O, Saadoun D, Abriol J, Dodille M, Piette JC, Cacoub P, Klatzmann D: CD4+CD25+ regulatory T-cell deficiency in patients with hepatitis C-mixed cryoglobulinemia vasculitis. Blood 2004;103:3428–3430.

29 Fields ML, Hondowicz BD, Metzgar MH, Nish SA, Wharton GN, Picca CC, Caton AJ, Erikson J: CD4+CD25+ regulatory T cells inhibit the maturation but not the initiation of an autoantibody response. J Immunol 2005;175: 4255–4264.

30 Lim HW, Hillsamer P, Kim CH: Regulatory T cells can migrate to follicles upon T cell activation and suppress GC-Th cells and GC-Th cell-driven B cell responses. J Clin Invest 2004;114:1640–1649.

31 Lim HW, Hillsamer P, Banham AH, Kim CH: Cutting edge: direct suppression of B cells by CD4+CD25+ regulatory T cells. J Immunol 2005;175:4180–4183.

32 Janssens W, Carlier V, Wu B, VanderElst L, Jacquemin MG, Saint-Remy JM: CD4+CD25+ T cells lyse antigen-presenting B cells by Fas-Fas ligand interaction in an epitope-specific manner. J Immunol 2003;171:4604–4612.

33 Zhao DM, Thornton AM, DiPaolo RJ, Shevach EM: Activated CD4+CD25+ T cells selectively kill B lymphocytes. Blood 2006;107:3925–3932.

34 Reichardt P, Dornbach B, Rong S, Beissert S, Gueler F, Loser K, Gunzer M: Naive B cells generate regulatory T cells in the presence of a mature immunologic synapse. Blood 2007; 110:1519–1529.

35 Yang ZZ, Novak AJ, Ziesmer SC, Witzig TE, Ansell SM: CD70+ non-Hodgkin lymphoma B cells induce Foxp3 expression and regulatory function in intratumoral CD4+CD25− T cells. Blood 2007;110:2537–2544.

36 Ring S, Schafer SC, Mahnke K, Lehr HA, Enk AH: CD4+CD25+ regulatory T cells suppress contact hypersensitivity reactions by blocking influx of effector T cells into inflamed tissue. Eur J Immunol 2006;36:2981–2992.

37 Uhlig HH, Coombes J, Mottet C, Izcue A, Thompson C, Fanger A, Tannapfel A, Fontenot JD, Ramsdell F, Powrie F: Characterization of Foxp3+CD4+CD25+ and IL-10-secreting CD4+CD25+ T cells during cure of colitis. J Immunol 2006;177:5852–5860.

38 You S, Leforban B, Garcia C, Bach JF, Bluestone JA, Chatenoud L: Adaptive TGF-β-dependent regulatory T cells control autoimmune diabetes and are a privileged target of anti-CD3 antibody treatment. Proc Natl Acad Sci USA 2007; 104:6335–6340.

39 Joetham A, Takeda K, Taube C, Miyahara N, Matsubara S, Koya T, Rha YH, Dakhama A, Gelfand EW: Naturally occurring lung CD4+CD25+ T cell regulation of airway allergic responses depends on IL-10 induction of TGF-β. J Immunol 2007;178:1433–1442.

40 Hara M, Kingsley CI, Niimi M, Read S, Turvey SE, Bushell AR, Morris PJ, Powrie F, Wood KJ: IL-10 is required for regulatory T cells to mediate tolerance to alloantigens in vivo. J Immunol 2001;166:3789–3796.

41 Taylor A, Verhagen J, Blaser K, Akdis M, Akdis CA: Mechanisms of immune suppression by interleukin-10 and transforming growth factor-β: the role of T regulatory cells. Immunology 2006;117:433–442.

42 Read S, Greenwald R, Izcue A, Robinson N, Mandelbrot D, Francisco L, Sharpe AH, Powrie F: Blockade of CTLA-4 on CD4+CD25+ regulatory T cells abrogates their function in vivo. J Immunol 2006;177:4376–4383.

43 Oida T, Xu L, Weiner HL, Kitani A, Strober W: TGF-β-mediated suppression by CD4+CD25+ T cells is facilitated by CTLA-4 signaling. J Immunol 2006;177:2331–2339.

44 Siegmund K, Feuerer M, Siewert C, Ghani S, Haubold U, Dankof A, Krenn V, Schon MP, Scheffold A, Lowe JB, Hamann A, Syrbe U, Huehn J: Migration matters: regulatory T-cell compartmentalization determines suppressive activity in vivo. Blood 2005;106:3097–3104.

45 Lehmann J, Huehn J, de la Rosa M, Maszyna F, Kretschmer U, Krenn V, Brunner M, Scheffold A, Hamann A: Expression of the integrin αEβ7 identifies unique subsets of CD25+ as well as CD25− regulatory T cells. Proc Natl Acad Sci USA 2002;99:13031–13036.

46 Schwarz A, Maeda A, Schwarz T: Alteration of the migratory behavior of UV-induced regulatory T cells by tissue-specific dendritic cells. J Immunol 2007; 178:877–886.

Karsten Mahnke, PhD
Department of Dermatology, University Hospital Heidelberg
Vosstrasse 11, DE–69115 Heidelberg (Germany)
Tel. +49 6221 56 8170, Fax +49 6221 56 1617
E-Mail Karsten.mahnke@med.uni-heidelberg.de

Blaser K (ed): T Cell Regulation in Allergy, Asthma and Atopic Skin Diseases.
Chem Immunol Allergy. Basel, Karger, 2008, vol 94, pp 40–47

Mucosal Regulatory T Cells in Airway Hyperresponsiveness

Deborah H. Strickland · Matthew E. Wikstrom ·
Debra J. Turner · Patrick G. Holt

Telethon Institute for Child Health Research and Centre for Child Health Research,
School of Paediatrics and Child Health, The University of Western Australia, Perth, WA, Australia

Abstract

Interest in regulatory T cells (Treg) and their role in immune regulation has grown almost exponentially over the last 10 years, though the notion of a suppressive population of T cells has been in existence since the early 1970s. Recent reports have highlighted the potential role of populations of Treg in control of T-cell-mediated inflammation in tissues, including the lung. In particular, there is now evidence to suggest that Treg form a fundamental part of the regulatory axis operating within the respiratory mucosa and that the number of Treg recruited to the airways may be crucial for the inhibition of airways hyperresponsiveness associated with exacerbations of asthma. A discussion of these concepts is the focus of this chapter.   Copyright © 2008 S. Karger AG, Basel

Respiratory Tolerance

The respiratory mucosal surface is chronically exposed to a plethora of non-pathogenic environmental antigens, some of which are potential triggers for allergic disease. In order to protect against the immunopathological consequences of continuously responding to these ubiquitous stimuli, the local 'default' immune response takes the form of non-inflammatory low-level T-helper 2 (Th2) immunity [1–4] and/or a form of T-cell-mediated immunological tolerance [5]. Our laboratory was the first to describe this process of respiratory tract tolerance [6], which protects against sensitization (and ensuing IgE production) to aeroallergens. We demonstrated contributions from a variety of T-cell populations with regulatory properties and more recent evidence has implicated regulatory T cells (Treg) as mediators of this form of tolerance [7]. Of note, a hallmark feature of respiratory tract tolerance is that it can only be induced in immunologically naive animals – once CD4+ T-helper (Th) cell priming has been initiated, recirculating Th memory cells are resistant to this form of tolerance and ongoing aerosol exposure instead slowly expands this memory population [5]. Thus early oral or nasal therapy may be effective in preventing the development of airways hyperresponsiveness (AHR) in children that are at a high risk of allergic sensitization, and indeed, clinical trials are underway to test this possibility [8].

The mechanism(s) underlying this protective default are only partially understood, but it appears that this immunological rheostat is set via the activity of local dendritic cell (DC) subsets [7]. Immature DC, such as those found within the respiratory mucosa, have been shown to play a role in the development of respiratory tolerance by the induction of Treg populations [7]. In this way, the capacity for local activation of sensitized Th2 memory cells in airway tissue is normally constrained by the immature functional status of resident DC.

Asthma

Asthma is a deviation from the normal state of respiratory immunological tolerance. It is a chronic inflammatory disorder of the airways in which many cells and cellular elements play a role. In pathological terms, asthma is defined as a disease of the airways characterized by chronic inflammation with infiltration of lymphocytes, eosinophils, and mast cells, with epithelial desquamation and thickening and disorganization of the tissues of the airway wall including the basement membrane [9]. Clinically, asthma is defined as a disease of the airways that makes the airway excessively prone to narrowing in response to a variety of provoking stimuli. Although a precise definition of asthma has been difficult to formulate over the years, there are three primary defining characteristics associated with this disease, namely inflammation, AHR, and reversible airway obstruction [9]. These features are thought to account for most of the clinical manifestations of asthma, and are presumably interrelated, although the precise links have not been established. The duration of AHR following asthma exacerbation is highly variable, and is one of the most important determinants of disease severity. In the most severe forms of chronic asthma, AHR can develop into an essentially continuous state, resulting in markedly reduced respiratory function.

Measuring AHR
Bronchoconstrictor challenge tests are used to confirm the diagnosis of asthma. AHR to histamine or methacholine (the most commonly used stimuli) is identifiable in virtually all currently symptomatic asthmatics and about 5% of non-asthmatics [10]. Measurements of lung function, at set time intervals following inhalation of increasing doses of a bronchoconstrictor from a nebulizer, are used to generate a dose-response curve (DRC). Hyperresponsiveness is characterized by both a leftward and an upward shift of the DRC that is the result of an increase in the capacity to induce bronchoconstriction, and an increase in the magnitude of bronchoconstriction, respectively [11].

AHR in Asthma
Despite a vast number of studies and ongoing research, the mechanisms of AHR in asthma remain essentially unknown. AHR can occur in two distinct phases and the likely mechanisms also appear to be distinct. In atopic asthmatics, aeroallergen challenge initially triggers a rapid and short-lived bronchoconstriction reaction (early phase response) mediated predominantly by IgE-armed mast cells. This is followed by a later and more sustained late phase response (LPR) driven by Th2 cells activated locally in the airway mucosa [12]. Damage to local airway mucosal tissues during the LPR, in particular by infiltrating eosinophils, activated via Th2-derived cytokines such as IL-5, results in the ensuing development of AHR to inhaled irritants. Although the exact mechanism is not known, airway inflammation appears to be crucial for the development of AHR. Chronic inflammation leads to remodelling of the airways in asthma, resulting in several pathological features that can contribute to excessive airway narrowing, namely: increases in smooth muscle and bronchial blood vessels, tissue oedema, goblet cell and mucus gland hyperplasia, thickening of collagen layers, and decreased distensibility of the airways [13].

Studying AHR in Animal Models

We and others have been able to develop mouse and rat models of allergic airways disease that exhibit shifts in DRC to bronchoconstrictor

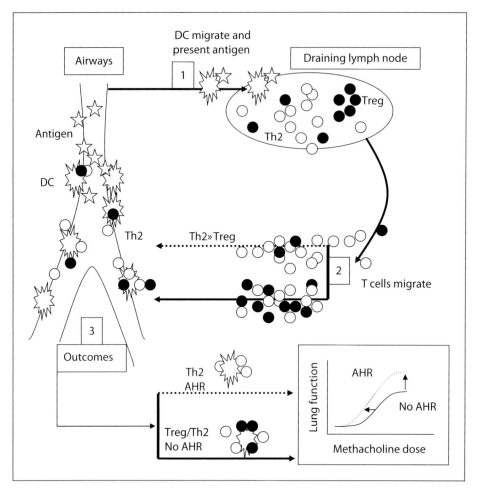

Fig. 1. Recruitment of Treg to the airways in sufficient numbers is required for the inhibition of AHR. Upon inhalation, allergens are captured from the airways by AMDC. (1) AMDC migrate out of the mucosa with the allergen and process it for presentation to T cells in the draining lymph nodes, generating a large proportion of Th2 effector cells and a smaller proportion of Treg. (2) Recently generated Th2 effectors and Treg are destined to migrate to the airway mucosa where they will interact with AMDC. (3) When there are insufficient numbers of Treg, AHR will result upon the next encounter with allergen in the airways.

challenge that are comparable to those seen in aeroallergen challenge studies in human atopic asthmatics [14]. Allergic sensitization is typically induced by systemic immunization with a model allergen (e.g., hen egg ovalbumin), followed by one or more challenges via the airways. AHR is accompanied in these models by an increase in airway inflammation driven by Th2 cells and a hallmark increase in eosinophils in bronchoalveolar lavage fluid and airway tissues [14].

Working with these rodent models, we have accumulated evidence that indicate local DC (airway mucosal dendritic cells, AMDC) are ideally positioned to drive activation of the aeroallergen-specific Th cells which are responsible for the LPR component of asthma exacerbations (fig. 1).

We have shown that a network of AMDC exists within the conducting airway epithelium and underlying the submucosa of experimental animals [15] and recently demonstrated a sequence of cellular interactions which occur in situ within the airway mucosa during the first few hours following challenge of sensitized animals with aerosolized allergen [16]. The crucial observation in these studies was the demonstration that AMDC are in virtually continuous communication (via short-term clustering) with Th memory cells transiting through the airway mucosa. We have demonstrated that the triggering step in the asthma LPR is the cognate interaction between allergen-bearing AMDC and incoming Th memory T cells, leading to transient upregulation of local APC activity followed by Th cell activation [16]. This in turn stimulates their mobilization and emigration to draining lymph nodes over the ensuing 12–24 h, but during the emigration process further interactions occur within the mucosa with other incoming Th memory cells, resulting in reactivation of the latter in situ, and subsequent development of AHR [16].

Inhibiting AHR in Animal Models

Allergen-specific tolerance can be induced in animals that have already been sensitized to an allergen, i.e. desensitization. These experiments are more relevant to SIT (see below), since human therapy normally commences after the onset of allergy. Thus, in some experimental models, sensitized mice that repeatedly inhale or ingest allergen exhibit a reduction in serum IgE levels, airway inflammation, and AHR [17]. In some instances, allergen-specific tolerance is induced more effectively via the nasal route than other routes [17], while other studies have found that inhaled allergen can exacerbate the allergic reaction in the airways [18]. In this case, the number of inhaled doses appears to be crucial: a short course of exposure is likely to elicit an allergic reaction in the airways, while a longer course will attenuate the reaction [3].

Our studies have shown that after triggering an initial round of AMDC activation and a subsequent burst of local Th cell activation, exposed animals rapidly become refractory to further aeroallergen exposure. In particular, local AMDC activation is not evident following more than three consecutive daily OVA aerosol exposures. This 'desensitized' state is maintained in the face of at least 10 consecutive daily aerosol challenges, and is paralleled by waning of AHR, which returns to baseline beyond day 3. Our earlier experiments [16] indicated that AMDC, which acquired OVA during the initial aerosol exposure and emigrated from the airway mucosa by the 24-hour time point, are replaced in the mucosa by incoming immature DC precursors. The failure of the latter to respond (by CD86 upregulation) to the second round of OVA aerosol exposure suggests that either the airway mucosal OVA-specific Th2 memory cell population in these animals had become anergized, or that a downregulatory control mechanism which prevents AMDC responding to activation signal(s) from CD4+ Th2 memory cells had been triggered within the mucosa.

Treg Populations

For the purposes of this chapter, we will consider Treg in the broader categories of natural and induced. Both of these Treg populations share some phenotypic and functional characteristics (table 1). However, there is a lot of variation in the phenotype and function of induced Treg that may be related to the variety of conditions that give rise to them. The most important distinction between these two types of Treg is that induced Treg arise as a consequence of antigen (or allergen) exposure. It is not yet clear how inducible Treg are generated or whether they are derived from natural Treg, though it is possible to generate Treg from conventional T cells (i.e., CD4+CD25−FoxP3−) in vitro and in vivo [19]. The origins of inducible

Table 1. Characteristics of natural and induced Treg

Natural Treg	Induced Treg
CD4+CD25+	CD4+CD25−/+
Express high levels of FoxP3	May express FoxP3
Generated in the thymus	Generated in the periphery
Slow turnover	Rapid turnover
Antigen-independent	Antigen-dependent
Regulatory activity can be attributed, at least in part, to cell contact and soluble mediators such as TGF-β and IL-10	Regulatory activity can be attributed, at least in part, to secretion of IL-10 and/or TGF-β

Treg will remain unclear until a specific marker for these cells can be identified and their phenotype more exclusively defined.

Role of Treg in Inhibiting AHR

CD4+ Treg expressing CD2 and FoxP3 can regulate peripheral T-cell responses via a variety of mechanisms including IL-10 and/or TGF-β [20]. Over the years, a variety of mechanisms have been proposed for oral and nasal tolerance, and while work in this field is ongoing, it is apparent that a variety of Treg derived from various means and possibly acting via different mechanisms can act to limit the allergic reaction to inhaled allergen. For example, Treg induced by inhaled allergen in naive mice were found to be effective, in an IL-10- and ICOS-dependent manner, at diminishing AHR in sensitized mice after adoptive transfer [2]. Several other studies have also found inducible Treg producing IL-10 are able to suppress allergic disease in the airways [20], especially when nasal tolerance is induced after sensitization. However, natural Treg can also inhibit AHR, by suppressing either the initial phase of sensitization [21] or the allergic reaction to inhaled allergen [22]. In our studies, we have shown that a regimen of repeated aerosol challenge induces a population of Treg in the draining lymph nodes and airways, coinciding with a decrease in DC activation, AHR and other allergic symptoms. The number of Treg declined upon cessation of the aerosols then increased again with further rounds of allergen exposure, all with concomitant modulation of DC activation and AHR [3]. Importantly, transfer of Treg derived from these repeatedly challenged animals could inhibit the development of AHR in previously sensitized animals, and since this effect depended on the number of Treg transferred [D.H. Strickland and P.G. Holt, unpubl. observations], we believe suppression of AHR in our studies depends on the number of Treg recruited to the airways. Such a scenario also provides a plausible explanation for the intermittent pattern of asthma exacerbations in the majority of human atopic asthmatics.

While our understanding of the role of Treg in experimental models of allergen-specific tolerance is growing, a number of limitations should be acknowledged. First, only a few studies have attempted to measure the function of Treg induced by allergen in vivo; and second, the mechanism of suppression is only poorly understood. Indeed, the targets of Treg need to be identified in vivo before more work on the mechanisms is carried out.

Role of Treg in Human AHR

While it is not possible to directly test the role of Treg in human AHR, there is some evidence to suggest they are important, and indeed, the number of Treg might determine the development of allergic disease and AHR in human asthma. Firstly, the number of Treg is reduced in bronchoalveolar lavage fluid samples from children compared with healthy controls [23]. Smaller reductions in Treg numbers have been reported for the blood of asthmatic children [23] and adults [24] although other studies have failed to find a difference [25, and M.E. Wikstrom and P.G. Holt, unpubl. observations]. These studies with peripheral blood are limited though, because they do not directly examine the number of Treg in the airway tissue. Furthermore, atopic asthmatics may not suffer from an absolute deficit in Treg; rather the deficit may occur in relation to the ratio of allergen-specific T cells producing Th2 cytokines to the number of locally available Treg, and indeed, there is evidence to support this notion [26].

Therapeutic Means of Inhibiting AHR in Asthma

Glucocorticoids (GC) are the most effective anti-inflammatory treatment used in allergic diseases, and for a significant proportion of asthmatics, they are effective at limiting AHR. A large number of studies have demonstrated that GC affect the immune system, including modulation of cytokine production, altering trafficking and function of effectors cells. Additionally, these steroids have been shown to increase Treg populations in vitro and in vivo [23], particularly IL-10-producing Treg. Since the induction of IL-10 appears to be closely associated with the effectiveness of steroid treatment for asthma [27], an increase in the number of Treg in airway tissue may explain at least some of the effects of inhaled steroids on human asthma. Alternatively, or perhaps in addition, inhaled steroids have been shown to act on Treg to increase their suppressive activity in vitro [28], and thus, improvements in the function of Treg may also explain the effects of inhaled steroids on human asthma. However, GC are not effective in permanent disease modification per

se, as cessation of treatment almost invariably results in return of symptomatology.

Ideally, the ultimate strategy would be to *prevent* asthma and AHR exacerbations, a concept that has been embraced in allergen-specific immunotherapy (SIT). SIT was first performed in humans at the beginning of the 20th century, when small doses of grass pollen were injected subcutaneously to alleviate the symptoms of hay fever. Today, SIT strategies most commonly employ small subcutaneous doses over a period of years to reduce allergic reactions in the skin, nasal passages, and the airways [29]. SIT is an important therapy because it can prevent AHR without any further need for medication. While SIT promises long-lasting relief, it is not always successful, and there is a danger of anaphylaxis for the duration of treatment. Recently, a less traumatic form of SIT has been introduced in the form of sublingual immunotherapy, which has proven efficacious in a number of large-scale trials [8]. This involves allergen stimulation of the lymph nodes draining the oropharynx via repeated application of drops containing allergen to the buccal surface under the tongue.

While the mechanisms have yet to be fully elucidated, it is clear that SIT, in its various forms, has many effects on the immune system [see 29 for a thorough review]. One of the most important effects of SIT is to reduce the high IgE level and the strong Th2 cytokine response that characterizes the allergic phenotype via the induction of allergen-specific tolerance. The phenomenon of allergen-specific tolerance has been intensively studied in a variety of animal models, and while a number of mechanisms have been proposed over the years, Treg have emerged in recent years as one of the strongest candidates.

Conclusions

In the past it has been proposed that the balance between the Th1 and Th2 cellular subsets is one of the factors dictating an allergic versus non-allergic response, and more recently a role for Th17 cells has been implicated in the control of respiratory immunological tolerance versus responsiveness. However, it is becoming increasingly clear that an important regulatory axis operating within the respiratory mucosa is dependent upon the balance that is achieved between the Th2 and Treg components. Ongoing studies in animal models of allergic sensitization and tolerance induction have shown cumulatively that the restoration and subsequent maintenance of immunological homeostasis in the airway mucosa following an experimental asthma exacerbation is a dynamic allergen-driven process involving interplay between populations of allergen-specific Th cells, AMDC, and Treg. These studies have demonstrated that Treg can act at different times to inhibit allergic sensitization or directly suppress AHR. For the latter, data is emerging to suggest the number of Treg recruited to the airways is an important step in the regulation of AHR, and may explain at least some of the effects of inhaled steroids on human AHR. Moreover, and with important ramifications in the context of therapies such as SIT, our recent findings [3] demonstrate that ongoing protection of airway tissues in sensitized animals via Treg relies absolutely on continuation of allergen exposure, as withdrawal of stimulation restores susceptibility to the Th2-dependent AHR inducing effects of aeroallergen challenge. Whether or not prolonged stimulation of Treg via continuous therapeutic administration of allergen can eventually exhaust respective target Th2 memory cell populations and establish potentially permanent protection against allergy, remains to be established. Further investigation of this concept and the mechanisms responsible will ultimately guide the development of new therapeutic strategies.

References

1 Herrick CA, Bottomly K: To respond or not to respond: T cells in allergic asthma. Nat Rev Immunol 2003;3: 405–412.

2 Akbari O, Freeman GJ, Meyer EH, Greenfield EA, Chang TT, Sharpe AH, Berry G, DeKruyff RH, Umetsu DT: Antigen-specific regulatory T cells develop via the ICOS-ICOS-ligand pathway and inhibit allergen-induced airway hyperreactivity. Nat Med 2002; 8:1024–1032.

3 Strickland DH, Stumbles PA, Zosky GR, Subrata LS, Thomas JA, Turner DJ, Sly PD, Holt PG: Reversal of airway hyperresponsiveness by induction of airway mucosal CD4+CD25+ regulatory T cells. J Exp Med 2006;203: 2649–2660.

4 Stumbles PA, Thomas JA, Pimm CL, Lee PT, Venaille TJ, Proksch S, Holt PG: Resting respiratory tract dendritic cells preferentially stimulate T-helper cell type 2 (Th2) responses and require obligatory cytokine signals for induction of Th1 immunity. J Exp Med 1998;188:2019–2031.

5 Holt PG: Immunoprophylaxis of atopy: light at the end of the tunnel? Immunol Today 1994;15:484–489.

6 Holt PG, Batty JE, Turner KJ: Inhibition of specific IgE responses in mice by pre-exposure to inhaled antigen. Immunology 1981;42:409–417.

7 Umetsu DT, DeKruyff RH: The regulation of allergy and asthma. Immunol Rev 2006;212:238–255.

8 Baena-Cagnani CE, Passalacqua G, Gomez M, Zernotti ME, Canonica GW: New perspectives in the treatment of allergic rhinitis and asthma in children. Curr Opin Allergy Clin Immunol 2007;7:201–206.

9 Woolcock A: Definitions and clinical classification; in Barnes PJ, Grunsyein MM, Leff AR, Woolcock AJ (eds): Asthma. Philadelphia, Lippincott-Raven, 1997, pp 27–32.

10 Cockcroft D, Berscheid B, Murdoch K, Gore B: Sensitivity and specificity of histamine PC20 measurements in a random selection of young college students. J Allergy Clin Immunol 1992;89:23–30.

11 Woolcock A, Salome C, Yan K: The shape of the dose-response curve to histamine in asthmatic and normal subjects. Am Rev Respir Dis 1984;130: 71–75.

12 Wills-Karp M: Immunologic basis of antigen-induced airway hyperresponsiveness. Annu Rev Immunol 1999;17: 255–281.

13 James A, Pare P, Hogg J: The mechanics of airway narrowing in asthma. Am Rev Respir Dis 1989;139:242–246.

14 Zosky G, Sly P, Turner D: Mouse models of asthma: what physiological evidence are they based on? Allergy Clin Immunol Int: J World Allergy Org 2006; 18:76–79.

15 Schon-Hegrad MA, Oliver J, McMenamin PG, Holt PG: Studies on the density, distribution, and surface phenotype of intraepithelial class II major histocompatibility complex antigen (Ia)-bearing dendritic cells in the conducting airways. J Exp Med 1991; 173:1345–1356.

16 Huh JC, Strickland DH, Jahnsen FL, Turner DJ, Thomas JA, Napoli S, Tobagus I, Stumbles PA, Sly PD, Holt PG: Bidirectional interactions between antigen-bearing respiratory tract dendritic cells (DCs) and T cells precede the late phase reaction in experimental asthma: DC activation occurs in the airway mucosa but not in the lung parenchyma. J Exp Med 2003;198: 19–30.

17 Takabayashi K, Libet L, Chisholm D, Zubeldia J, Horner AA: Intranasal immunotherapy is more effective than intradermal immunotherapy for the induction of airway allergen tolerance in Th2-sensitized mice. J Immunol 2003;170:3898–3905.

18 Janssen EM, van Oosterhout AJM, Nijkamp FP, van Eden W, Wauben MHM: The efficacy of immunotherapy in an experimental murine model of allergic asthma is related to the strength and site of T cell activation during immunotherapy. J Immunol 2000;165:7207–7214.

19 Shevach EM: From vanilla to 28 flavors: multiple varieties of T regulatory cells. Immunity 2006;25:195–201.

20 Hawrylowicz CM, O'Garra A: Potential role of interleukin-10-secreting regulatory T cells in allergy and asthma. Nat Rev Immunol 2005;5:271–283.

21 Lewkowich IP, Herman NS, Schleifer KW, Dance MP, Chen BL, Dienger KM, Sproles AA, Shah JS, Kohl J, Belkaid Y, Wills-Karp M: CD4+CD25+ T cells protect against experimentally induced asthma and alter pulmonary dendritic cell phenotype and function. J Exp Med 2005;202:1549–1561.

22 Kearley J, Barker JE, Robinson DS, Lloyd CM: Resolution of airway inflammation and hyperreactivity after in vivo transfer of CD4+CD25+ regulatory T cells is interleukin-10 dependent. J Exp Med 2005;202:1539–1547.

23 Hartl D, Koller B, Mehlhorn AT, Reinhardt D, Nicolai T, Schendel DJ, Griese M, Krauss-Etschmann S: Quantitative and functional impairment of pulmonary CD4+CD25^{hi} regulatory T cells in pediatric asthma. J Allergy Clin Immunol 2007;119:1258–1266.

24 Ling EM, Smith T, Nguyen XD, Pridgeon C, Dallman PM, Arbery J, Carr VA, Robinson DS: Relation of CD4+CD25+ regulatory T-cell suppression of allergen-driven T-cell activation to atopic status and expression of allergic disease. Lancet 2004;363: 608–615.

25 Hoffmann HJ, Malling TM, Topcu A, Ryder LP, Nielsen KR, Varming K, Dahl R, Omland O, Sigsgaard T: CD4^{dim}CD25^{bright} Treg cell frequencies above a standardized gating threshold are similar in asthmatics and controls. Cytometry A 2007;71A:371–378.

26 Akdis M, Verhagen J, Taylor A, Karamloo F, Karagiannidis C, Crameri R, Thunberg S, Deniz G, Valenta R, Fiebig H, Kegel C, Disch R, Schmidt-Weber CB, Blaser K, Akdis CA: Immune responses in healthy and allergic individuals are characterized by a fine balance between allergen-specific T regulatory 1 and T-helper-2 cells. J Exp Med 2004;199:1567–1575.

27 Xystrakis E, Kusumakar S, Boswell S, Peek E, Urry Z, Richards DF, Adikibi T, Pridgeon C, Dallman M, Loke T-K, Robinson DS, Barrat FJ, O'Garra A, Lavender P, Lee TH, Corrigan C, Hawrylowicz CM: Reversing the defective induction of IL-10-secreting regulatory T cells in glucocorticoid-resistant asthma patients. J Clin Invest 2006;116:146–155.

28 Dao Nguyen X, Robinson DS: Fluticasone propionate increases CD4+CD25+ T regulatory cell suppression of allergen-stimulated CD4+CD25− T cells by an IL-10-dependent mechanism. J Allergy Clin Immunol 2004;114:296–301.

29 Larche M, Akdis CA, Valenta R: Immunological mechanisms of allergen-specific immunotherapy. Nat Rev Immunol 2006;6:761–771.

Deborah H. Strickland
Telethon Institute for Child Health Research and Centre for Child Health Research
School of Paediatrics and Child Health, The University of Western Australia
PO Box 855, West Perth, WA 6872 (Australia)
Tel. +61 8 9489 7777, Fax +61 8 9489 7700, E-Mail deborahs@ichr.uwa.edu.au

Blaser K (ed): T Cell Regulation in Allergy, Asthma and Atopic Skin Diseases.
Chem Immunol Allergy. Basel, Karger, 2008, vol 94, pp 48–57

Natural Killer Cells in Allergic Inflammation

Gaye Erten · Esin Aktas · Gunnur Deniz

Department of Immunology, Institute of Experimental Medicine (DETAE),
Istanbul University, Istanbul, Turkey

Abstract

Natural killer (NK) cells are large granular lymphocytes of the innate immune system that exert a potent function against infected and tumor cells. Although NK cells were originally defined by their capacity to lyse target cells and produce interferon-γ without prior activation, recent studies showed that NK cells also display a potent regulatory function. They are activated or inhibited through the ligation of germline-encoded receptors and are involved in mediating cytotoxicity, producing cytokines and providing costimulation to cells of the adaptive immune system. NK cells play important roles in viral infections, autoimmunity, pregnancy, cancer and bone marrow transplantation, but little is known about the role of NK cells in allergy. Recent developments in the understanding of the role of human NK cells in allergy are overviewed.

Copyright © 2008 S. Karger AG, Basel

Human Natural Killer Cell Subtypes

Natural killer (NK) cells are bone marrow-derived large granular lymphocytes playing an important role in the innate immunity, especially against viruses and tumor cells, and they form 10–15% of the total lymphocyte population. NK cells have the ability to lyse cells without specific antigen recognition, and these cells may be considered as effector cells, especially in the innate immune system. Peripheral NK cells have been identified in humans as a discrete lymphocyte subset expressing the low-affinity receptor for the Fc portion of IgG (FcγRIIIA, CD16) or CD56 and CD161 (NKR-P1A) in the absence of T-cell receptor and its associated CD3 complex.

Recent studies have identified at least 48 distinct NK cell subsets, whose significance and function is largely uncertain [1]. A few NK cell subsets have been well defined. The expression of CD56 on NK cells is not believed to serve any specific function but allows the division of NK cells into two major functional subsets according to intensity of CD56 expression (CD56^{bright} and CD56^{dim}) [2]. CD56^{dim} NK cells comprise the majority of peripheral blood NK cells (approx. 90%) and express high levels CD16 as well as perforin. As a result, these cells are effective killers. CD56^{bright} NK cells are considered as immunoregulatory cells and CD56^{dim} NK cells as cytotoxic cells [3] (fig. 1). NK cells express CD56 and CD16 at different levels, 90% of NK cells express CD16 in high levels (CD16^{bright}) and CD56 in low levels (CD56^{dim}) and approximately 10% of NK cells express CD16 in low levels (CD16^{dim}) and CD56 in high levels (CD56^{bright}). CD56 expression level influences the effect of NK cells, and it

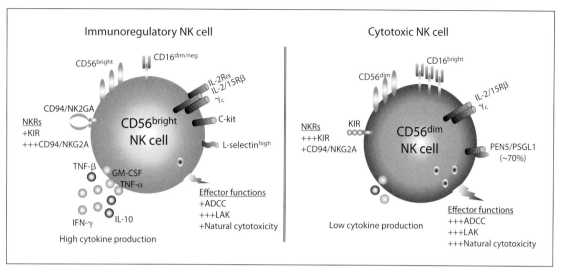

Fig. 1. NK cell subsets: NK cells are divided into two different subsets according to CD56 and CD16 expressions resulting in different functions [from 3, with permission].

has been found to identify an isoform of the neural cell adhesion molecule (NCAM). NCAM is a member of the immunoglobulin superfamily of cell adhesion molecules and it contains polysialic acid, which appears to regulate binding avidity of NCAM and other cell adhesion processes [4]. These two subsets of NK cells differ in cytotoxic activity and cytokine production. CD56^{bright} immunoregulatory NK cells have the ability to secrete high levels of cytokines such as interferon-γ (IFN-γ), interleukin (IL)-10, tumor necrosis factor-α (TNF-α) and granulocyte macrophage-colony stimulating factor (GM-CSF). CD16^{bright} NK cells are much more involved in cytotoxicity. Both NK cell subsets constitutively express similar levels of intermediate affinity IL-2 receptor, but exposure to exogenous IL-2 induces tenfold greater proliferation of CD56^{bright} cells compared to CD56^{dim} cells, because only CD56^{bright} NK cells express the high-affinity IL-2 receptor [5]. There is also a difference in IL-2 receptor expression among the CD56^{bright} NK cell population. CD56^{bright} NK cells

either lack CD16 (CD56^{bright} CD16$-$) or express it at low density (CD56^{bright} CD16^{dim}). Both the CD56^{bright} CD16$-$ and CD56^{bright} CD16^{dim} NK subsets express the high-affinity IL-2 receptor. But each CD56^{bright} NK cell subset has distinct functional responses to IL-2. Activation of the high-affinity IL-2 receptor on CD56^{bright} CD16$-$ NK cells induces a proliferative response that is significantly weaker than that observed in the CD56^{bright} CD16^{dim} NK cell subset. The distinct functional response to IL-2 of both CD56^{bright} NK subsets suggests that each phenotype may identify a discrete stage of NK cell differentiation [6]. NK cells also differ in chemokine receptor expressions. Freshly isolated primary NK cells were found to express CXCR1, CXCR3, and CXCR4, and to contain subsets expressing CCR1, CCR4, CCR5, CCR6, CCR7, CCR9, CXCR5, and CXCR6. With the exception of CCR4, these chemokine receptors were expressed at higher percentages by CD56^{bright} NK cells than by CD56^{dim} NK cells. In particular, CCR7 is expressed by almost all CD56^{bright} NK cells but was not detected on CD56^{dim} NK cells indicating that within both the CD56^{bright} and CD56^{dim} NK cell populations, subsets with the capacity for differential trafficking programs exist, which likely influence their functions in innate and adaptive immunity [7].

Lysis by NK Cells

NK cells possess large numbers of cytolytic granules, lysosomes containing mainly perforins and various granzymes. NK cells can also kill in a perforin-independent manner utilizing FAS ligand, TNF or TNF-related apoptosis-inducing ligand (TRAIL). Human NK cells use inhibitory and activating killer cell immunoglobulin-like receptors (KIR) for recognition of the healthy and infected cells. The inhibitory KIRs recognize human leukocyte antigen (HLA) class I molecules on cells and trigger signals that stop NK killing. The activating KIRs recognize determinants associated with infections and tumors, and trigger activating signals for NK cells to kill. Therefore, the effector function of a given NK cell depends upon the receptors that it expresses and ligands that it recognizes on the targets [8]. KIRs play a critical role in recognizing self class I major histocompatibility complex (MHC) molecules and thus protect healthy host cells from NK targeted lysis. In contrast, both NKG2D and CD16 are activating NK receptors that trigger the NK cell lysis of various tumor and virally infected cells through either direct ligand engagement or antibody-dependent cellular cytotoxicity [9].

In humans, a major component of NK cell target recognition depends mainly on the surveillance of HLA class I molecules by KIR belonging to the immunoglobulin superfamily. Different KIRs can transmit inhibitory or activatory signals to the cell, and effector function is considered to result from the balance of these contributing signals [10]. KIRs have two (KIR2D) or three (KIR3D) immunoglobulin-like extracellular domains with either a long (KIR2DL or KIR3DL) or a short (KIR2DS or KIR3DS) cytoplasmic tail. While short tails have immunoreceptor tyrosine-based activating motif (ITAM) on the cytoplasmic domain, long tails are associated with immunoreceptor tyrosine-based inhibitory motif (ITIM) resulting in activation or inhibition of the NK cell killing, respectively [11]. The KIR family predominantly recognizes classical HLA class I molecules and different family members interact with discrete HLA class I allotypes [12].

The next receptor family expressed on NK cells belongs to the heterodimeric C-type lectin receptors containing CD94 which is associated with C-type lectin NKG2 family [13]. The CD94/NKG2 family of receptors is composed of members with activating or inhibitory potential. These receptors are expressed predominantly on NK cells and a subset of CD8+ T cells, and they have been shown to play an important role in regulating responses against infected and tumorigenic cells [14]. The lectin-like CD94/NKG2 receptors specifically interact with the non-classical class I molecule, HLA-E [12].

The third receptor family expressed on NK cells are the natural cytotoxic receptors (NCR), and these receptors deliver activatory signals for NK cells to recognize and lyse tumor cells. Three novel, NK-specific, triggering surface molecules (NKp46, NKp30, and NKp44) have been identified. They represent the first members of a novel emerging group of receptors collectively termed NCR [15]. Among these, the NKp46 receptor is considered to be the major lysis receptor for NK cells. The viral hemagglutinin protein was recently identified as the ligand for the NKp46 receptor [16]. Activatory and inhibitory receptors of NK cells are summarized in table 1.

NK Cells and Cytokines

Although NK cells were originally defined by their capacity to lyse target cells, they also produce

Table 1. Activatory and inhibitory receptors of NK cells [from 35, with permission]

Function	Receptors	Ligand(s)	Species
Activation	CD94/NKG2C	HLA-E/Q^a-1^b	H, M
	NKG2D	MICA/B, ULBPs	H, M
	NKG2E	HLA-E/Q^a-1^b	H, M
	NKp30	Unknown	H
	NKp44	Unknown	H
	NKp46	Unknown	H, M
	NKR-P1A	Unknown	H, M
	NKR-P1C	Unknown	M
	NKR-P1F	Unknown	M
	Ly49C	H-2D/H-2K	M
	Ly49D	H-2D	M
	Ly49H	MCMV m157	M
	KIR2DS1, KIR2DS2	HLA-C	H
Inhibition	CD94/NKG2A	HLA-E/Q^a-1^b	H, M
	NKRP1B	Unknown	M
	NKRP1D	Unknown	M
	Ly49A	H-2D	M
	Ly49E	Unknown	M
	Ly49G	H-2D	H
	KIR2DL1, KIR2DL2	HLA-C	H
	KIR3DL1	HLA-Bw4	H
	KIR3DL3	HLA-A	H
	2B4	CD48	H, M

MIC = MHC class I chain-related antigens; ULBPs = UL16-binding protein; KIR = killer immunoglobulin-like receptor; HLA = human leukocyte antigen; H = human; M = mouse.

IFN-γ and the other cytokines without prior activation. As shown in figure 2, ex vivo CD56^{dim} cells contain detectable perforin and thus are expected to mediate cytotoxicity. In contrast, the CD56^{bright} NK cells express low levels of perforin (and CD16) but express high levels of cytokines and are thought to be an important inflammatory or regulatory subset [17]. NK cells exert their activity by producing high amounts of IFN-γ, that activates a strong inflammatory response. Other than IFN-γ, NK cells are able to produce many other important cytokines and chemokines, including myeloid differentiation and activation factors such as IL-3, GM-CSF, CSF-1, TNF-α, IL-5, IL-13.

NK cells express receptors for numerous monokines constitutively, and produce IFN-γ and other NK-derived cytokines rapidly in response to stimulation by monokines [18, 19]. Freshly isolated CD56^{bright} human NK cells are the primary source of NK cell-derived immunoregulatory cytokines, including IFN-γ, TNF-β (lymphotoxin), IL-10, IL-13 and GM-CSF, whereas the CD56^{dim} NK-cell subset produces consistently negligible amounts of these cytokines following stimulation with recombinant monokines in vitro [20]. The production of cytokines by NK cell subsets was investigated following activation with phorbol esters (e.g. phorbol 12-myristate 13-acetate (PMA)) and ionomycin,

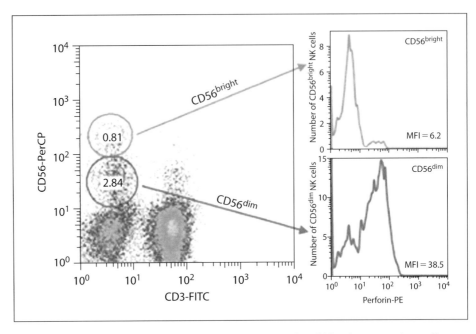

Fig. 2. Perforin expression in NK cell subsets. Normal peripheral blood mononuclear cells were isolated, stained for CD56 using a PerCP-conjugated antibody and CD3 using a FITC-conjugated antibody, then fixed, permeabilized and stained for intracellular perforin using a PE-conjugated antibody. The dot plot displays CD3 on the X-axis and CD56 on the Y-axis. The CD56[bright] and CD56[dim] subpopulations of NK cells are encircled by the orange and red gates, respectively. Perforin content within these populations is depicted in the histograms (CD56[bright] top, CD56[dim] bottom). The CD56 [bright] NK cells are largely perforin-negative, while the CD56[dim] NK cells (which also express CD16) are the ones with detectable perforin demonstrating their ability to mediate cytotoxicity [from 17, with permission].

non-specific activators of lymphocytes that are not dependent on specific monokine receptors. Again, CD56[bright] NK cells produced significantly more of all the cytokines induced by this combination, including IFN-γ, TNF-β and GM-CSF, than did identically cultured CD56[dim] cells [21]. Therefore, CD56[bright] NK cells appear to have an intrinsic capacity for high-level production of cytokines compared with CD56[dim] NK cells. These data suggest that the major function of CD56[bright] NK cells during the innate immune response in vivo might be to provide macrophages and other antigen-presenting cells with early IFN-γ and other cytokines, promoting a positive cytokine feedback loop and efficient control of infection. T and NK cells are also developmentally related. However, unlike T cells, many of the details of NK cell development are poorly characterized. IL-2 is a major growth factor for NK cells. NK cells proliferate, secrete other cytokines and show expanded cytolytic activity by IL-2 stimulation [22]. IL-15 is also able to activate NK cells via IL-2Rβ and γ$_c$ subunits and its own α chain (IL-15Rα) for high-affinity binding, although it has no sequence homology with IL-2 [23]. Infection or other damage induces local production of distinct cytokines by tissue cells and antigen-presenting cells initiating the differentiation of T cells into either type 1 or type 2 cells [23]. IL-12 drives naive T cells towards a type 1 phenotype and IL-4 drives towards type 2. The production of IFN-γ by NK cells has been demonstrated to be enhanced by IL-12, and inhibited by IL-4 [24]. Recently, it was shown that in the presence of IL-12 or IL-4, human NK cells can differentiate into NK cell subsets secreting distinct cytokine patterns similar to T cells. The authors have shown that NK cells grown in IL-12 (NK1) produce IL-10 and IFN-γ, whereas NK cells grown in IL-4 (NK2) produce IL-5 and IL-13 [25, 26]. Although these NK cell subsets do not differ in cytotoxic activity, NK1 cells express higher levels of cell surface CD95 (Fas) antigen than NK2 cells and are more sensitive to Ab or chemically induced apoptosis. NK1 cells accumulate much higher levels of the IL-12Rβ_2-chain mRNA and are significantly more responsive to IL-12 than NK2 cells at the level of activation of STAT4 transcription factor. The identification of NK cell subsets that are analogous to T-cell subsets suggests a new role for NK cells in innate inflammatory responses and in their effect on adaptive immunity [25].

NK Cells in Allergy

Many studies concerning the role of T cells and cytokines in allergy have been performed, but little is known about the role of NK cells. Numerous studies demonstrated increased frequency of allergen-specific Th2 cells producing increased IL-4, IL-5 and IL-13 in the peripheral blood of atopic dermatitis patients [27, 28]. However, the role of NK cells in allergic diseases has so far gained little attention. In response to allergenic antigens, CD4+ T-cell clones from atopic subjects produce IL-4 and IL-5, whereas non-atopic CD4+ T-cell clones produce Th1 cytokines [29]. Atopic subjects have a higher frequency of IL-4-producing T cells than healthy subjects and T-cell clones generated from cord blood lymphocytes of newborns with atopic parents produce higher IL-4 concentrations than neonatal lymphocytes

of newborns with non-atopic parents [30, 31]. It is well recognized that type 2 cytokines are not only produced by CD4+ T cells but also by CD8+ Tc cells, dendritic cells (DCs), and NK cells, and those cells are called Tc2 (type II cytotoxic T lymphocyte), DC2, or NK2 on the basis of secretion of type 2 cytokines [32, 33]. The ratio of IL-4+CD56+ NK2 cells in PBMCs of asthmatic patients was found to be higher than in healthy individuals. NK cell clones were then obtained by means of limited dilution, and the average mean of the relative intensity signal transducer and activator of transcription 6, a key transcript factor of type 2 phenotype, was constitutively activated in NK2 clones from asthmatic patients. The percentage of IFN-γ+CD56+ NK1 cells in the peripheral blood of asthmatic patients was remarkably increased, but that of IL-4+CD56+ NK2 cells was significantly decreased [33].

The in vivo existence of human NK cell subsets similar to Th1 and Th2 cells was demonstrated in freshly isolated IFN-γ-secreting and IFN-γ-non-secreting NK cells. The IFN-γ-secreting NK subset showed a typical cytokine pattern with predominant expression of IFN-γ, but almost no IL-4, IL-5 and IL-13. In contrast, the IFN-γ-non-secreting NK subset was composed of IL-4, IL-5 and IL-13-producing NK cells. In vitro differentiation of NK cells led to distinct patterns of cytokine production similar to freshly-purified IFN-γ-positive or IFN-γ-negative NK cell subsets. NK cells stimulated with IL-12 produced increased levels of IFN-γ and decreased levels of IL-4. In contrast, stimulation of NK cells with IL-4 inhibited IFN-γ, but increased IL-13 production. Freshly-purified IFN-γ-positive and IFN-γ-negative or in vitro differentiated NK1 and NK2 subsets showed similar cytotoxicity to K562 cells. These results demonstrate that circulating NK cells retain effector subsets in humans with distinct cytokine profiles and may display different inflammatory properties [34].

Accordingly, the expression of costimulatory, inhibitory and apoptosis receptors, cytokine

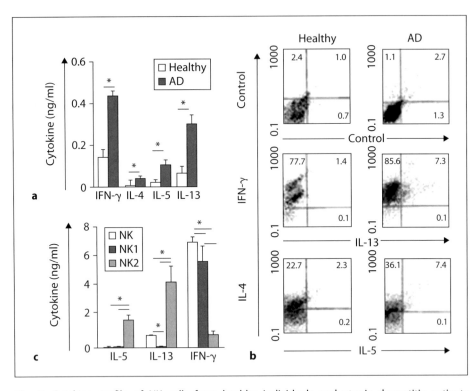

Fig. 3. Cytokine profile of NK cells from healthy individuals and atopic dermatitis patients. **a** Intracytoplasmic cytokines were determined by flow cytometry. NK cells from AD patients spontaneously released significantly more IL-4, IL-5, IL-13 and IFN-γ than those of controls, demonstrating an in vivo activation of NK cells in atopic patients. **b** To determine their full capacity to synthesize these cytokines, NK cells were stimulated and intracytoplasmic cytokines were analyzed. High percentages of IL-5- and IL-13-producing NK cells were detected in allergic patients, whereas very few IL-5- and IL-13-producing NK cells were found in healthy individuals. **c** NK1 and NK2 cell subsets were differentiated from freshly isolated NK cells of AD patients. IL-5 and IL-13 release were increased in NK2 cells compared to NK1 and NK cells. In contrast, IFN-γ was higher in NK1 cell subsets compared to NK and NK2 cells. NK1 cells did not show any IL-13, but released significantly high amounts of IFN-γ. The above results suggest that NK cells might influence the overall inflammatory network in allergy by increased IL-4, IL-5, IL-13 and IFN-γ release [from 34, with permission]. *p < 0.01.

profiles and their effect on immunoglobulin isotypes were investigated in polyallergic atopic dermatitis patients with hyperimmunoglobulin E (IgE) and healthy individuals. Atopic dermatitis patients showed significantly decreased peripheral blood NK cells compared to healthy individuals: freshly isolated NK cells by IL-12 and neutralizing anti-IL-4 monoclonal antibodies (mAb), and to NK2 cells by IL-4 and neutralizing

anti-IL-12 mAb. Following IL-12 stimulation, NK cells produced increased levels of IFN-γ and decreased IL-4. In contrast, stimulation of NK cells with IL-4 inhibited IFN-γ but increased IL-13 production (fig. 3).

The effect of NK cell subsets on IgE regulation was examined in cocultures of in vitro differentiated NK cells with peripheral blood mononuclear cells or B cells. NK1 cells significantly inhibited

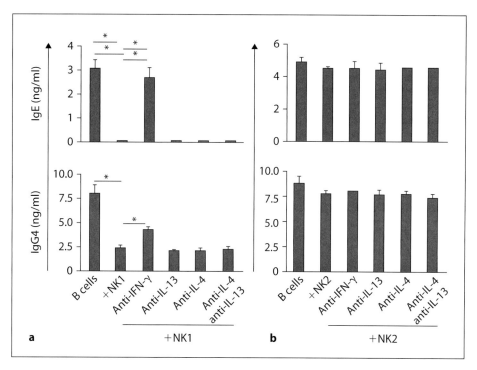

Fig. 4. Suppression of IgE production by NK1 cells is mediated by IFN-γ. To investigate the mechanism of IgE inhibition by NK1 cells, in vitro differentiated NK1 cells were cocultured with purified B cells in the presence of neutralizing anti-IFN-γ, anti-IL-4 and anti-IL-13 mAbs. **a** Inhibition of IgE and IgG4 by NK1 cells was significantly blocked by neutralization of IFN-γ (*p < 0.001 and p < 0.02, respectively). There was no influence in neutralization of IL-4 and IL-13 on NK1 cell-mediated IgE suppression. **b** Unlike Th2 cells, NK2 cells did not induce IgE in B cell cocultures [from 34, with permission].

IL-4- and soluble CD40-ligand-stimulated IgE production; however, NK2 cells did not have any effect. The inhibitory effect of NK1 cells on IgE production was blocked by neutralization of IFN-γ (fig. 4) [34].

Except for CD40, NK cell subsets showed different expression of killer-inhibitory receptors and costimulatory molecules between the polyallergic and healthy subjects. The study demonstrates that human NK cells comprise distinct receptor-expressing and cytokine-producing subsets similar to Th1 and Th2 cells. These subsets of NK cells show differences in surface KIR receptors and costimulatory receptors and interfere with immunoglobulin regulation [34].

Concluding Remarks

Even though remarkable progress has been made in understanding the biology of NK cells, many questions remain to be answered. NK cells did not receive much attention until the last decade when their multiple functions as killers, cytokine producers and potential regulators of adaptive immunity began to emerge. In humans, NK cells appear to play important roles in viral infection, cancer immunity, transplantation, pregnancy and autoimmunity. Recent studies support the role of NK cell subsets in allergic diseases. NK cells need to be evaluated whenever an allergy investigation is undertaken.

References

1　Jonges L-E, Albertsson P, van Vlierberghe RL, Ensink NG, Johansson BR, van de Velde CJ, Fleuren GJ, Nannmark U, Kuppen PJ: The phenotypic heterogeneity of human natural killer cells: presence of at least 48 different subsets in the peripheral blood. Scand J Immunol 2001;53:103–110.

2　Cooper M-A, Fehniger TA, Caligiuri MA: The biology of human natural killer-cell subsets. Trends Immunol 2001;22:633–640.

3　Frag S-S, Caligiuri MA: Human natural killer cell development and biology. Blood Rev 2006;20:123–137.

4　Kern W-F, Spier CM, Miller TP, Grogan TM: NCAM (CD56)-positive malignant lymphoma. Leuk Lymphoma 1993;12:1–10.

5　Baume D-M, Robertson MJ, Levine H, Manley TJ, Schow PW, Ritz J: Differential responses to interleukin-2 define functionally distinct subsets of human natural killer cells. Eur J Immunol 1992;22:1–6.

6　Carson W-E, Fehniger TA, Caligiuri MA: CD56[bright] natural killer cell subsets: characterization of distinct functional responses to interleukin-2 and the c-kit ligand. Eur J Immunol 1997;27:354–360.

7　Berahovich R-D, Lai NL, Wei Z, Lanier LL, Schall TJ: Evidence for NK cell subsets based on chemokine receptor expression. J Immunol 2006;177:7833–7840.

8　Rajalingam R: Killer cell immunoglobulin-like receptors influence the innate and adaptive immune responses. Iran J Immunol 2007;4:61–78.

9　Sun P-D: Structure and function of natural-killer-cell receptors. Immunol Res 2003;27:539–548.

10　Boyton R-J, Altmann DM: Natural killer cells, killer immunoglobulin-like receptors and human leucocyte antigen class I in disease. Clin Exp Immunol 2007;149:1–8.

11　Middleton D, Curran M, Maxwell L: Natural killer cells and their receptors. Transpl Immunol 2002;10:147–164.

12　Brooks A-G, Boyington JC, Sun PD: Natural killer cell recognition of HLA class I molecules. Rev Immunogenet 2000;2:433–448.

13　Ogasawara K, Lanier LL: NKG2D in NK and T-cell-mediated immunity. J Clin Immunol 2005;25:534–540.

14　Borrego F, Masilamani M, Marusina AI, Tang X, Coligan JE: The CD94/NKG2 family of receptors: from molecules and cells to clinical relevance. Immunol Res 2006;35:263–278.

15　Moretta A, Bottino C, Vitale M, Pende D, Cantoni C, Mingari MC, Biassoni R, Moretta L: Activating receptors and coreceptors involved in human natural killer cell-mediated cytolysis. Annu Rev Immunol 2001;19:197–223.

16　Mandelboim O, Porgador A: NKp46. Int J Biochem Cell Biol 2001;33:1147–1150.

17　Orange J-S, Ballas ZK: Natural killer cells in human health and disease. Clin Immunol 2006;118:1–10.

18　Carson W-E, Giri JG, Lindemann MJ, Linett ML, Ahdieh M, Paxton R, Anderson D, Eisenmann J, Grabstein K, Caligiuri MA: Interleukin (IL)-15 is a novel cytokine that activates human natural killer cells via components of the IL-2 receptor. J Exp Med 1994;180:1395–1403.

19　Fehniger T-A, Shah MH, Turner MJ, VanDeusen JB, Whitman SP, Cooper MA, Suzuki K, Wechser M, Goodsaid F, Caligiuri MA: Differential cytokine and chemokine gene expression by human NK cells following activation with IL-18 or IL-15 in combination with IL-12: implications for the innate immune response. J Immunol 1999;162:4511–4520.

20　Aste-Amezaga M, D'Andrea A, Kubin M, Trinchieri G: Cooperation of natural killer cell stimulatory factor/interleukin-12 with other stimuli in the induction of cytokines and cytotoxic cell-associated molecules in human T and NK cells. Cell Immunol 1994;156:480–492.

21　Cooper M-A, Fehniger TA, Turner SC, Chen KS, Ghaheri BA, Ghayur T, Carson WE, Caligiuri MA: Human natural killer cells: a unique innate immunoregulatory role for the CD56[bright] subset. Blood 2001;97:3146–3151.

22　Itoh K, Tilden AB, Kumagai K, Balch CM: Leu11a+ lymphocytes with natural killer activity are precursors of recombinant interleukin-2-induced activated killer cells. J Immunol 1985;134:802–807.

23　Mosmann T-R, Sad S: The expanding universe of T cell subsets: Th1, Th2 and more. Immunol Today 1996;17:142–146.

24　Chan S-H, Perussia J, Gupta W, Kobayashi M, Pospisil M, Young HA, Wolf SF, Young D, Clark SC, Trichieri G: Induction of IFN-γ production by NK cell stimulatory factor: characterization of the responder cells and synergy with other inducers. J Exp Med 1991;173:869–879.

25　Peritt D, Robertson S, Gri G, Showe L, Aste-Amezaga M, Trinchieri G: Differentiation of human NK cells into NK1 and NK2 subsets. J Immunol 1998;161:5821–5824.

26　Deniz G, Akdis M, Aktas E, Blaser K, Akdis CA: Human NK1 and NK2 subsets determined by purification of IFN-γ-secreting and IFN-γ-nonsecreting NK cells. Eur J Immunol 2002;32:879–884.

27　Akdis M, Akdis CA, Weig lL, Disch R, Blaser K: Skin homing, CLA+ memory T cells are activated in atopic dermatitis and regulate IgE by an IL-13-dominated cytokine pattern. IgG4 counter-regulation by CLA+ memory T cells. J Immunol 1997;159:4611–4619.

28　Akdis M, Simon HU, Weigl L, Kreyden O, Blaser K, Akdis AC: Skin homing CLA+ CD8+ T cells respond to superantigen and contribute to eosinophilia and IgE production in atopic dermatitis. J Immunol 1999;163:466–475.

29　Parronchi P, De Carli M, Manetti R, Simonelli C, Piccinni MP, Macchia D, Maggi E, Del Prete G, Ricci M, Romagnani S: Aberrant interleukin (IL)-4 and IL-5 production in vitro by CD4+ helper T cells from atopic subjects. Eur J Immunol 1992;22:1615–1620.

30　Chan S-C, Brown MA, Willcox TM, Li SH, Stevens SR, Tara D, Hanifin JM: Abnormal IL-4 gene expression by atopic dermatitis T lymphocytes is reflected in altered nuclear protein interactions with IL-4 transcriptional regulatory element. J Invest Dermatol 1996;106:1131–1136.

31 Piccinni M-P, Beloni L, Giannarini L, Livi C, Scarselli G, Romagnani S, Maggi E: Abnormal production of T-helper 2 cytokines interleukin-4 and interleukin-5 by T cells from newborns with atopic parents. Eur J Immunol 1996;26:2293–2298.

32 Vukmanovic-Stejic M, Vyas B, Gorak-Stolinska P, Noble A, Kemeny DM: Human Tc1 and Tc2/Tc0 CD8 T-cell clones display distinct cell surface and functional phenotypes. Blood 2000;95:231–240.

33 Wei H, Zhang J, Xiao W, Feng J, Sun R, Tian Z: Involvement of human natural killer cells in asthma pathogenesis: natural killer 2 cells in type 2 cytokine predominance. J Allergy Clin Immunol 2005;115:841–847.

34 Aktas E, Akdis M, Bilgic S, Disch R, Falk CS, Blaser K, Akdis C, Deniz G: Different natural killer receptor expression and immunoglobulin E regulation by NK1 and NK2 cells. Clin Exp Immunol 2005;140:301–309.

35 Yoon SR, Chung JW, Choi I: Development of NK cells from hemotopoietic stem cells. Mol Cells 2007;24:1–8.

Gunnur Deniz, PhD
Department of Immunology, Istanbul University
Institute of Experimental Medicine (DETAE)
Vakif Gureba Cad., TR–34280 Sehremini/Istanbul (Turkey)
Tel. +90 212 414 2232, Fax +90 212 532 4171, E-Mail gdeniz@istanbul.edu.tr

Blaser K (ed): T Cell Regulation in Allergy, Asthma and Atopic Skin Diseases.
Chem Immunol Allergy. Basel, Karger, 2008, vol 94, pp 58–66

Mast Cells and Mast Cell-Derived Factors in the Regulation of Allergic Sensitization

Christian Taube[a] · Michael Stassen[b]

[a]Third Medical Clinic and [b]Institute for Immunology, Johannes Gutenberg University, Mainz, Germany

Abstract

Mast cells have been mainly regarded as effector cells in IgE-dependent mucosal immunity, including the host response to helminthic parasites but also the formidable and sometimes fatal anaphylactic reactions to inhaled or ingested allergens. Work performed mostly within the last decade revealed novel functions for mast cells as critical initiators of fast inflammatory reactions upon IgE-independent activation. Thus, their role as a sentinel in innate immunity also suggests that mast cells are able to bridge innate and adaptive immunity. Herein, we will summarize the accumulating evidence that mast cells are also able to promote and to modulate the development of adaptive immune reactions with emphasis on their role in allergic sensitization in skin and lung. Based on murine data published so far, it is becoming apparent that mast cells and their mediators are of critical relevance for allergen sensitization under conditions which more closely resemble physiological contact with allergens. Yet, the function of mast cells can sometimes be bypassed using vigorous sensitization protocols, a finding which should be taken into account when animal models for complex human diseases are investigated.   Copyright © 2008 S. Karger AG, Basel

Mast cells have for a long time been regarded as mere effector cells in acute allergic and anaphylactic reactions. Indeed, mast cells can be quickly activated following crosslinking of high-affinity IgE receptor (FcεRI) through allergen-specific IgE and allergen, which leads to degranulation, production of biologically highly active lipid mediators, chemokines and cytokines [1]. However, in recent years, important functions of mast cells in innate immune responses have also been described and the underlying non-IgE-dependent pathways of mast cell activation have been analyzed in detail. Models of acute septic peritonitis and infection with *Klebsiella pneumoniae* have identified mast cells as indispensable for efficient defense against infections [2, 3]. The ability of mast cells to respond to microbial challenges is due to the expression of different pattern recognition receptors (PAMPs), including Toll-like receptors (TLRs), complement receptors and CD48 [4, 5]. This IgE-independent activation of mast cells also leads to the release of mediators which promote the migration of antigen presenting cells (APCs) from skin or mucosa to the regional lymph nodes (LNs), where APCs can interact with the cells of the adaptive branch of the immune system to induce specific T-cell and B-cell responses. There is now growing evidence that mast cells directly contribute to the sensitization phase to antigens by influencing APCs to mount adequate immune responses. Herein, we summarize recent work showing a pivotal role of mast cells for sensitization to allergens. These murine studies include skin models for priming of adaptive and allergic immune responses as well as models of allergic airway disease. Furthermore, a novel insight into the mechanisms of how mast cells exacerbate allergic reactions in sensitized individuals will be presented. Specific roles for basophils in chronic allergic inflammation and shaping of immune responses will also be discussed.

Skin Models Implicate a Role for Mast Cells in Priming of Adaptive Immune Responses and Allergic Sensitization

Investigating a murine model for hapten-induced contact hypersensitivity (CHS), a potential role for mast cells in the induction of an adaptive response was reported by Wang et al. [6]. In response to sensitization with the hapten 2,4-dinitrofluorobenzene (DNFB), it was shown that skin mast cells degranulate, and that local skin mast cell numbers decrease by half accompanied by a fivefold increase of mast cells in the draining LNs. Using fluorescent-labeled mast cells, the authors demonstrated migration of these cells from the DNFB-treated skin to the regional LNs. Importantly, mast cells were found to produce the chemokine MIP-1β in LNs which was shown to boost T-cell recruitment, a finding which was corroborated by an additional report [7]. These studies were substantiated by the observation that mast cells also strongly promote hypertrophy of LNs following bacterial infection. Mast cell-dependent LN hypertrophy was shown to depend on mast cell-derived TNF-α, which also represents an important trigger for the recruitment of circulating T cells to LNs [8]. In the latter study, the authors did not see any increase in nodal mast cell numbers, suggesting that mast cell-derived TNF-α is not produced locally but drains into LNs via afferent lymphatics within a few hours following mast cell activation. Thus, depending on the model, migration of mast cells to the draining LNs seems not to be a necessity for hypertrophy to occur. However, as LNs serve as a platform for the interaction of APCs with cells of the adaptive immune system, the above-mentioned studies already proposed critical roles for mast cells and mast cell-derived products with respect to the initiation of adaptive responses.

These reports were supplemented by the work of Bryce et al. [9] who demonstrated crucial functions for both IgE and mast cells during the sensitization phase to the chemical hapten oxazolone. Both mast cells and IgE have to be present for efficient sensitization to the hapten, irrespective of the antigen specificity of IgE. Yet, only mast cells are required and IgE is dispensable upon re-exposure to the antigen. Importantly, the authors of this study demonstrated that emigration of Langerhans' cells (LCs) out of the epidermis following hapten exposure is impaired in both IgE- and mast cell-deficient animals. LCs are important APCs in the skin due to their ability to deliver antigen to the draining LN. Thus, this finding strongly proposed that mast cells participate in the development of an adaptive immune response by promoting the migration of antigen-laden APCs.

In a model for passive cutaneous anaphylaxis, IgE-mediated activation of mast cells was also shown to provide an important signal for migration of LCs to the LNs [10]. Blockade of H_2 histamine receptor in mice impaired migration of LCs, but injection of histamine alone in order to mimic the local effects of mast cells had no effect on LC migration, suggesting that additional mast cell-derived factors are necessary. However, the results of this study imply that IgE/allergen-activated mast cells may facilitate the development of additional allergic IgE responses by triggering the migration of antigen-laden LCs.

Topical application of the contact allergen FITC was also reported to initiate emigration of LCs in a mast cell-dependent manner [11]. Mast cell-derived TNF-α was shown to promote migration of LC 24 h after application of FITC, but LC migration reached comparable levels in wild-type, mast cell-deficient and TNF-α-deficient mice 48–72 h after application of FITC. Thus, mast cells accelerate migration of APCs in this study but their presence is not a prerequisite for migration to occur. In line with this, 6 days following hapten exposure, identical levels of T-cell proliferation induced upon restimulation of LN cell suspensions with FITC ex vivo were measured in wild-type, mast cell- and TNF-α-deficient mice [11]. Thus, mast cells, at least in this model, are not required for the development of an efficient T-cell response, although they are able to accelerate the migration of LCs.

With respect to the role of TNF-α for LN hypertrophy, Jawdat et al. [12] recently reported that peptidoglycan (PGN), a cell wall component of Gram-positive bacteria, induces mast cell-dependent LN hypertrophy independent of TNF-α, whereas hypertrophy induced by crosslinking IgE on mast cells requires TNF-α. In line with this, injection of PGN also promotes mast cell-dependent migration of LC which only partly depends on TNF-α, whereas migration induced by IgE-mediated activation is TNF-α-dependent. The apparent discrepancies with respect to the role of TNF-α for both LN hypertrophy and LC migration are most likely due to the release of a distinct panel of mast cell mediators under specific activation conditions. The authors of the latter study showed that treatment of bone marrow-derived mast cells (BMMCs) with PGN in vitro does not induce production of TNF-α, which is in sharp contrast to crosslinking of IgE which causes the production of large amounts of this cytokine. Notably, neither hypertrophy of LNs nor migration of LCs require TLR2 or the adapter molecule MyD88 but depend on complement component C3, indicating that PGN acts

via activation of the complement cascade independent of TLR signaling in vivo.

Taken together, the studies cited above strongly suggest that mast cells can contribute to the sensitization phase of acquired immune responses by virtue of their ability to produce mediators that can promote migration of APCs. Furthermore, mast cells prepare LNs to become the meeting point of antigen-laden APCs and T cells (fig. 1).

A recent paper establishes a link between mast cells and the ability of mice to mount a peptide-specific cytotoxic T lymphocyte (CTL) response following transcutaneous immunization [13]. Immunization was carried out by topical application of the MHC class I-restricted CTL peptide SIINFEKL in combination with the synthetic TLR7 agonist imiquimod as adjuvant. Mast cells activated via TLR7 induce a fast inflammatory skin reaction and they also promote the migration of LCs to the draining LNs as well as LN hyperplasia. For the initiation of an early inflammation, both mast cell-derived IL-1 and TNF-α were required, whereas migration of LC partly depends on mast cell-derived IL-1. In addition, hypertrophy of regional LNs is driven by mast cell-derived TNF-α. Consequently, the ability to elicit a peptide-specific CTL response following transcutaneous immunization is severely impaired in mast cell-deficient mice. These findings demonstrate that, under certain conditions, mast cells are able to bridge innate and adaptive immune reactions (fig. 1). However, immunization with mature peptide-loaded DCs mounts a potent CTL response in both mast cell-deficient and wild-type mice [13]. Thus, the function of mast cells can be bypassed using vigorous immunization protocols, a phenomenon which is also of critical relevance for murine models of allergic airway diseases, which will be discussed later.

The ability of mast cells to promote and even to shape acquired immune responses was further corroborated by Maurer et al. [14] investigating host defense mechanisms in *Leishmania major*

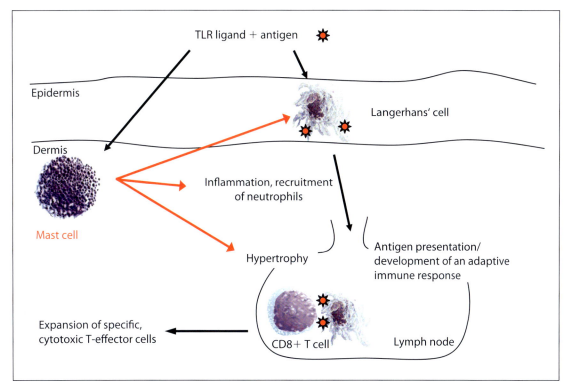

Fig. 1. Mast cells bridge innate and adaptive immunity. Activation of mast cells by TLR ligands induces a fast local inflammatory response. Mast cell-derived mediators also promote the migration of antigen-laden LCs from the skin to the regional LNs, where a specific adaptive immune response is induced.

infections. Compared to wild-type littermates, mast cell-deficient mice infected with this parasite develop larger skin lesions and recruitment of inflammatory cells including DC is impaired. In line with this, the appearance of parasite-specific T cells is significantly delayed. Notably, in mast cell-deficient mice the T-cell response skewed toward non-protective Th2 priming. CD11c+ infected DCs are crucial for the initiation of a protective Th1 driven immune response against *L. major*, therefore the impaired local recruitment of IL-12 producing DCs is supposedly responsible for the delayed and shifted T-cell response.

Besides their influence on APCs, evidence accumulates that mast cells are also able to directly enhance the activity of T cells. This was reported to require mast cell–T-cell contact and TNF-α produced by both T cells and mast cells [15]. In a CHS model, activated mast cells were also found to act synergistically with T cells in vivo [15]. In addition, mast cells display various ligands for costimulatory molecules expressed on the surface of T cells, and it was demonstrated that the application of neutralizing antibodies to OX40L reduces mast cell-mediated enhancement of T-cell activity [16].

As described so far, mast cells were found to exacerbate immune reactions, including allergic responses. A recent paper shows that mast cells are also critical to limit pathology in a murine CHS model, including the reduction of infiltrating cells, epidermal hyperplasia, and necrosis

[17]. Mast cells influence the long-term consequences and the resolution of CHS beginning 3 days after challenge of sensitized animals with DNFB or urushiol. Production of the immunosuppressive cytokine IL-10 by mast cells strongly contributed to these late anti-inflammatory effects of mast cells. Thus, this example demonstrates for the first time that mast cells are able to truly modulate – and not only to promote – allergic responses.

Mast Cells Initiate and Modulate T-Cell Responses during Allergic Airway Inflammation

Allergic asthma is an inflammatory disease of the small airways characterized by cellular infiltration of lung tissue (mainly with eosinophils and T cells), excessive mucus production and airway hyperresponsiveness (AHR) to cholinergic agonists, e.g. methacholine, leading to bronchoconstriction. It is well established that mast cells release their preformed mediators shortly after exposure to an allergen triggering the ligation of antigen-specific IgE bound to FcεRI receptors. This translates into acute bronchoconstriction following allergen exposure described as early phase reactions. In addition to these acute effects, the role of mast cells for the initiation of allergic sensitization and modulation of airway disease has been a matter of debate and especially murine models have shown varying results. It seems apparent now that the role and function of mast cells during the initiation of allergic airway disease is critically dependent on the mode of sensitization. Models of allergic airway disease using systemic sensitization with adjuvant have repeatedly shown a similar degree of AHR and airway inflammation in mast cell- or IgE-deficient mice compared to respective wild-type mice. In contrast, a prominent role for mast cells in the development of allergic airway disease has emerged using sensitization protocols without an additional adjuvant or only inhaled exposures [18]. In these models, the presence of mast cells was necessary for the initiation of airway inflammation and AHR (fig. 2). Further studies, using mast cell reconstitution protocols, revealed that the expression of the Fc receptor γ chain in mast cells [19], necessary for the surface expression of the Fcγ receptor I, Fcγ receptor III and FcεRI receptor, is pivotal for the induction of most features of allergen-induced lung pathology [20]. The main effect of mast cells in these models seems to be a result of mast cell mediator release. Several mediators and their effects on the development of airway disease have been studied. Indeed, histamine and the expression of histamine receptor 1 on T cells induce T-cell migration and are associated with the development of allergic airway disease [21]. A second mast cell-released mediator involved in allergic inflammation seems to be TNF-α. Following allergen exposure, sensitized mast cell-deficient mice express lower levels of TNF-α in BAL fluid, and reconstitution with BMMCs restored BAL fluid levels of TNF-α and AHR [22]. Mast cell-reconstitution experiments further underscore the relevance of TNF-α produced mast cells for the induction of airway inflammation and AHR [23, 24].

The local release of TNF-α from mast cells in this setting might influence several different cell types. Migration of dendritic cells to regional LNs, an essential process during the development of airway inflammation, could be influenced by mast cell-derived TNF-α [11]. As already mentioned above, mast cell-produced TNF-α might also directly affect lymphocytes [15, 16], including the optimal activation of Th2-polarized T cells [25]. These recent studies advance our understanding that mast cells are not only mere effector cells during acute allergic responses, but also initiate the development of allergic airway disease. This might be mediated by regulation of dendritic cell activation and migration from the lung to regional LNs and by optimal T-cell stimulation.

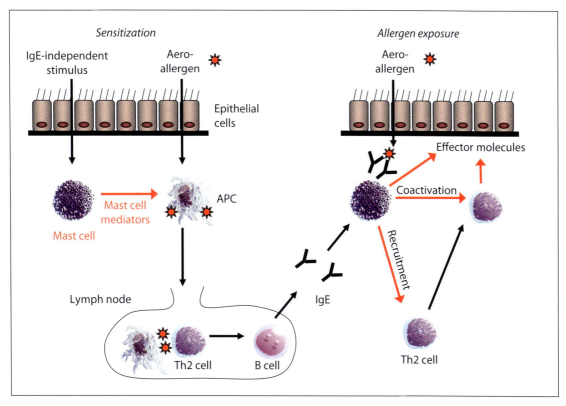

Fig. 2. Dual role of mast cells in sensitization to aeroallergen and challenge. During sensitization with an aeroallergen, combined exposure with the allergen and an alternative/IgE-independent mast cell-activating stimulus leads to increased migration of antigen-laden DCs to the regional LNs. Consequently, a Th2 response and allergen-specific IgE production are induced. During allergen exposure of a sensitized host, IgE-dependent mast cell activation leads to increased T-cell chemotaxis and promotes local T-cell activation.

There is also an emerging amount of evidence suggesting a direct involvement of mast cells and mast cell activation for the induction of specific T-cell responses to aeroallergens. Following exposure to aeroallergens the usual outcome of their inhalation is tolerance, because most allergens are immunological inert proteins and inflammation does not develop even following chronic exposure. Resident pulmonary DCs are usually in a state specialized to internalize foreign antigens, but not able to activate naive T cells. Stimulation of DCs with additional factors like ligands for TLRs eventually leads to their activation, migration to the regional lymphatic tissue and induction of a specific T-cell response by antigen presentation and increased expression of CD40, CD80 and CD86 [26]. Therefore, a modulation of the lung micromilieu, leading to activation of DCs, seems to be necessary to induce a specific T-cell response to inhaled allergens (fig. 2). There is increasing evidence in vitro that activation of mast cells can modulate DCs to a Th2-biased phenotype by histamine and prostaglandin secretion [27, 28]. In vivo several studies also suggest an involvement of mast cells in T-cell priming following inhaled allergen exposure. Studies from the group of Kim Bottomly [29, 30] show that additional to the administration of a protein allergen, low doses of bacterial lipopolysaccharide (LPS) can induce sensitization to the allergen. This is mediated by TLR-4 and production of TNF-α, which leads to increased migration of DCs from the lung to the regional LNs. Interestingly, mast cells express TLR-4 on their surface and also release TNF-α following exposure to LPS [31]. To further investigate this matter, Nigo et al. [32] treated mast cell-deficient and respective wild-type mice intranasally with allergen in conjunction with low-dose LPS and rechallenged the animals 2 weeks later. This protocol elicits eosinophilic airway inflammation in wild-type mice. In contrast, mast cell-deficient mice display a markedly decreased number of eosinophils in the lung compared to the wild-type animals. In several reconstitution experiments, only transfer of BMMCs expressing TLR-4 on their surface but not TLR-4-deficient BMMCs reconstituted airway inflammation in the mast cell-deficient animals and their IgE-independent activation is involved in the initiation of a T-cell response following inhaled allergen exposure.

In contrast to other protein allergens, house dust mite allergen (Der p, Der f) has the potential to directly induce rapid IgE-independent release and de novo synthesis of mast cell mediators [33, 34]. In vitro assays of Der f-stimulated mast cells show that their supernatants chemoattract monocytes and T cells, support T-cell proliferation and promote Th2 cell development. In this context it is not surprising that inhalative exposure to house dust mite can directly induce Th2 sensitization and an influx of activated Th2 effector cells into the lung in vivo [35]. Further supporting a role of mast cells in this process, administration of sodium cromoglycate, a mast cell stabilizer, during repeated house dust mite allergen exposure not only suppresses production of acute mast cell mediators but also attenuates airway inflammation following repeated Der f exposure [34].

Novel and Distinct Roles for Basophils in Allergy

The work described above sheds new light on the roles of mast cells in allergic diseases and immunity in general, but the function of a closely related cell, the basophil, remains obscure. Unlike tissue-resident mast cells, basophils enter the circulation as mature cells but are able to enter inflamed tissues. Basophils are scarce (<0.5% of blood leukocytes) and detailed analyses of their biology has been hampered by the lack of specific antibodies or appropriate animal models, such as basophil-deficient mice [reviewed in 36]. Recently, a monoclonal antibody (mAb) was established that specifically depletes murine basophils in vivo [37]. Interestingly, treatment of mice with this mAb did not impair allergic reactions such as systemic anaphylaxis, passive cutaneous anaphylaxis and CHS. Yet, it abolished the development of IgE-mediated chronic allergic dermatitis independently of the presence of mast cells. In this model, mast cells were previously shown to be critical for immediate and late phase skin responses, but dispensable for the development of delayed/chronic dermatitis [38]. In contrast, elimination of basophils from the skin lesions led to a strong reduction of infiltrating neutrophils and eosinophils and abolished the development of the chronic phase [37]. Furthermore, basophils are proposed to be an important and early source of IL-4 upon parasitic infection in vivo and may thereby contribute to the development of type 2 immunity [reviewed in 39].

Although there are more questions than answers with respect to the function of basophils so far, there is increasing evidence for specific roles of these cells in allergy and infection.

Conclusion

The work summarized herein extends our view on the role of mast cells not only in allergic disorders but in immunity in general. As known so far, this is mostly due to their ability to produce a variety of proinflammatory and immunomodulatory mediators. IgE-independent activation of mast cells makes it possible to initiate fast inflammatory reactions in a variety of settings. Upon their ability to promote both the migration of antigen-laden APCs and the hyperplasia of LNs, mast cells can link innate and adaptive branches of the immune response. Consequently, mast cells, at least under certain conditions, are able to strongly promote the development of specific T-cell responses and are also able to shape them. Furthermore, mast cells were repeatedly found to be able to exacerbate acquired responses including allergic reactions. Yet, evidence is also emerging that mast cells are critical to limit inflammatory responses which sheds new light on their dual role as true modulators – promoters and suppressors – of immune responses. However, we also learned that the role of mast cells can be bypassed using very robust experimental settings in animal models for complex human diseases, which should always be considered with respect to the physiological relevance of animal models.

Taken together, these findings clearly demonstrate that mast cells are not only mere effector cells during allergic reactions, but also have a complex role in the induction and regulation of adaptive immune responses. In regard to allergic sensitization, the activation of mast cells seems to be an important regulatory step for the development of specific T-cell responses to the allergen. Therefore, modulation of mast cell activation could be a potential therapeutic strategy for the prevention of allergic sensitization.

Acknowledgements

Our work was supported by grants from the Deutsche Forschungsgemeinschaft, SFB 548 (projects A10, A11), and STA984/1-1.

References

1 Metcalfe DD, Baram D, Mekori YA: Mast cells. Physiol Rev 1997;77:1033–1079.
2 Echtenacher B, Mannel DN, Hultner L: Critical protective role of mast cells in a model of acute septic peritonitis. Nature 1996;381:75–77.
3 Malaviya R, Ikeda T, Ross E, Abraham SN: Mast cell modulation of neutrophil influx and bacterial clearance at sites of infection through TNF-α. Nature 1996;381:77–80.
4 Stassen M, Hultner L, Schmitt E: Classical and alternative pathways of mast cell activation. Crit Rev Immunol 2002;22:115–140.
5 Marshall JS: Mast-cell responses to pathogens. Nat Rev Immunol 2004;4:787–799.
6 Wang HW, Tedla N, Lloyd AR, Wakefield D, McNeil PH: Mast cell activation and migration to lymph nodes during induction of an immune response in mice. J Clin Invest 1998;102:1617–1626.

7 Tedla N, Wang HW, McNeil HP, et al: Regulation of T lymphocyte trafficking into lymph nodes during an immune response by the chemokines macrophage inflammatory protein (MIP)-1α and MIP-1β. J Immunol 1998;161:5663–5672.
8 McLachlan JB, Hart JP, Pizzo SV, et al: Mast cell-derived tumor necrosis factor induces hypertrophy of draining lymph nodes during infection. Nat Immunol 2003;4:1199–1205.
9 Bryce PJ, Miller ML, Miyajima I, Tsai M, Galli SJ, Oettgen HC: Immune sensitization in the skin is enhanced by antigen-independent effects of IgE. Immunity 2004;20:381–392.
10 Jawdat DM, Albert EJ, Rowden G, Haidl ID, Marshall JS: IgE-mediated mast cell activation induces Langerhans cell migration in vivo. J Immunol 2004;173:5275–5282.

11 Suto H, Nakae S, Kakurai M, Sedgwick JD, Tsai M, Galli SJ: Mast cell-associated TNF promotes dendritic cell migration. J Immunol 2006;176:4102–4112.
12 Jawdat DM, Rowden G, Marshall JS: Mast cells have a pivotal role in TNF-independent lymph node hypertrophy and the mobilization of Langerhans' cells in response to bacterial peptidoglycan. J Immunol 2006;177:1755–1762.
13 Heib V, Becker M, Warger T, et al: Mast cells are crucial for early inflammation, migration of Langerhans cells, and CTL responses following topical application of TLR7 ligand in mice. Blood 2007;110:946–953.
14 Maurer M, Lopez KS, Siebenhaar F, et al: Skin mast cells control T cell-dependent host defense in *Leishmania major* infections. FASEB J 2006;20:2460–2467.
15 Nakae S, Suto H, Kakurai M, Sedgwick JD, Tsai M, Galli SJ: Mast cells enhance T cell activation: importance of mast cell-derived TNF. Proc Natl Acad Sci USA 2005;102:6467–6472.

16 Nakae S, Suto H, Iikura M, et al: Mast cells enhance T cell activation: importance of mast cell costimulatory molecules and secreted TNF. J Immunol 2006;176:2238–2248.

17 Grimbaldeston MA, Nakae S, Kalesnikoff J, Tsai M, Galli SJ: Mast cell-derived interleukin-10 limits skin pathology in contact dermatitis and chronic irradiation with ultraviolet B. Nat Immunol 2007;8:1095–1104.

18 Taube C, Dakhama A, Gelfand EW: Insights into the pathogenesis of asthma utilizing murine models. Int Arch Allergy Immunol 2004;135:173–186.

19 Yu M, Tsai M, Tam SY, Jones C, Zehnder J, Galli SJ: Mast cells can promote the development of multiple features of chronic asthma in mice. J Clin Invest 2006;116:1633–1641.

20 Taube C, Wei X, Swasey CH, et al: Mast cells, FcεRI, and IL-13 are required for development of airway hyperresponsiveness after aerosolized allergen exposure in the absence of adjuvant. J Immunol 2004;172:6398–6406.

21 Bryce PJ, Mathias CB, Harrison KL, Watanabe T, Geha RS, Oettgen HC: The H_1 histamine receptor regulates allergic lung responses. J Clin Invest 2006;116:1624–1632.

22 Kim YS, Ko HM, Kang NI, et al: Mast cells play a key role in the development of late airway hyperresponsiveness through TNF-α in a murine model of asthma. Eur J Immunol 2007;37:1107–1115.

23 Reuter S, Heinz A, Sieren M, et al: Mast cell-derived tumour necrosis factor is essential for allergic airway disease. Eur Respir J 2008;31:773–782.

24 Nakae S, Ho LH, Yu M, et al: Mast cell-derived TNF contributes to airway hyperreactivity, inflammation, and Th2 cytokine production in an asthma model in mice. J Allergy Clin Immunol 2007;120:48–55.

25 Nakae S, Lunderius C, Ho LH, Schafer B, Tsai M, Galli SJ: TNF can contribute to multiple features of ovalbumin-induced allergic inflammation of the airways in mice. J Allergy Clin Immunol 2007;119:680–686.

26 Hammad H, Lambrecht BN: Recent progress in the biology of airway dendritic cells and implications for understanding the regulation of asthmatic inflammation. J Allergy Clin Immunol 2006;118:331–336.

27 Gosset P, Pichavant M, Faveeuw C, Bureau F, Tonnel AB, Trottein F: Prostaglandin D_2 affects the differentiation and functions of human dendritic cells: impact on the T cell response. Eur J Immunol 2005;35:1491–1500.

28 Kitawaki T, Kadowaki N, Sugimoto N, et al: IgE-activated mast cells in combination with pro-inflammatory factors induce Th2-promoting dendritic cells. Int Immunol 2006;18:1789–1799.

29 Eisenbarth SC, Zhadkevich A, Ranney P, Herrick CA, Bottomly K: IL-4-dependent Th2 collateral priming to inhaled antigens independent of Toll-like receptor 4 and myeloid differentiation factor 88. J Immunol 2004;172:4527–4534.

30 Eisenbarth SC, Piggott DA, Huleatt JW, Visintin I, Herrick CA, Bottomly K: Lipopolysaccharide-enhanced, toll-like receptor 4-dependent T-helper cell type 2 responses to inhaled antigen. J Exp Med 2002;196:1645–1651.

31 Stassen M, Hultner L, Schmitt E: Classical and alternative pathways of mast cell activation. Crit Rev Immunol 2002;22:115–140.

32 Nigo YI, Yamashita M, Hirahara K, et al: Regulation of allergic airway inflammation through Toll-like receptor 4-mediated modification of mast cell function. Proc Natl Acad Sci USA 2006;103:2286–2291.

33 Machado DC, Horton D, Harrop R, Peachell PT, Helm BA: Potential allergens stimulate the release of mediators of the allergic response from cells of mast cell lineage in the absence of sensitization with antigen-specific IgE. Eur J Immunol 1996;26:2972–2980.

34 Yu CK, Chen CL: Activation of mast cells is essential for development of house dust mite Dermatophagoides farinae-induced allergic airway inflammation in mice. J Immunol 2003;171:3808–3815.

35 Cates EC, Fattouh R, Wattie J, et al: Intranasal exposure of mice to house dust mite elicits allergic airway inflammation via a GM-CSF-mediated mechanism. J Immunol 2004;173:6384–6392.

36 Falcone FH, Zillikens D, Gibbs BF: The 21st century renaissance of the basophil? Current insights into its role in allergic responses and innate immunity. Exp Dermatol 2006;15:855–864.

37 Obata K, Mukai K, Tsujimura Y, et al: Basophils are essential initiators of a novel type of chronic allergic inflammation. Blood 2007;110:913–920.

38 Mukai K, Matsuoka K, Taya C, et al: Basophils play a critical role in the development of IgE-mediated chronic allergic inflammation independently of T cells and mast cells. Immunity 2005;23:191–202.

39 Min B, Paul WE: Basophils and type 2 immunity. Curr Opin Hematol 2008;15:59–63.

Dr. Michael Stassen
Institute for Immunology, Johannes Gutenberg University
Hochhaus am Augustusplatz, DE–55131 Mainz (Germany)
Tel. +49 6131 393 3350, Fax +49 6131 393 5688
E-Mail stassenm@uni-mainz.de

Blaser K (ed): T Cell Regulation in Allergy, Asthma and Atopic Skin Diseases.
Chem Immunol Allergy. Basel, Karger, 2008, vol 94, pp 67–82

Regulatory Effects of Histamine and Histamine Receptor Expression in Human Allergic Immune Responses

Cezmi A. Akdis[a] · Marek Jutel[b] · Mübeccel Akdis[a]

[a]Swiss Institute of Allergy and Asthma Research (SIAF), Davos, Switzerland, and
[b]Department of Internal Medicine and Allergology, Wroclaw Medical University, Wroclaw, Poland

Abstract

Histamine influences several immune/inflammatory and effector functions in addition to its dominant role in type I hypersensitivity reactions. Histamine can selectively recruit the major effector cells into tissue sites and affect their maturation, activation, polarization, and other functions leading to chronic inflammation. Histamine also regulates monocytes, dendritic cells, T cells and B cells, as well as related antibody isotype responses. The diverse effects of histamine on immune regulation appear to be due to differential expression and regulation of four types of histamine receptors and their distinct intracellular signals. In addition, differences in affinities of these receptors for histamine are highly decisive for the biological effects of histamine and drugs that target histamine receptors.   Copyright © 2008 S. Karger AG, Basel

Molecular Basis for Action

Histamine (2-[4-imidazole]ethylamine) is a low-molecular-weight amine synthesized from L-histidine exclusively by histidine decarboxylase. It is produced by various cells throughout the body, including central nervous system neurons, gastric mucosa parietal cells, mast cells, basophils and lymphocytes [1–4]. Since its discovery as a uterine stimulant more than 100 years ago it has become one of the most intensely studied molecules in medicine. The name *histamine* was given after the Greek word for tissue, *histos*, after it was isolated first from liver and lung tissue, and then from several other sites. Its smooth muscle-stimulating and vasodepressor action was demonstrated in the first experiments by Dale and Laidlaw [5], who also found that the effects of histamine mimicked those occurring during anaphylaxis.

Histamine is involved in the regulation of many physiological functions including cell proliferation and differentiation, hematopoiesis, embryonic development, regeneration, and wound healing. Within the central nervous system it affects cognition and memory, the regulation of cycle of sleeping and waking, energy and endocrine homeostasis [6]. In human pathology, histamine triggers acute symptoms due to its very rapid activity on vascular endothelium and bronchial and smooth muscle cells leading to the development of such symptoms as acute rhinitis, bronchospasm, cramping, diarrhea or cutaneous wheal-and-flare responses. In addition to these effects on the immediate-type response, histamine significantly regulates the immune response and a number of chronic phase inflammatory events [1, 2]. For example, histamine is increased in bronchoalveolar lavage fluid (BALF) from patients with allergic asthma and this increase negatively correlates with airway function [7]. An increase in histamine levels has been noted in the skin and plasma of patients with atopic dermatitis [8] and in chronic urticaria [9]. Histamine levels are also increased in multiple sclerosis [10] and in psoriatic skin [11]. Both plasma and synovial fluid of patients with rheumatoid arthritis and plasma of patients with psoriatic arthritis have increased histamine levels [12]. Consequently, the antihistamines should be viewed as systemic antiallergic agents and immunoregulators.

Histamine Receptors

The pleiotropic effects of histamine are triggered by activating on one or several of histamine membrane receptors on different cells. Four subtypes of receptors (histamine receptor (HR)1, HR2, HR3, and HR4) have been described (table 1). All of these receptors belong to the G-protein-coupled receptor family. They are heptahelical transmembrane molecules that transduce extracellular signal by using G proteins and intracellular second messenger systems [1, 2]. The active and inactive states of HRs exist in equilibrium. However, it has been shown in recombinant systems that HRs can trigger downstream events in the absence of receptor occupancy by an agonist, which accounts for constitutive spontaneous receptor activity [13].

HR agonists stimulate the active state in the receptor and inverse agonists, the inactive one. An agonist with a preferential affinity for the active state of the receptor stabilizes the receptor in its active conformation leading to a continuous activation signal. An inverse agonist with a preferential affinity for the inactive state stabilizes the receptor in this conformation and consequently induces an inactive state, which is characterized

by blocked signal transduction via the HR [13]. In reporter gene assays, constitutive HR1-mediated nuclear factor (NF)-κB activation has been shown to be inhibited by many of the clinically used H_1 antihistamines, indicating that these agents are inverse HR1 agonists [13]. Constitutive activity has now been shown for all four HRs [13].

Specific activation or blockade of HRs showed that they differ in expression, signal transduction or function and improved the understanding of the role of histamine in physiology and disease mechanisms. It has long been recognized that most positive effects of histamine are mediated by HR1, while HR2 is mostly involved in its suppressive activities. The human $G_{q/11}$-coupled HR1 is encoded by a single exon gene located on the distal short arm of chromosome 3p25b and contains 487 amino acids. The HR1 is expressed in numerous cells including airway and vascular smooth muscle cells, hepatocytes, chondrocytes, nerve cells, endothelial cells, dendritic cells (DCs), monocytes, neutrophils, T and B cells [1, 2]. Histamine binds to transmembrane domains 3 and 5. Activation of the HR1-coupled $G_{q/11}$ stimulates the inositol phospholipid signaling pathways resulting in formation of inositol-1,4,5-triphosphate and diacylglycerol and an increase in intracellular calcium [14]. The rise in intracellular calcium accounts for nitric oxide production and liberation of arachidonic acid from phospholipids increased cyclic AMP. The HR1 also activates phospholipase D and phospholipase A_2 and the transcription factor NF-κB through $G_{q/11}$ and $G_{\beta\gamma}$ upon agonist binding. Constitutive activation of NF-κB occurs only through $G_{\beta\gamma}$ [14]. The HR1 is responsible for the development of many symptoms of allergic disease. Targeted disruption of the H_1-receptor gene in mice results in the impairment of neurologic functions such as memory, learning, locomotion, and nociperception, and in aggressive behavior. Immunologic abnormalities have also been described in HR1-deleted mice, with impairment

Table 1. Histamine receptors, expression, activated intracellular signals, and coupled G proteins

Histamine receptors	Expression	Activated intracellular signals	G proteins
Histamine H_1 receptor	Nerve cells, airway and vascular smooth muscles, hepatocytes, chondrocytes, endothelial cells, epithelial cells, neutrophils, eosinophils, monocytes, DC, T and B cells	Ca^{2+}, cGMP, phospholipase D, phospholipase A_2, NF-κB	$G_{q/11}$
Histamine H_2 receptor	Nerve cells, airway and vascular smooth muscles, hepatocytes, chondrocytes, endothelial cells, epithelial cells, neutrophils, eosinophils, monocytes, DC, T and B cells	Adenylate cyclase, cAMP, c-Fos, c-Jun, PKC, p70S6K	$G\alpha_s$
Histamine H_3 receptor	Histaminergic neurons, eosinophils, DC, monocytes Low expression in peripheral tissues	Enhanced Ca^{2+}, MAP kinase, inhibition of cAMP	$G_{i/o}$
Histamine H_4 receptor	High expression on bone marrow and peripheral hematopoietic cells, eosinophils, neutrophils, DC, T cells, basophils, mast cells Low expression in nerve cells, hepatocytes peripheral tissues, spleen, thymus, lung, small intestine, colon and heart	Enhanced Ca^{2+}, inhibition of cAMP	$G_{i/o}$

of both T- and B-cell responses [15]. Activation of HR1 is responsible for many symptoms of allergic disease.

In humans the intronless gene encoding HR2 is located on chromosome 5. The human HR2 is a protein of 359 amino acids coupled to both adenylate cyclase and phosphoinositide second messenger systems by separate GTP-dependent mechanisms including $G\alpha_s$ and also induces activation of c-Fos, c-Jun PKC and p70S6 kinase [16]. Studies in different species and several human cells demonstrated that inhibition of characteristic features of the cells by primarily cAMP formation dominates in HR2-dependent effects of histamine.

Human HR3 encoded by a gene, which consists of four exons on chromosome 20, was demonstrated in 1987 and cloned recently [17]. HR3 has initially been identified in the central and peripheral nervous system as presynaptic receptors controlling the release of histamine and other neurotransmitters (dopamine, serotonin, noradrenaline, GABA, and acetylocholine). HR3 signal transduction involves $G_{i/o}$ of G proteins leading to inhibition of cAMP and accumulation of Ca^{2+} and activation of the mitogen-activated protein kinase pathway. R-α-methyhistamine and imetit are agonists, thioperamide and clobenpropit are antagonists of HR3. The control of mast cells by histamine acting on HR3 involves neuropeptide-containing nerves and might be related to a local neuron-mast cell feedback loop controlling neurogenic inflammation. Dysregulation of this feedback loop may lead to excessive inflammatory responses and suggests a novel therapeutic approach by using HR3 agonists. Probably more than one HR3 subtype exists, which differ in central nervous system localization and signaling pathways.

Human HR4, which is encoded by a gene containing three exons, separated by two large introns located in chromosome 18q11.2. It has 37–43% homology to HR3 (58% in the transmembrane region). HR4 is functionally coupled to G-protein $G_{i/o}$, inhibiting forskolin-induced cAMP formation like the HR3 [14]. HR4 shows high expression in the bone marrow and peripheral hematopoietic cells, neutrophils, eosinophils and T cells, basophils and mast cells, and moderate expression in spleen, thymus, lung, small intestine, colon, and heart [18]. Until now, relatively little is known about the biological function of HR4. It seems to be involved in the immune regulatory functions including chemotaxis and cytokine secretion [1, 2]. H4 HR is expressed in cells of the innate immune system, which include NK cells, monocytes, and DCs [19].

HRs form dimers and even oligomers, which allow cooperation between HRs and other G-protein-coupled receptors. Thus, the effects of histamine upon receptor stimulation can be very complex.

Synthesis and Metabolism of Histamine

The classical cellular sources of histamine are mast cells and basophils, gastric enterochromaffin-like cells, platelets and histaminergic neurons. Interestingly the cells in the immune system, which do not store histamine, show high HDC activity and are capable of production of high amounts of histamine, which is secreted immediately after synthesis [20]. These cells include platelets, monocytes/macrophages, DCs, neutrophils, and T and B lymphocytes.

Histamine is synthesized by decarboxylation of histidine by L-histidine decarboxylase (HDC), which is dependent on the cofactor pyridoxal-5′-phosphate [21]. Mast cells and basophils are the major source of granule-stored histamine, where it is closely associated with the anionic proteoglycans and chondroitin-4-sulfate. Histamine is released when these cells degranulate in response to various immunologic and non-immunologic stimuli. In addition, several myeloid and lymphoid cell types (DCs and T cells), which do not

store histamine, show high HDC activity and are capable of production of high amounts of histamine [20]. HDC activity is modulated by cytokines, such as interleukin (IL)-1, IL-3, IL-12, IL-18, GM-CSF, macrophage colony-stimulating factor, TNF-α and calcium ionophore, in vitro [22]. HDC activity has been demonstrated in vivo in conditions such as LPS stimulation, infection, inflammation, and graft rejection [14]. The generation of HDC-deficient mice provided histamine-free systems to study the role of endogenous histamine in a broad range of normal and disease processes. These mice show decreased numbers of mast cells and significantly reduced granule content, which suggests that histamine might affect the synthesis of mast cell granule proteins [23]. IgE binding to the FcεRI on IL-3-dependent mouse bone marrow-derived mast cells induces the expression of HDC through a signaling pathway distinct to that operating during antigen-stimulated FcεRI activation [24]. More than 97% of the histamine is metabolized in two major pathways before excretion [25]. Histamine N-methyltransferase metabolizes the majority of histamine to N-methylhistamine, which is further metabolized to the primary urinary metabolite N-methylimidazole acetic acid by monoamine oxidase. Diamine oxidase metabolizes 15–30% of histamine to imidazole acetic acid.

Histamine in Chronic Inflammatory Responses

Chronic inflammatory response is one of the hallmarks of allergic diseases. Over the course of pollen season, there might be even a tenfold increase in numbers of nasal epithelial submucosal mast cells. Histamine released from these cells might not only induce acute allergic symptoms but also be crucial for sustaining this response into a chronic phase, as increasing evidence suggests that it influences several immune/inflammatory and effector functions (table 2) [2].

Table 2. Histamine receptors in allergic inflammation and immune modulation

	Histamine H$_1$ receptor	Histamine H$_2$ receptor	Histamine H$_3$ receptor	Histamine H$_4$ receptor
Histamine function in allergic inflammation and immune modulation	Increases release of histamine and other mediators Increases cellular adhesion molecule expression and chemotaxis of eosinophils and neutrophils Increases antigen-presenting cell capacity, costimulatory activity on B cells Increases cellular immunity (Th1), IFN-γ, auto-immunity Decreases humoral immunity and IgE production	Decreases eosinophil and neutrophil chemotaxis Decreases IL-12 by DCs Increases IL-10 and induces development of Th2 or tolerance-inducing DCs Increases humoral immunity Decreases cellular immunity Suppresses Th2 cells and cytokines Role in allergy, autoimmunity, malignancy, graft rejection	Probably involved in control of neurogenic inflammation through local neuron-mast cell feedback loops Increases proinflammatory activity and antigen-presenting cells capacity	Increases calcium flux in human eosinophils Increases eosinophil chemotaxis Increases IL-16 production (H$_2$ receptor also involved)

Histamine contributes to the progression of allergic-inflammatory responses by enhancement of the secretion of proinflammatory cytokines like IL-1α, IL-1β, IL-6 as well as chemokines like RANTES or IL-8, both in several cell types and local tissues [26–29]. Endothelial cells express functional HR1 and HR2 and increased adhesion molecule expression such as ICAM-1, VCAM-1 and P-selectin was demonstrated by histamine infusion via HR1 [30–32]. Histamine regulates the expression of its own receptors on endothelial cells and influences the overall inflammatory reaction [33].

Histamine regulates granulocyte accumulation to tissues in distinct ways. Allergen-induced accumulation of eosinophils in the skin, nose and airways is potently inhibited by H$_1$ antihistamines [34]. The effect of histamine on eosinophil migration may differ according to the dose. Whereas high doses inhibit eosinophil chemotaxis via

HR2, low doses enhance eosinophil chemotaxis via HR1 [35]. Recently, it has been shown that the HR responsible for the selective recruitment of eosinophils is HR4 [36]. Histamine possesses all the properties of a classical leukocyte chemoattractant (i.e., agonist-induced actin polymerization, mobilization of intracellular calcium, alteration in cell shape, and upregulation of adhesion molecule expression). Eosinophil's chemoattractive ability of histamine is weak, when compared to the potent CCR3-binding chemokines, eotaxin and eotaxin-2 [36–38]. Histamine possesses all the properties of a classical leukocyte chemoattractant, including: agonist-induced actin polymerization, mobilization of intracellular calcium, alteration in cell shape, and upregulation of adhesion molecule expression. In vivo, allergen-specific wild-type, but not histamine H$_1$-receptor-deficient CD4+ T cells were recruited to the lungs of naive recipients following inhaled allergen challenge [39]. Histamine inhibits neutrophil chemotaxis due to histamine H_2-receptor triggering, which is mimicked by impromidine (histamine H_2-receptor agonist), but not by betahistine (histamine H_1-receptor agonist) [40]. Histamine contributes to the progression of allergic-inflammatory responses by enhancement of the secretion of proinflammatory cytokines such as IL-1α, IL-1β, IL-6 as well as chemokines such as RANTES or IL-8, in several cell types and local tissues [27, 28, 41, 42]. Histamine induces the CC chemokines, monocyte chemotactic protein 1 and 3, RANTES, and eotaxin in explant cultures of human nasal mucosa via histamine H_1 receptor, suggesting a prolonged inflammatory cycle in allergic rhinitis between the cells that release histamine and their enhanced migration to nasal mucosa [43].

However, histamine upon activation of the HR4 induces enhanced migration of eosinophils towards eotaxin and eotaxin-2 [44]. On the other hand, the potential of histamine alone to act as an eosinophil chemoattractant in vivo might be augmented by other factors, such as growth factors or cytokines like IL-5, the cytokine specific for the differentiation, activation, and survival of eosinophils [36]. Triggering of HR4 also induces chemotaxis of mast cells [45]. Experiments in mice showed that mast cells from wild-type and HR3-receptor-deleted mice migrated in response to histamine, while mast cells from the HR4-deleted mice did not. Thus, chemotaxis of eosinophils and mast cells via histamine is triggered mainly through the HR4. The HR4-mediated chronic inflammatory effects of histamine may be aborted by administration of HR4 antagonists and combination therapies with the HR1 antagonists are a promising approach.

Histamine inhibits neutrophil chemotaxis due to HR2 triggering, which is mimicked by impromidine (HR2 agonist), but not by betahistine (HR1 agonist). In addition, histamine inhibits neutrophil activation, superoxide formation and degranulation via HR2 [40]. Downregulation of NF-κB, which acts as a potent transcription factor in initiating inflammation, may represent a possible mechanism for H_1 antihistamines to inhibit inflammatory cell accumulation [46]. Low concentrations of H_1 antihistamines, cetirizine and azelastine, have been demonstrated to downregulate NF-κB expression in parallel to inhibition of proinflammatory cytokines [47]. A recent study with HDC-deficient and mast cell-deficient mice demonstrated that histamine mainly derived from non-mast cells plays an essential role in angiogenesis and the generation of inflammatory granulation [48]. The pretreatment of the nasal mucosa and the conjunctivae with topical H_1 antihistamines has been shown to downregulate the inflammation locally after an allergen challenge [49]. Decreased macrophage IL-6 production and in DCs decreased expression of CD86 and decreased IL-8 production was shown [50, 51].

These findings open a new therapeutic window for antihistamines as systemic antiallergic agents. Although the use of H_1 antihistamine in persistent asthma is currently not recommended, some recent evidence might finally lead to reevaluation of this approach. Histamine has been found in the airways of asthma patients even during asymptomatic periods [52, 53]. An increased number of degranulated mast cells and basophils have been detected in biopsies of asthmatic airways long after an acute asthma attack [54]. The level of histamine in BALF has been found to correlate with the severity of asthma and airway hyperresponsiveness [55].

Inhaled and intravenous histamine causes bronchoconstriction as one of the first recognized properties of histamine, which is inhibited by H_1 antihistamines. As a manifestation of airway hyperresponsiveness, asthmatic individuals are more sensitive to the bronchoconstrictor effect of histamine than normal individuals. In addition, in vitro studies have shown increased histamine release in basophils and mast cells obtained from asthmatic subjects compared with cells obtained from persons without asthma [52]. In lavage fluid of the patients treated with H_1 antihistamines, decreased levels of proinflammatory cytokines and mediators (e.g., histamine, leukotrienes, prostaglandin), cell adhesion molecules (e.g., intercellular adhesion molecules and vascular cell adhesion molecules), cells (e.g., eosinophils and neutrophils), and plasma exudation along with a reduced symptom score have been found [56].

The potential efficacy of H_1 antihistamines in asthma has been intensively investigated [56]. It has been shown that inhalation, intravenous or oral administration of clemastine or chlorpheniramine induced significant bronchodilatation. However, second-generation H_1 antihistamines induce only a very limited increase of FEV_1 (5–10% over baseline) by recommended doses [57, 58]. There is a variable effect on allergen challenge or exercise-induced bronchospasm. Only terfenadine with 3 times recommended dose inhibited early and late bronchoconstrictor response [58]. Terfenadine, cetirizine and loratadine with 2–5 times the usual dose appeared to improve asthma symptoms in mild seasonal or perennial asthma, but did not block development of bronchial hyperresponsiveness in seasonal pollen asthma or show apparent benefit in patients with more severe asthma [57, 58]. In patients with concurrent symptoms of allergic rhinitis and asthma, treatment with H_1 antihistamine results in significant decrease in symptoms of both rhinitis and asthma, decrease in use of β_2 agonists, and some improvement of airway function [59]. Montelukast sodium, a leukotriene receptor antagonist, showed similar effect as desloratadine [59].

The mechanisms of the beneficial effect of HR1 antihistamines in asthma have been investigated in a mice model. Fexofenadine was found to suppress allergic immune/inflammatory responses in sensitized mice [60]. Treatment with fexofenadine diminished Th2-like response that typically follows sensitization and challenge with allergen. Decreased secretion of IL-4, IL-5, prevention of allergen-specific IgE increase and reduced eosinophilia in lung tissue and BALF as well as normalization of airway response to metacholine was observed.

Importantly, in an adoptive transfer model it was demonstrated that the target mechanism was T-cell-mediated. Lung T cells from sensitized mice, when transferred to naive recipient mice, triggered airway hyperresponsiveness and allergic inflammatory features after allergen challenge. In contrast, naive mice which received T cells from sensitized mice treated before with fexofenadine showed no such responses to allergen challenge [60]. The inability of T cells from HR1 antihistamine-treated allergen-sensitized mice to transfer allergic sensitivity to naive recipients resulted from an alteration in the cytokine production profile of the transferred cells.

Consistently, histamine-induced concentration-dependent release of IL-6 and β-glucuronidase from macrophages isolated from the human lung parenchyma was inhibited by fexofenadine but not by ranitidine, an H_2-receptor antagonist [61]. Thus long-term treatment with H_1 antihistamines can alter disease progression in patients with respiratory allergy associated with tissue damage/remodeling mediated by macrophage and Th2 cell activation. It has been shown that treatment with cetirizine over period of 18 months delayed the onset of asthma in some young children with atopic dermatitis [62]. Although H_1 antihistamines clearly show weaker anti-inflammatory effects than corticosteroids but they may in a subtle way modulate the immune response by modulating the balance between Th1, Th2 and Treg cells and suppressing the accumulation of inflammatory cells. Although previous studies suggested a basal tone of smooth muscle mediated by histamine binding to HR1, currently constitutive intrinsic activity of the HR1 without any occupation by histamine could be more relevant. Histamine also induces proliferation of cultured airway smooth muscle cells [63].

Difference in histamine response between species has been reported indicating a role for HR2-mediated bronchodilatation in cat, rat, rabbit, sheep and horse [64]. However, in humans, H_2 antihistamines such as cimetidine and ranitidine do not cause bronchoconstriction in normal or asthmatic individuals [65]. Although there is no direct evidence that it plays a role in disease pathogenesis, HR2-mediated gastric secretion is impaired in asthma [66]. Histamine may play an important role in the modulation of the cytokine network in the lung via HR2, HR3 and HR4 that are expressed in distinct cells and cell subsets. Apparently, due to the same signal transduction patterns, β_2-adrenergic receptors may function similar to HR2 in humans. The role of histamine and other redundant G-protein-coupled receptors in the regulation of immune/inflammatory pathways in the lung remain to be intensely focused in future studies.

Role of Histamine in the Regulation of Immune Response

Antigen-Presenting Cells

DCs are often located in the vicinity of various histamine sources such as connective tissue mast cells. They are potent antigen-presenting and cytokine-producing cells. Therefore, histamine may effectively influence the immune response through DC. These professional antigen-presenting cells mature from monocytic and lymphoid precursors, and acquire DC1 and DC2 phenotypes, which in turn facilitate the development of Th1 and Th2 cells, respectively. Endogenous histamine is actively synthesized during cytokine-induced DC differentiation, which acts in an autocrine and paracrine fashion and modifies DC markers [67]. Histamine actively participates in functions and activity of DC precursors as well as their immature and mature forms (fig. 1). Immature and mature DCs express all four HRs, however comparison of their levels of expression has not yet been studied. In the differen-

tiation process of DC1 from monocytes, HR1 and HR3 act as positive stimulants that increase antigen-presentation capacity and proinflammatory cytokine production and Th1 priming activity. In contrast, HR2 acts as a suppressive molecule for antigen-presentation capacity, enhances IL-10 production and induces IL-10-producing T cells or Th2 cells (table 2) [68, 69].

In monocytes stimulated with Toll-like receptor-triggering bacterial products, histamine inhibits the production of proinflammatory IL-1-like activity, TNF-α, IL-12 and IL-18, but enhances IL-10 secretion, through HR2 stimulation [26, 69]. Histamine also downregulates CD14 expression via H_2 receptors on human monocytes [70]. The inhibitory effect of histamine via H_2 receptor appears through the regulation of ICAM-1 and B7.1 expression, leading to the reduction of innate immune response stimulated by LPS [71].

Histamine induces intracellular Ca^{2+} flux, actin polymerization, and chemotaxis in immature DCs due to stimulation of HR1 and HR3 subtypes. Maturation of DCs results in loss of these responses. In maturing DCs, however, histamine dose-dependently enhances intracellular cAMP levels and stimulates IL-10 secretion, while inhibiting production of IL-12 via HR2 [16]. Interestingly, although human monocyte-derived dendritic cells have both histamine H_1 and H_2 receptors and can induce CD86 expression by histamine, human epidermal Langerhans' cells express neither H_1 nor H_2 receptors [72].

Effect of Histamine on T Cells and Antibody Isotypes

Histamine has been shown to intervene in the Th1, Th2, Treg cell balance and consequently antibody formation. Differential patterns of HR expression on Th1 and Th2 cells determine reciprocal T-cell responses following histamine stimulation (table 2; fig. 1) [73]. Th1 cells show predominant, but not

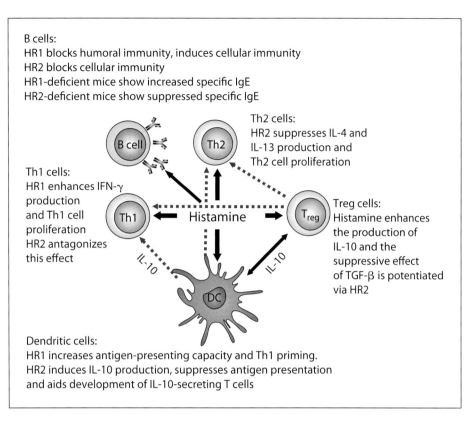

B cells:
HR1 blocks humoral immunity, induces cellular immunity
HR2 blocks cellular immunity
HR1-deficient mice show increased specific IgE
HR2-deficient mice show suppressed specific IgE

Th2 cells:
HR2 suppresses IL-4 and
IL-13 production and
Th2 cell proliferation

Th1 cells:
HR1 enhances IFN-γ
production
and Th1 cell
proliferation
HR2 antagonizes
this effect

Treg cells:
Histamine enhances
the production of
IL-10 and the
suppressive effect
of TGF-β is potentiated
via HR2

Dendritic cells:
HR1 increases antigen-presenting capacity and Th1 priming.
HR2 induces IL-10 production, suppresses antigen presentation
and aids development of IL-10-secreting T cells

Fig. 1. Histamine regulates monocyte, dendritic cell, T cells and B-cell functions. Monocytes and DCs express all four HRs. Activation of HR1 and HR3 triggers proinflammatory events and increases antigen-presenting cell capacity. HR2 plays a suppressive role on monocytes and monocyte-derived dendritic cells (DCs). Th1 cells show predominant, but not exclusive, expression of HR1, whereas Th2 cells show upregulation of HR2. Histamine induces increased proliferation and IFN-γ production in Th1 cells. Th2 cells express predominant HR2, which acts as the negative regulator of proliferation, IL-4 and IL-13 production. Histamine enhances Th1-type responses by triggering the HR1, whereas both Th1- and Th2-type responses are negatively regulated by HR2, showing an essential role for immune regulation for this receptor. Distinct effects of histamine suggest roles of HR1 and HR2 on T cells for autoimmunity and peripheral tolerance, respectively. Histamine also modulates antibody production. Histamine directly effects B-cell antibody production as a costimulatory receptor on B cells. HR1 predominantly expressed on Th1 cells may block humoral immune responses by enhancing Th1-type cytokine IFN-γ. In contrast, HR2 enhances humoral immune responses. Allergen-specific IgE production is differentially regulated in HR1- and HR2-deficient mice. HR1-deleted mice show increased allergen-specific IgE production, whereas HR2-deleted mice show suppressed IgE production.

exclusive expression of HR1, while Th2 cells show increased expression of HR2. Histamine enhances Th1-type responses by triggering the HR1, whereas both Th1- and Th2-type responses are negatively regulated by HR2, due to activation of different biochemical intracellular signals [73]. In mice, deletion of HR1 results in suppression of IFN-γ and dominant secretion of Th2 cytokines (IL-4 and

IL-13). HR2-deleted mice show upregulation of both Th1 and Th2 cytokines. *Bphs*, a non-major histocompatibility complex-linked gene involved in the susceptibility to many autoimmune diseases, has been identified as HR1 gene in mice. HR1-deleted mice showed delayed disease onset and decreased disease severity when immunized to develop experimental allergic encephalomyelitis [74]. It has also been shown that histamine stimulation induced IL-10 secretion through HR2 [1, 2]. Increased IL-10 production in both DC and T cells may account for an important regulatory mechanism in the control of inflammatory functions through histamine. Various cytokines regulate the production of histamine and its receptor expression. IL-3 stimulation significantly increases HR1 expression on Th1, but not on Th2 cells [73].

In mice, histamine enhances anti-IgM-induced proliferation of B cells, which is abolished in HR1-deleted mice. In HR1-deleted mice, antibody production against a T-cell-independent antigen-TNP-Ficoll is decreased [15], suggesting an important role of HR1 signaling in responses triggered from B-cell receptors. Antibody responses to T-cell-dependent antigens like ovalbumin (OVA) show a different pattern [15]. HR1-deleted mice produced high OVA-specific IgG1 and IgE in comparison to wild-type mice. In contrast, HR2-deleted mice showed decreased serum levels of OVA-specific IgE in comparison to wild-type mice and HR1-deficient mice. Although T cells of HR2-deficient mice secreted increased IL-4 and IL-13, OVA-specific IgE was suppressed in the presence of highly increased IFN-γ. Thus, HR1 and related Th1 response may play a dominant role in the suppression of humoral immune response.

Role of Histamine and H$_1$ Antihistamines during Allergen-SIT

The rationale for the use of H$_1$ antihistamines during SIT is diverse and may include both the reduction of side effects, which may develop immediately after the shots of vaccine and providing help in the long-term induction of allergen tolerance induced by vaccination. Pretreatment with antihistamines was proposed as early as in the 1980s as an effective approach to reduce the side effects of allergen immunotherapy [75]. It has been confirmed in a number of studies that administration of high doses of second-generation H$_1$R antihistamines before vaccine shots of insect venom or grass pollen is effective in reduction of local allergic reactions and generalized symptoms of the urticaria and angioedema type [76–78]. Unfortunately, this modality is much less effective in the reduction of more severe systemic symptoms [76–78].

The effect of pretreatment with terfenadine on the long-term protection from honeybee stings during rush immunotherapy with honeybee venom was analyzed in a double-blind, placebo-controlled trial [79]. After an average of 3 years, 41 patients were re-exposed to honeybee stings. Surprisingly, none of 20 patients, who had been given HR1 antihistamine premedication, but 6 of 21 given placebo, had a systemic allergic reaction to the re-exposure by either a field sting or a sting challenge. This highly significant difference suggests that H$_1$ antihistamine premedication during the initial dose-increase phase may have enhanced the long-term efficacy of immunotherapy. This indicates a positive role of histamine in immune regulation during SIT [80]. Similarly, in the ETAC (early treatment of the atopic child) study – a double-blind placebo-controlled trial aiming at the determination of the preventative effect of cetirizine on the development of asthma which included 830 children with atopic dermatitis aged 12–24 months – it has been shown that treatment with cetirizine reduced the relative risk of developing asthma in children sensitized to grass pollen or house dust mite [81]. These findings indicate the immunoregulatory and anti-inflammatory effects of H_1 antihistamines. The underlying mechanisms are not fully elucidated. On one side, treatment with H_1R antagonists also results in H_2R predominance. Moreover, the expression of HR1 on T lymphocytes is strongly reduced during ultra-rush immunotherapy, which may lead to a dominant expression of HR2.

Peripheral T-cell tolerance characterized by immune deviation to regulatory/suppressor T cells represents a key event in the control of specific immune response during allergen-specific immunotherapy [82]. Although multiple suppressor factors including contact-dependent or -independent mechanisms might be involved, IL-10 and TGF-β predominantly produced by allergen-specific T cells play an essential role [83, 84]. Histamine interferes with the peripheral tolerance induced during SIT in several pathways. Histamine induces the production of IL-10 by DCs [85]. In addition, histamine induces IL-10 production by Th2 cells [86]. Furthermore, histamine enhances the suppressive activity of TGF-β on T cells [87]. All three of these effects are mediated via HR2, which is relatively highly expressed on Th2 cells and suppresses IL-4 and IL-13 production and T-cell proliferation. Apparently, these recent findings suggest that HR2 may represent an essential receptor that participates in peripheral tolerance or active suppression of inflammatory/immune responses. Although the selective activation of H_2R might be a more promising approach as compared to the use of H_1 antihistamines, so far it has not been investigated in vivo.

However, selective HR2 antagonists have attracted interest because of their potential immune response-modifying activity [88]. Most data suggest that cimetidine has a stimulatory effect on the immune system, possibly by blocking the receptors on subsets of T lymphocytes and inhibiting HR2-induced immunosuppression. Cimetidine has also been used successfully to restore immune functions in patients with malignant disorders, hypogammaglobulinemia and AIDS-related complexes.

Use of H_1 Antihistamines in Asthma

Histamine administered intravenously or by inhalation causes bronchoconstriction, which is inhibited by HR1 antihistamines. Individuals with asthma are more sensitive to the bronchoconstrictor effect of histamine than healthy individuals. Although current evidence does not support the use of H_1 antihistamines in persistent asthma, some investigators have shown a significant decrease in asthma symptoms and improvement in pulmonary function after H_1 antihistamine treatment [3, 62, 89–91]. Treatment with the H_1 antihistamine cetirizine over a period of 18 months was reported to delay the onset of asthma in some young children with atopic dermatitis who were at high risk for the disease, however this observation requires confirmation [3, 62, 89–91]. In sensitized mice, treatment with the H_1 antihistamine fexofenadine before allergen challenge prevented airway hyperresponsiveness. Decreases in BALF and tissue eosinophilia, lymphocyte numbers, and Th2 cytokine production were also observed in this model [60]. Another HR1 antihistamine, desloratadine, given at the time of allergen exposure, inhibited the induction of allergic inflammation in the airways and bronchial hyperresponsiveness [92].

Histamine-induced, concentration-dependent release of IL-6 and β-glucuronidase from macrophages isolated from human lung parenchyma can be consistently inhibited by fexofenadine but not by ranitidine, an H_2 antihistamine [61]. Thus, long-term treatment with HR1 antihistamines might potentially alter disease progression in patients with respiratory allergy associated with tissue damage/remodeling mediated by macrophage and Th2 cell activation.

Although previous studies suggested a basal tone of smooth muscle mediated by histamine binding to HR1, constitutive intrinsic activity of the HR1 without any occupation by histamine might be more relevant. Histamine also induces proliferation of cultured airway smooth muscle cells [63].

Species differences in the response to histamine have been reported. HR2-mediated bronchodilatation occurs in cats, rats, rabbits, sheep and horses [64]; however, in healthy and asthmatic humans, H_2 antihistamines such as cimetidine and ranitidine do not cause bronchoconstriction [65, 93]. Although there is no direct evidence that it plays a role in disease pathogenesis, HR2-mediated gastric secretion may be impaired in asthma [66]. H_2 antihistamines, given for the treatment of gastroesophageal reflux, improve asthma symptoms [94]; whether this is an indirect effect due to downregulation of gastric acid secretion, or whether it is a direct effect remains to be elucidated. In addition, recent studies suggest that histamine may play an important role in the modulation of the cytokine network in the lung via HR2, HR3 and HR4 that are expressed in distinct cells and cell subsets [95, 96]. Apparently, due to the same signal transduction patterns, β_2-adrenergic receptors may function similar to HR2 in humans [97]. Future research should focus on the role of histamine and other redundant G-protein-coupled receptors in the regulation of immune/inflammatory pathways in the lung.

In particular, the discovery of a fourth HR (H4) and its expression on numerous immune and inflammatory cells has prompted a re-evaluation of the actions of histamine, suggesting a new potential for H_4-receptor antagonists and a possible synergy between H_1- and H_4-receptor antagonists in targeting various inflammatory conditions [98].

Conclusions

The emerging pattern of immune regulation by histamine is very complex and calls for further investigation. Histamine and four different HRs constitute a multifaceted system with distinct functions of receptor types due to their differential expression, which changes according to the stage of cell differentiation and influences of the microenvironment. The diverse effects of histamine on immune regulation appear to be due to differential expression and regulation of four types of HRs and their distinct intracellular signals. In addition, the differences in affinities of these receptors for histamine are highly decisive for the biological effects of histamine and drugs that target HRs. The cells involved in the regulation of immune response and hematopoiesis express HRs and also secrete histamine. Histamine can selectively recruit the major effector cells into tissue sites and affect their maturation, activation, polarization, and other functions leading to chronic inflammation. Histamine also regulates DCs, T cells and B cells, as well as related antibody isotype responses. Although contrasting findings have been reported, HR1 stimulates the immune system cells by potentiating their proinflammatory activity for increased migration to the area of inflammation as well as increased effector functions. In addition, acting through its receptor 2, histamine positively interferes with the peripheral antigen tolerance induced by T regulatory cells in several pathways. The data on the role of HR3 and HR4 in immune regulation are limited. The observation that H4R activation promotes the accumulation of inflammatory cells at sites of allergic inflammation opens a new window of therapeutic opportunity based on concurrent H_1 antihistamine and H_4 antihistamine administration, or development of selective dual H_1/H_4 antihistamines. Whether such treatment will provide additional suppression of allergic inflammatory responses compared with that observed after H_1 antihistamine treatment alone remains to be elucidated.

Acknowledgments

The authors' laboratory is sponsored by Swiss National Science Foundation Grants and Global Allergy and Asthma European Network (GA2LEN).

References

1 Akdis CA, Blaser K: Histamine in the immune regulation of allergic inflammation. J Allergy Clin Immunol 2003; 112:15–22.

2 Jutel M, Watanabe T, Akdis M, Blaser K, Akdis CA: Immune regulation by histamine. Curr Opin Immunol 2002; 14:735–740.

3 Simons FE: Advances in H$_1$ antihistamines. N Engl J Med 2004;351: 2203–2217.

4 Akdis CA, Simons FE: Histamine receptors are hot in immunopharmacology. Eur J Pharmacol 2006;533:69–76.

5 Dale HH, Laidlaw PP: The physiological action of β-imidazolylethylamine. J Physiol (Lond) 1910;41:318–344.

6 Haas H, Panula P: The role of histamine and the tuberomamillary nucleus in the nervous system. Rev Neurosci 2003;4:121–130.

7 Casale TB, Wood D, Richerson HB, Zehr B, Zavala D, Hunninghake GW: Direct evidence of a role for mast cells in the pathogenesis of antigen-induced bronchoconstriction. J Clin Invest 1987; 80:1507–1511.

8 Johnson HH Jr, Deoreo GA, Lascheid WP, Mitchell F: Skin histamine levels in chronic atopic dermatitis. J Invest Dermatol 1960;34:237–238.

9 Kaplan AP, Horakova Z, Katz SI: Assessment of tissue fluid histamine levels in patients with urticaria. J Allergy Clin Immunol 1978;61:350–354.

10 Tuomisto L, Kilpelainen H, Riekkinen P: Histamine and histamine-N-methyltransferase in the CSF of patients with multiple sclerosis. Agents Actions 1983; 13:255–257.

11 Petersen LJ, Hansen U, Kristensen JK, Nielsen H, Skov PS, Nielsen HJ: Studies on mast cells and histamine release in psoriasis: the effect of ranitidine. Acta Derm Venereol 1998;78:190–193.

12 Frewin DB, Cleland LG, Jonsson JR, Robertson PW: Histamine levels in human synovial fluid. J Rheumatol 1986;13:13–14.

13 Leurs R, Church MK, Taglialatela M: H$_1$-antihistamines: inverse agonism, anti-inflammatory actions and cardiac effects. Clin Exp Allergy 2002;32: 489–498.

14 Leurs R, Smit MJ, Timmerman H: Molecular and pharmacological aspects of histamine receptors. Pharmacol Ther 1995;66:413–463.

15 Banu Y, Watanabe T: Augmentation of antigen receptor-mediated responses by histamine H$_1$ receptor signaling. J Exp Med 1999;189:673–682.

16 Del Valle J, Gantz I: Novel insights into histamine H$_2$ receptor biology. Am J Physiol 1997;273:G987–G996.

17 Lovenberg TW, Roland BL, Wilson SJ, Jiang X, Pyati J, Huvar A, Jackson MR, Erlander MG: Cloning and functional expression of the human histamine H$_3$ receptor. Mol Pharmacol 1999;55: 1101–1107.

18 Nakamura K, Kitani A, Strober W: Cell contact-dependent immunosuppression by CD4+CD25+ regulatory T cells is mediated by cell surface-bound transforming growth factor-β. J Exp Med 2001;194:629–644.

19 Damaj BB, Becerra CB, Esber HJ, Wen Y, Maghazachi AA: Functional expression of H4 histamine receptor in human natural killer cells, monocytes, and dendritic cells. J Immunol 2007; 179:7907–7915.

20 Kubo Y, Nakano H: Regulation of histamine in mouse CD4+ and CD8+ lymphocytes. Infamm Res 1999;48:149–153.

21 Endo Y: Simultaneous induction of histidine and ornithine decarboxylases and changes in their product amines following the injection of Escherichia coli lipopolysaccharide into mice. Biochem Pharmacol 1982;31:1643–1647.

22 Yoshimoto T, Tsutsui H, Tominaga K, Hoshino K, Okamura H, Akira S, Paul WE, Naknushi K: IL-18, although antiallergic when administered with IL-12, stimulates IL-4 and histamine release by basophils. Proc Natl Acad Sci USA 1999;96:13962–13966.

23 Ohtsu H, Tanaka S, Terui T, Hori Y, Makabe-Kobayashi Y, Pejler G: Mice lacking histidine decarboxylase exhibit abnormal mast cells. FEBS Lett 2001; 502:53–56.

24 Tanaka S, Takasu Y, Mikura S, Satoh N, Ichikawa A: Antigen-independent induction of histamine synthesis by immunoglobulin E in mouse bone marrow-derived mast cells. J Exp Med 2002;196:229–235.

25 Abe Y, Ogino S, Irifune M, Imamura I, Fukui H, Wada H, Matsunaga T: Histamine content, synthesis and degradation in human nasal mucosa. Clin Exp Allergy 1993;23:132–136.

26 Vannier E, Dinarello CA: Histamine enhances interleukin (IL)-1-induced IL-1 gene expression and protein synthesis via H$_2$ receptors in peripheral blood mononuclear cells. Comparison with IL-1 receptor antagonist. J Clin Invest 1993;92:281–287.

27 Meretey K, Falus A, Taga T, Kishimoto T: Histamine influences the expression of the interleukin-6 receptor on human lymphoid, monocytoid and hepatoma cell lines. Agents Actions 1991;33: 189–191.

28 Jeannin P, Delneste Y, Gosset P, Molet S, Lassalle P, Hamid Q, Tsicopoulos A, Tonnel AB: Histamine induces interleukin-8 secretion by endothelial cells. Blood 1994;84:2229–2233.

29 Bayram H, Devalia JL, Khair OA, Abdelaziz MM, Sapsford RJ, Czarlewski W, Campbell AM, Bousquet J, Davies RJ: Effect of loratadine on nitrogen dioxide-induced changes in electrical resistance and release of inflammatory mediators from cultured human bronchial epithelial cells. J Allergy Clin Immunol 1999;104:93–99.

30 Lo WW, Fan TP: Histamine stimulates inositol phosphate accumulation via the H$_1$ receptor in cultured human endothelial cells. Biochem Biophys Res Commun 1987;148:47–53.

31 Kubes P, Kanwar S: Histamine induces leukocyte rolling in post-capillary venules. A P-selectin-mediated event. J Immunol 1994;152:3570–3577.

32 Yamaki K, Thorlacius H, Xie X, Lindbom L, Hedqvist P, Raud J: Characteristics of histamine-induced leukocyte rolling in the undisturbed microcirculation of the rat mesentery. Br J Pharmacol 1998;123:390–399.

33 Schaefer U, Schmitz V, Schneider A, Neugebauer E: Histamine induced homologous and heterologous regulation of histamine receptor subtype mRNA expression in cultured endothelial cells. Shock 1999;12:309–315.

34 Fadel R, Herpin-Richard N, Rihoux JP, Henocq E: Inhibitory effect of cetirizine 2HCl on eosinophil migration in vivo. Clin Allergy 1987;17:373–379.

35 Clark RA, Sandler JA, Gallin JI, Kaplan AP: Histamine modulation of eosinophil migration. J Immunol 1977;118: 137–145.

36 O'Reilly M, Alpert R, Jenkinson S, Gladue RP, Foo S, Trim S, Peter B, Trevethick M, Fidock M: Identification of a histamine H4 receptor on human eosinophils – role in eosinophil chemotaxis. J Recept Signal Transduct Res 2002;22:431–448.

37 Buckland KF, Williams TJ, Conroy DM: Histamine induces cytoskeletal changes in human eosinophils via the H4 receptor. Br J Pharmacol 2003;140:1117–1127.

38 Ling P, Ngo K, Nguyen S, Thurmond RL, Edwards JP, Karlsson L, Fung-Leung WP: Histamine H4 receptor mediates eosinophil chemotaxis with cell shape change and adhesion molecule upregulation. Br J Pharmacol 2004;142:161–171.

39 Bryce PJ, Mathias CB, Harrison KL, Watanabe T, Geha RS, Oettgen HC: The H_1 histamine receptor regulates allergic lung responses. J Clin Invest 2006;116:1624–1632.

40 Seligmann BE, Fletcher MP, Gallin JI: Histamine modulation of human neutrophil oxidative metabolism, locomotion, degranulation, and membrane potential changes. J Immunol 1983;130:1902–1909.

41 Vannier E, Dinarello CA: Histamine enhances interleukin (IL)-1-induced IL-1 gene expression and protein synthesis via H_2 receptors in peripheral blood mononuclear cells. Comparison with IL-1 receptor antagonist. J Clin Invest 1993;92:281–287.

42 Bayram H, Devalia JL, Khair OA, Abdelaziz MM, Sapsford RJ, Czarlewski W, Campbell AM, Bousquet J, Davies RJ: Effect of loratadine on nitrogen dioxide-induced changes in electrical resistance and release of inflammatory mediators from cultured human bronchial epithelial cells. J Allergy Clin Immunol 1999;104:93–99.

43 Fujikura T, Shimosawa T, Yakuo I: Regulatory effect of histamine H_1 receptor antagonist on the expression of messenger RNA encoding CC chemokines in the human nasal mucosa. J Allergy Clin Immunol 2001;107:123–128.

44 Buckland KF, Williams TJ, Conroy DM: Histamine induces cytoskeletal changes in human eosinophils via the H(4) receptor. Br J Pharmacol 2003;140:1117–1127.

45 Gantz I, Schaffer M, DelValle J: Molecular cloning of a gene encoding the histamine H_2 receptor. Proc Natl Acad Sci USA 1991;88:5937.

46 Oda T, Morikawa N, Saito Y, Masuho Y, Matsumoto S: Molecular cloning and characterization of a novel type of histamine receptor preferentially expressed in leukocytes. J Biol Chem 2000;275:36781–36786.

47 Yoneda K, Yamamoto T, Ueta E, Osaki T: Suppression by azelastine hydrochloride of NF-κB activation involved in generation of cytokines and nitric oxide. Jpn J Pharmacol 1997;73:145–153.

48 Ghosh AK, Hirasawa N, Ohtsu H, Watanabe T, Ohuchi K: Defective angiogenesis in the inflammatory granulation tissue in histidine decarboxylase-deficient mice but not in mast cell-deficient mice. J Exp Med 2002;195:973–982.

49 Simons FER: Antihistamines; in Adkinson NF Jr, Yunginger JW, Busse WW, Bochner BS, Holgate ST, Simons FER (eds): Middleton's Allergy: Principles & Practice. St Louis, Mosby, 2003, pp 834–869.

50 Paolieri F, Battifora M, Riccio AM: Terfenadine and fexofenadine reduce in vitro ICAM-1 expression on human continuous cell lines. Ann Allergy Asthma Immunol 1988;81:601–607.

51 Caron G, Delneste Y, Roelandts E: Histamine induces CD86 expression and chemokine production by human immature dendritic cells. J Immunol 2001;166:6000–6006.

52 Casolaro V, Gale D: Functional comparisons of cells obtained from peripheral blood, lung parenchyma, bronchoalveolar lavage in asthmatics. Am Rev Respir Dis 1989;139:1375–1382.

53 Wenzel SE, Fowler AA, Schwartz LB: Activation of pulmonary mast cells by bronchoalveolar allergen challenge: in vivo release of histamine and tryptase in atopic subjects with and without asthma. Am Rev Respir Dis 1988;137:1002–1008.

54 Crimi E, Chiaramondia M, Milanese M: Increase of mast cell numbers in mucosa after the late-phase asthmatic response to allergen. Am Rev Respir Dis 1991;144:1282–1286.

55 Nakamura T, Itadani H, Hidaka Y, Ohta M, Tanaka K: Molecular cloning and characterization of a new human histamine receptor, HH4R. Biochem Biophys Res Commun 2000;279:615–620.

56 Milligan G, Bond R, Lee M: Inverse agonism: pharmacological curiosity or potential therapeutic strategy? Trends Pharmacol Sci 1995;16:10–13.

57 Malick A, Grant JA: Antihistamines in the treatment of asthma. Allergy 1997;52:55–66.

58 Town GI, Holgate ST: Comparison of the effect of loratadine on the airway and skin responses to histamine, methacholine, and allergen in subjects with asthma. J Allergy Clin Immunol 1990;86:886–893.

59 Baena-Cagnani CE, Berger WE, DuBuske LM: Comparative effects of desloratadine versus montelukast on asthma symptoms and use of β_2 agonists in patients with seasonal allergic rhinitis and asthma. Int Arch Allergy Immunol 2003;130:307–313.

60 Gelfand EW, Cui ZH, Takeda K, Kanehiro A, Joetham A: Fexofenadine modulates T-cell function, preventing allergen-induced airway inflammation and hyperresponsiveness. J Allergy Clin Immunol 2002;110:85–95.

61 Triggiani M, Gentile M, Secondo A, Granata F, Oriente A, Taglialatela M, Annunziato L, Marone G: Histamine induces exocytosis and IL-6 production from human lung macrophages through interaction with H_1 receptors. J Immunol 2001;166:4083–4091.

62 Warner JO: A double-blind, randomized, placebo-controlled trial of cetirizine in preventing the onset of asthma in children with atopic dermatitis: 18 months' treatment and 18 months' post-treatment follow-up. J Allergy Clin Immunol 2001;108:929–937.

63 Panettieri RA, Yadvish PA, Kelly AM, Rubinstein NA, Kotlikoff MI: Histamine stimulates proliferation of airway smooth muscle and induces c-fos expression. Am J Physiol 1990;259:L365–L371.

64 Chand N, Eyre P: Classification and biological distribution of histamine receptor subtypes. Agents Actions 1975;5:277–295.

65 Thomson NC, Kerr JW: Effect of inhaled H_1 and H_2 receptor antagonist in normal and asthmatic subjects. Thorax 1980;35:428–434.

66 Gonzales H, Ahmed T: Suppression of gastric H_2-receptor-mediated function in patients with bronchial asthma and ragweed allergy. Chest 1986;89: 491–496.

67 Szeberenyi JB, Pallinger E, Zsinko M, Pos Z, Rothe G, Orso E, et al: Inhibition of effects of endogenously synthesized histamine disturbs in vitro human dendritic cell differentiation. Immunol Lett 2001;76:175–182.

68 Mazzoni A, Young HA, Spitzer JH, Visintin A, Segal DM: Histamine regulates cytokine production in maturing dendritic cells, resulting in altered T cell polarization. J Clin Invest 2001; 108:1865–1873.

69 Van der Pouw Kraan TC, Snijders A, Boeije LC, de Groot ER, Alewijnse AE, Leurs R, Aarden LA: Histamine inhibits the production of interleukin-12 through interaction with H_2 receptors. J Clin Invest 1998;102: 1866–1873.

70 Takahashi HK, Morichika T, Iwagaki H, Tamura R, Kubo S, Yoshino T, et al: Histamine downregulates CD14 expression via H_2 receptors on human monocytes. Clin Immunol 2003;108: 274–281.

71 Morichika T, Takahashi HK, Iwagaki H, Yoshino T, Tamura R, Yokoyama M, et al: Histamine inhibits lipopolysaccharide-induced tumor necrosis factor-α production in an intercellular adhesion molecule-1- and B7.1-dependent manner. J Pharmacol Exp Ther 2003;304:624–633.

72 Ohtani T, Aiba S, Mizuashi M, Mollah ZU, Nakagawa S, Tagami H: H_1 and H_2 histamine receptors are absent on Langerhans' cells and present on dermal dendritic cells. J Invest Dermatol 2003;121:1073–1079.

73 Jutel M, Watanabe T, Klunker S, Akdis M, Thomet OAR, Malolepszy J, et al: Histamine regulates T-cell and antibody responses by differential expression of H_1 and H_2 receptors. Nature 2001;413:420–425.

74 Ma RZ, Gao J, Meeker ND, Fillmore PD, Tung KS, Watanabe T, et al: Identification of Bphs, an autoimmune disease locus, as histamine receptor H_1. Science 2002;297:620–623.

75 Jarisch R, Goetz M, Aberer W, Sidl R, Stabel A, Zajc J, Fordos A: Reduction of side effects of specific immunotherapy by premedication with antihistamines and reduction of maximal dosage to 50,000 SQ-U/ml. Arbeiten aus dem Paul-Ehrlich Institut 1988;82:163–175.

76 Berchtold E, Maibach R, Muller UR: Reduction of side effects from rush-immunotherapy with honey bee venom by pretreatment with terfenadine. Clin Exp Allergy 1992;22:59–65.

77 Nielsen L, Johnsen CR, Mosbech H, Poulsen L, Malling HJ: Antihistamine premedication in specific cluster immunotherapy: a double-blind placebo-controlled study. J Allergy Clin Immunol 1996;97:1207–1213.

78 Reimers A, Hari Y, Muller UR: Reduction of side effects from ultra-rush immunotherapy with honey bee venom by pretreatment with fexofenadine: a double-blind, placebo-controlled trial. Allergy 2000;55:484–488.

79 Muller U, Hari Y, Berchtold E: Premedication with antihistamines may enhance efficacy of specific-allergen immunotherapy. J Allergy Clin Immunol 2001;107:81–86.

80 Jutel M, Zak-Nejmark T, Wrzyyszcz M, Malolepszy J: Histamine receptor expression on peripheral blood CD4+ lymphocytes is influenced by ultrarush bee venom immunotherapy. Allergy 1997;52(suppl 37):88.

81 Diepgen TL: Long-term treatment with cetirizine of infants with atopic dermatitis: a multi-country, double-blind, randomized, placebo-controlled trial (the ETAC trial) over 18 months. Pediatr Allergy Immunol 2002;13:278–286.

82 Akdis CA, Blaser K, Akdis M: Genes of tolerance. Allergy 2004;59:897–913.

83 Akdis CA, Blesken T, Akdis M, Wüthrich B, Blaser K: Role of IL-10 in specific immunotherapy. J Clin Invest 1998;102:98–106.

84 Jutel M, Akdis M, Budak F, Aebischer-Casaulta C, Wrzyszcz M, Blaser K, Akdis C: IL-10 and TGF-β cooperate in the regulatory T cell response to mucosal allergens in normal immunity and specific immunotherapy. Eur J Immunol 2003;33:1205–1214.

85 Mazzoni A, Young HA, Spitzer JH, Visintin A, Segal DM: Histamine regulates cytokine production in maturing dendritic cells, resulting in altered T cell polarization. J Clin Invest 2001; 108:1865–1873.

86 Osna N, Elliott K, Khan MM: Regulation of interleukin-10 secretion by histamine in Th2 cells and splenocytes. Int Immunopharmacol 2001;1: 85–96.

87 Kunzmann S, Mantel P-Y, Wohlfahrt J, Akdis M, Blaser K, Schmidt-Weber C: Histamine enhances TGF-β_1-mediated suppression of Th2 responses. FASEB J 2003;17:1089–1095.

88 Gifford R, Schmidke J: Cimetidine-induced augmentation of human lymphocyte blastogenesis: comparison with levamisole in mitogen stimulation. Surg Forum 1979;30:113–115.

89 Simons FER: Allergic rhinobronchitis: the asthma/allergic rhinitis link. J Allergy Clin Immunol 1999;104: 543–537.

90 Simons FE: Is antihistamine (H_1-receptor antagonist) therapy useful in clinical asthma? Clin Exp Allergy 1999;29 (suppl 3):98–104.

91 Baena-Cagnani CE, Berger WE, DuBuske LM, Gurne SE, Stryszak P, Lorber R, Danzig M: Comparative effects of desloratadine versus montelukast on asthma symptoms and use of β_2 agonists in patients with seasonal allergic rhinitis and asthma. Int Arch Allergy Immunol 2003;130:307–313.

92 Bryce PJ, Geha R, Oettgen HC: Desloratadine inhibits allergen-induced airway inflammation and bronchial hyperresponsiveness and alters T-cell responses in murine models of asthma. J Allergy Clin Immunol 2003;112:149–158.

93 White JP, Mills J, Eiser NM: Comparison of the effects of histamine H_1- and H_2-receptor agonists on large and small airways in normal and asthmatic subjects. Br J Dis Chest 1987;81: 155–169.

94 Field SK, Sutherland LR: Does medical antireflux therapy improve asthma in asthmatics with gastroesophageal reflux? a critical review of the literature. Chest 1998;114:275–283.

95 Gantner F, Sakai K, Tusche MW, Cruikshank WW, Center DM, Bacon KB: Histamine h4 and h2 receptors control histamine-induced interleukin-16 release from human CD8+ T cells. J Pharmacol Exp Ther 2002;303: 300–307.

96 Sirois J, Menard G, Moses AS, Bissonnette EY: Importance of histamine in the cytokine network in the lung through H_2 and H_3 receptors: stimulation of IL-10 production. J Immunol 2000;164:2964–2970.

97 Benovic J: Novel β_2-adrenergic receptor signaling pathways. J Allergy Clin Immunol 2002;110:S229–S235.

98 Thurmond RL, Gelfand EW, Dunford PJ: The role of histamine H_1 and H_4 receptors in allergic inflammation: the search for new antihistamines. Nat Rev Drug Discov 2008;7:41–53.

Cezmi A. Akdis, MD
Swiss Institute of Allergy and Asthma Research (SIAF)
Obere Strasse 22, CH–7270 Davos (Switzerland)
Tel. +41 81 410 0848, Fax +41 81 410 0840
E-Mail akdisac@siaf.unizh.ch

Blaser K (ed): T Cell Regulation in Allergy, Asthma and Atopic Skin Diseases.
Chem Immunol Allergy. Basel, Karger, 2008, vol 94, pp 83–92

T-Cell Regulation in Asthmatic Diseases

Susetta Finotto

Laboratory of Cellular and Molecular Lung Immunology, First Medical Clinic,
Mainz, Germany

Abstract

Effector and regulatory T cells (Tregs) play a fundamental role in the airways in allergic asthma. Here, the role of T cells in the immunopathogenesis of human asthma as well as in animal models of allergic airway inflammation is reviewed. Recent data have shown that Th2 and Th17 effector T cells augment experimental airway inflammation, while Tregs have an important anti-inflammatory function. The local induction of Th2 cells is critically dependent on the balance between the transcription factors T-bet and GATA-3, while Th17 and Tregs require the transcription factors ROR-γt and Foxp3, respectively. Cytokine signaling controls the development and activation of all the above T-cell subsets. For instance, local blockade of the membrane-bound interleukin (IL)-6R results in induction of lung CD4+CD25+ Foxp3+ Tregs producing TGF-β and IL-10. In humans, it has been suggested that asthmatic patients have increased Th2 but decreased Tregs, however the role of Th17 cells in allergic asthma remains to be elucidated. However, the currently available data suggest that allergic asthma is a multifaceted disease that is actively controlled by T lymphocytes. A better understanding of effector and Treg activation will most likely lead to novel treatment strategies in the near future.

Copyright © 2008 S. Karger AG, Basel

In the last decade there has been increasing interest in the scientific community in T-cell-mediated immunosuppression or regulation as a mechanism of self-tolerance and immune regulation. To date, the most studied cellular component of this regulation is the CD4+ T-regulatory cell (Treg). Although originally described in the thymus as naturally occurring Tregs, this subset of CD4+ T cells has been described also in the periphery and therefore recognized as adaptive Tregs because they participate to adaptive responses. In addition to self-tolerance and autoimmunity, adaptive Tregs play an important role in tumor immunity and allergy.

Currently there are at least six Treg subtypes, including CD4+CD25+ naturally occurring (N-Tregs), inducible naive CD4+CD25− T cells (T_R1), T_R1 memory phenotype (CD127+), T-helper type 3 (Th3), CD4−CD25+DX5+ natural killer T cells (T_RNKT), and CD4−CD25+CD8+ cytotoxic T cells (T_RCTC). The development of Tregs is controversial as to whether they occur in the thymus or peripheral lymphoid tissue. Studies have shown that N-Tregs are generated in the thymus and T_R1 cells occur in the periphery Nevertheless, Tregs are recognized not only for their function but also for their surface markers such as CD3, CD25, CD62L, CD69, CD127, GITR, ICOS, neuroplin-1 (Nrp-1), and PD-1. However, the most definitive marker is forkhead winged-helix transcription factor (Foxp3).

New Molecular Target for Allergic Asthma

In some Western countries, every third child needs medical attention by the physician because of allergic disease. Although much effort has been devoted to understand this specific disease, an asthmatic episode is still treated with non-specific drugs. Allergic diseases such as allergic asthma follow a pathological immune response to an otherwise innocuous antigen and can be life-threatening.

In spite of its chronic condition, allergic asthma is characterized by a very fast immune response to a particular antigen. Therefore, intervention strategies include avoidance of the allergen through environmental controls aiming at reducing amounts of indoor allergens which can reduce the symptoms in atopic children, but such strategies have obvious limitations. More importantly, specific immunotherapy against pollen given to children 6–12 years of age has proven successful in decreasing the risk of progression from allergic rhinitis to atopic asthma. Thus the inhibition of the progression of the disease can probably be accomplished by redirecting dendritic cell (DC)-mediated responses also from sites distal to the lung. In this regard it has recently been described that DCs present in the nose-draining lymph nodes can stir the T-cell immune responses to induce tolerance to inhaled antigen [1]. The authors suggested that the level of the enzyme indoleamine 2,3-dioxygenase (IDO) in DCs present in the nose-draining lymph nodes allows the generation of a sufficient number of Tregs to control effector T cells. By contrast, blockade of IDO breaks this tolerance and induced pathological immune responses.

Th1 T cells with their signature cytokine interferon (IFN)-γ have been seen as a protective but functionally defective cell type in the airways of the asthmatic patients, although an overall analysis of IFN-γ production in immuno- and non-immunocompetent cells in the airways is still missing in humans. However, genetic studies suggest that IFN-γ production is highly relevant for the development of allergic asthma. In fact, the genetic risk for allergic sensitization during early life is associated with attenuated postnatal maturation of Th1 T-cell functions, possibly as a result of variations in key pattern-recognition genes such as CD14 [2] and TLR2 [3], and is also likely to involve developmental deficiencies in associated immune functions [4]. The risk of wheezing between 2 and 13 years was found to be significantly higher for subjects with low 9-month IFN-γ production as compared with those producing high levels of IFN-γ. These findings suggest that characteristics of the immune system present during the first year of life modulate the likelihood of development of episodes of airway obstruction characterized by wheezing at later time points [5].

IFN-γ-mediated immunity is also important in resistance to viral infection. IFN-γ production by CD11c+ lung cells plays a protective role in allergic responses [6], as shown in studies using EBI-3 (Epstein-Barr virus-induced protein-3)-deficient mice. EBI-3 is secreted by antigen presenting cells or B cells upon viral infection. It is therefore possible that there is an inhibition of the IFN-γ release by local antigen presenting cells during viral infections. In this case, strategies inducing IFN-γ levels would be favorable in asthma associated with virus infection.

Interleukin-6 as a Bridge between Innate and Adaptive Immune Responses

Interleukin (IL)-6 is a cytokine released by DCs upon activation. IL-6 plays a central role in host defense against infections and tissue injury. It binds to its receptor which comprises the binding component α chain and the signaling chain gp130. The binding of IL-6 to the α chain of the IL-6R induces gp130 recruitment and intracellular activation of a series of kinases (Janus kinases) bridging the extracellular events with the translocation of phosphorylated STAT-1/STAT-3 (signal transducers of activated T cells) into the nucleus of the target cell. The expression of the α chain of the IL-6R is restricted to cells of hematopoietic origin, whereas gp130 is ubiquitously expressed. Thus the IL-6R α chain expression identifies the immediate and unique target of IL-6 [7]. The gp130 element is shared by other family members of IL-6 such as oncostatin M and IL-11 [8–10]. As it is likely that IL-6 production by antigen presenting cells is increased in allergic asthma, IL-6 is an interesting cytokine for modulating immune cell function in asthma. Enhanced IL-6 release would inhibit directly Treg development [7, 11] and favor the development of pathological Th2 cells in the airways of patients with allergic asthma. Analysis of the cytokine spectrum in CD4+ T cells isolated from the lung of mice with asthma-like disease showed consistently increased Th2 cytokine profile release and decreased IFN-γ a signature cytokine of the protective Th1 response. This cytokine profile is consistent with the increase of IL-6 and the increased level of the soluble form of the IL-6 receptor in the airways of asthmatic subjects both spontaneously and after allergen challenge. In addition, sIL-6R levels positively correlated with the percentage of CD4+ Th2 cells in the bronchoalveolar lavage fluid of asthmatic subjects suggesting a direct relationship between the sIL-6R and the survival of Th2 cells in asthma. In a further analysis it was found that locally antagonizing IL-6R signaling using an antibody against the gp80 unit of the IL-6 receptor leads to decreased STAT-3 but not STAT-1 phosphorylation in the lung of treated mice as compared to control-treated mice. Anti-IL-6R antibody treatment also induced apoptosis of lung CD4+ effector T cells and this effect was induced by the presence of lung CD4+CD25+ Tregs, thereby contributing to the resolution of airway hyperresponsiveness in OVA-treated mice. Thus, blockade of IL-6 signaling in vivo inhibited signaling of IL-6 in CD4+CD25+/CD4+CD25+Foxp-3+ T cells and induced Th2 cell apoptosis. Additional studies demonstrated an increased suppressive function of the CD4+CD25+ cells isolated from mice treated intranasally with anti-IL-6R antibodies as compared to OVA-sensitized and OVA-challenged and untreated mice. This immunosuppression and anti-inflammatory function was also confirmed in vivo in immunodeficient mice reconstituted with CFSE labeled target CD4+CD25− cells and CD4+CD25+ cells isolated from mice treated with anti-IL-6R antibodies.

Subsequent studies tested the effect of selective blockade of the sIL-6R. Blockade of the sIL-6R by application of a chimeric protein (gp130-Fc) into the airways during the challenge phase, led to a downregulation of the effector CD4+ T cells in this disease without altering the number of Tregs [11]. Interestingly, blockade of the soluble IL-6R (sIL-6R) led to downregulation of all three Th2 cytokines IL-4, IL-5 and IL-13 and the Th2-associated transcription factor GATA-3. Taken together, these experimental data suggest a potential role of the sIL-6R in controlling the Th2 responses in the lung of patients with allergic asthma. Moreover, the parallel increase of IFN-γ and Tregs in the airways after blockade of the membrane-bound IL-6R α chain suggests either the possible presence of Tregs producing IFN-γ or alternatively, the possible induction of Th1 cells and Tregs as some tissue rejection disease is associated with a decrease in tolerogenic Tregs and decreased IFN-γ production by Th1 cells [12]. This combined beneficial effect on the T-cell responses makes the anti-IL-6R antibodies an attractive local therapy.

Interaction of Th2 and T-Regulatory Cells

The last two decades have witnessed numerous studies on the role of the T-helper CD4+ T cells in the onset of the asthmatic response. These studies led to the concept that CD4+ helper cells producing (Th)-type 2 cytokines play a key role in allergic responses in susceptible individuals. Moreover, while blockade of the Th2 cytokines IL-4 and IL-13 are still under consideration for a possible therapy for allergic disease, the anti-IL-5 human trial has shown little therapeutic effectiveness. Another possibility to target Th2 cells in asthma consists of a more upstream approach by targeting transcription factors controlling different cytokines at once. Specifically, targeting the major transcription factor of the Th2 cells, GATA-3, could ameliorate different pathological features of this disease, such as inflammation and airway hyperresponsiveness. Interestingly, after intranasal delivery of antisense to GATA-3, a major inhibition of IL-4 but not IL-5 production was noted [13, 14]. This observation was simultaneously confirmed in promoter study analyses describing binding of GATA-3 to the IL-4 promoter [15]. In addition, to date the increase of GATA-3 in the airways of asthmatic airways was confirmed in different studies leading to the design and synthesis of different and more updated therapeutic molecules that confirmed the above findings in the murine model of asthma [16, 17].

Immunotherapy may involve multi-antigen-specific challenge of DCs or other local antigen presenting cells to induce expansion and activation of a pool of regulatory cells inhibiting the pathological expanded Th2 cells specifically in the draining lymph nodes. This concept implies the upregulation of organ-specific distribution of different Tregs. Indication in this direction has also recently been suggested in an analysis of different Treg types in different sites of the intestine and in the lung [18, 19]. This study indicated an organ-specific distribution of Tregs with a certain profile of cytokine distribution and receptors interacting with well-defined sets of effector CD4+ T cells and therefore probably regulating their cell death. Apoptosis and other forms of cell death are common mechanisms for eliminating and selecting defined cell subtypes, thus redirecting lineage differentiation. Therefore, it must be possible to use specific Tregs that target the Th2 lineage. Direct interaction between Tregs and Th2 effector cells in the lung has been recently demonstrated in the lung. In this set of experiments it was demonstrated

that lung CD4+CD25− effector cells used as target for demonstrating the suppressor activity of CD4+CD25+ high do not undergo apoptosis. However, upon coincubation with CD4CD25+ T cells, the CD4+CD25− T cell underwent apoptosis.

The impaired production of IL-10 from Tregs has been proposed as a causal mechanism of asthma. Pulmonary exposure to innocuous aeroallergens is a common event leading to inhalation tolerance. Distinct subsets of pulmonary DCs and Tregs play critical roles in mediating and maintaining such tolerance. The mechanisms underlying the breakdown of inhalation tolerance, leading to the Th2-driven inflammation in rising numbers of asthmatic patients from industrialized countries remain elusive [20]. The mechanism of tolerance appears to be modulated by a specialized subset of T cells called regulatory T cells – Tregs. The suppression of N-Tregs occurs by cell-to-cell contact, and low levels of IL-10 and moderate levels of TGF-β, but the primary mechanism involves the sequestration and activation of neighboring naive CD4+CD25− T cells to become T_R1 cells. In contrast, T_R1 cells exert their suppressive properties by copious secretion of IL-10 and TGF-β. These suppressive mechanisms occur by the inhibition of IL-2 production and the promotion of cell cycle arrest. Therefore it is of interest to analyze conditions that favor a low level of IL-2 secretion by CD4+ T cells.

Do Th17 Cells Counteract T-Regulatory Cells in Allergic Asthma?

Upon activation, T cells undergo distinct developmental pathways, attaining specialized properties and effector functions. T-helper (Th) cells are traditionally thought to differentiate into Th1 and Th2 cell subsets. Th1 cells are necessary to clear intracellular pathogens and Th2 cells are important for clearing extracellular organisms. Recently, a subset of IL-17-producing Th17 cells distinct from Th1 or Th2 cells has been described and shown to have a crucial role in the induction of autoimmune tissue injury. In contrast, CD4+ CD25+Foxp3+ Tregs inhibit autoimmunity and protect against tissue injury. Transforming growth factor-$_1$ (TGF-β_1) is a critical differentiation factor for the generation of Tregs. By contrast, IL-6 is an acute phase protein induced during inflammation that completely inhibits the generation of Foxp3+ Tregs induced by TGF-β as well as other adaptive Tregs (fig. 1). Moreover, it has been recently demonstrated that IL-21 and/or TGF-β in the presence of IL-6 can differentiate naive CD4+ T cells into pathogenic helper T cells (Th17/Th [IL-17]) that produce IL-17A, IL-17F, IL-6, and TNF-α [21, 22]. These cells express the transcription factor ROR-γt, require IL-23 for the stabilization of their phenotype and are known to counteract the naturally occurring CD4+CD25+ Tregs leaving unanswered the question whether they can also inhibit adaptive Tregs.

As local blockade of IL-6R in the airways led to increased Tregs in the airways, it is interesting to understand whether IL-6-deficient mice have increased Tregs and whether in the absence of Treg Th17 cells would be expanded. A very recent paper answered this question and elegantly showed that IL-6-deficient (IL-6−/−) mice do not develop a Th17 response although their peripheral repertoire is dominated by Foxp3+ Tregs. However, deletion of Tregs leads to the reappearance of Th17 cells in IL-6−/− mice, suggesting an additional pathway by which Th17 cells might be generated in vivo. The authors showed that an IL-2 cytokine family member, IL-21, cooperates with TGF-β to induce Th17 cells in naive IL6−/− T cells and that IL-21-receptor-deficient T cells are defective in generating a Th17 response [23]. Thus the direct interaction between Tregs and Th17 cell is still unclear and must be further investigated.

Th2 cells selectively express IL-21 in addition to the classic Th2 cytokines IL-4, IL-5, and IL-13. In contrast to these clustered Th2 cell cytokine genes, the IL-21 gene resides on a different chromosome and is not coordinately regulated by the same locus control region that directs the expression of other Th2 cytokines. In this study the authors reported that the proximal promoter of IL-21 controls its Th-cell-subset-specific expression through the action of NFATc2 and T-bet. Whereas NFATc2 directly binds to and activates transcription of the IL-21 promoter in Th2 cells, T-bet represses IL-21 transcription by inhibiting the binding of NFATc2 to the promoter in Th1 cells. These data suggest that NFATc2 induces via IL-21 the Th17, whereas T-bet inhibits the IL-17 confirming previous data demonstrating increased Th17 cells in T-bet-deficient mice [24].

In another study the authors showed that suppression of T-bet ameliorates EAE by limiting the differentiation of autoreactive Th1 cells, as well as inhibiting pathogenic Th17 cells via regulation of IL-23R [25]. To make even more complicated the understanding of Th17 and allergic asthma, a recent paper described a pathogenetic role of Th17 cells at the beginning of allergic disease during antigen sensitization, by contrast in sensitized mice IL-17 attenuates the allergic response by inhibiting DCs and chemokine synthesis [26]. Thus the role of T-bet and NFATc2 on Th17 in disease has not been completely elucidated [27].

T-Bet Deficiency: Genetic and Epigenetic Control in Allergic Asthma

Inhaled corticosteroids mediate a variety of immunological actions and are commonly used in the treatment of allergic asthma [28]. However, not all patients respond well to this treatment and some are steroid-resistant. In a recent study, Tantisira et al. [29] described a new genetic nonsynonymous variation in TBX21 that encodes for the transcription factor T-bet (T-box expressed in T cells) associated with significant improvement of the airway hyperresponsiveness in children affected by allergic asthma [30]. Noteworthy, the

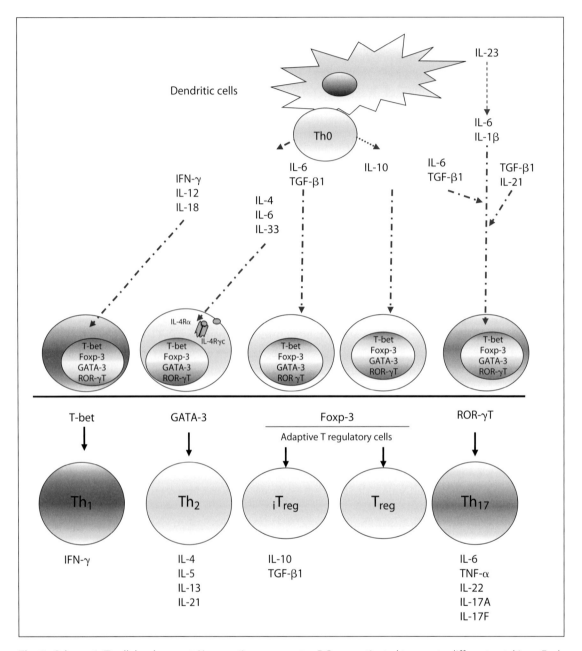

Fig. 1. Schematic T-cell development. Upon antigen encounter, DCs are activated to secrete different cytokines. Each cytokine or the combination of different cytokines can determine the cell type present in the airways of asthmatic subjects. Particularly complicated is the development of Th17 cells which can develop either upon IL-23 exposure and/or TGF-β a combined to IL-6. In the absence of IL-6, Th17 cells develop under the influence of TGF-β and IL-21. Under this latter condition, Th17 cells coexist with the Tregs.

improvement in the respiratory functions was linked to the use of inhaled corticosteroids. This variant thus could be an important marker to determine the pharmacogenetic response to the therapy of asthma with inhaled corticosteroids. It is possible thus that this mutated form of T-bet changes its binding with the corticosteroid receptor or and the binding of T-bet with other transcription factors (like NFAT) located in the proximity of T-bet on the IFN-γ promoter (fig. 2a, b).

Moreover, transcription factors play a crucial role during hematopoiesis by orchestrating lineage commitment and determining cellular fate. Although tight regulation of transcription factor expression appears to be essential, little is known about the epigenetic mechanisms involved in transcription factor gene regulation. Aberrant methylation of transcription factor genes is frequently observed in diffuse large B-cell lymphomas and might have a functional role during tumorigenesis [31]. T-bet is a transcription factor of the T-box family that regulates the expression of numerous immune system-associated genes; it directs the acquisition of the Th1-associated genetic program in differentiating CD4+ lymphocytes. Glucocorticoid-mediated (GCs) immunosuppression acts via regulation of several transcription factors, including activating protein (AP)-1, NF-κB, and NFAT/T-bet. The glucocorticoid receptor (GR) physically interacts with T-bet both in transfected cell lines and in primary splenocyte cultures with endogenous GR and T-bet (fig. 2a). This interaction also blocks GR-dependent transcription. The mechanism underlying T-bet inhibition further involves reduction of T-bet binding to DNA GCs additionally inhibit T-bet both at mRNA and protein expression levels, revealing another layer of GR action on T-bet. Finally, the functional consequence of GR/T-bet interaction is the inhibition of the transcriptional activity of T-bet on IFN-γ promoter. In view of the crucial role of T-bet in T-cell differentiation and inflammation,

GR inhibitory interaction with T-bet may be an important mechanism underlying the immunosuppressive properties of GCs [27]. It is therefore important to determine the footprint of T-cell-specific transcription factor expression and binding on the IFN-γ promoter in asthmatics, resulting in a closer classification of this disease. Allergic asthma is possibly a multifaceted disease that can be further better subclassified and therefore treated with different strategies.

Glucocorticoid Receptor and T-Cell-Specific Transcription Factors

It has been reported that human CD4+ Tregs secrete high levels of IL-10 when stimulated in the presence of dexamethasone and calcitriol (vitamin D_3). Xystrakis et al. [32] described the mechanism responsible for this, showing that vitamin D_3 induced GC expression in CD4+ T cells in patients with GC-resistant asthma. An independent observation pointed out that the transcription factor NFAT can induce CD4+ T-cell proliferation or suppression dependently from the transcription partner it chooses. In this respect it has been reported by Wu et al. [33] that NFATc can bind to Jun and Fos to induce proliferation but can repress cell proliferation after binding with Foxp-3. Moreover, it is possible that another suppression mechanism takes place without involving T regulation. In fact it has been reported that addition of vitamin D_3 induced vitamin D_3 receptor, thus repressing NFATc binding to the promoter (fig. 2c). This mechanism could be a non-specific mechanism working also for T-bet and other transcription factors, and would explain difficulties in finding differences in lineage T-cell-specific transcription in human asthma as compared to animal models. In fact, the use of transcription factor-deficient mice is useful to describe the function of a deleted gene but cannot address questions related to the genetic modulation. A back and forward proof of

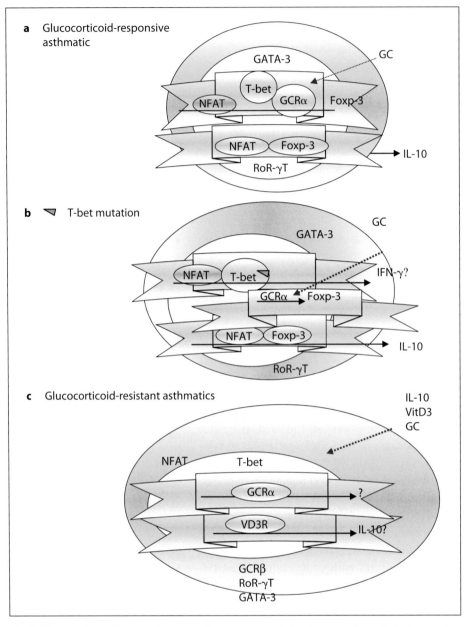

Fig. 2. Hypothetic distribution of some T-cell-specific transcription factor on the indicated promoters.
a Glucocorticoids inhibit T-bet binding to the DNA. T-bet interacts with glucocorticoid receptor (GCRα).
GCR induces Foxp-3 synthesis. Foxp-3 then binds to NFATc leading to IL-10 production. This possibility
would define the Tregs (Foxp-3+) producing IL-10 but not IFN-γ. **b** A second possibility is that mutations in T-bet do not change its concentration but inhibit GCRα binding to T-bet so that T-bet interacts
with NFATc thus driving the IFN-γ synthesis. In another genetic site NFATc can interact with Foxp-3 thus
promoting the IL-10 synthesis. **c** Asthmatics resistant to glucocorticoids can respond to glucocorticoids
when IL-10 and vitamin D₃ are added. In this case, vitamin D₃ replaces NFATc on the promoter. T-bet
analysis on these patients is unknown. GC induces Foxp-3. VD3 and Foxp-3 (?) interaction induce IL-10.
This last synthesis has not been scientifically demonstrated and thus is hypothetical.

principle between the human and experimental model is thus needed.

Conclusions

The onset of asthma might depend on both genetic and environmental components. In childhood the expression of IFN-γ is fundamental in determining the future T-cell development. In fact, defective IFN-γ early in life favors a Th2 cell development probably as a result of increased IL-6 production by DCs or mast cells and/or IL-4 production by natural killer or other cells. The increased GATA-3 expression in the lung of asthmatics points in this direction. The defect in T-bet or its genetic modification in asthmatics underlines the role of IFN-γ in this disease. The orchestration of the Th1/Th2 balance is probably mediated by the Tregs whose defect could lead to the pathological expansion of Th2 cells in allergic asthma. The genetic and posttranscriptional modification of different T-cell-specific transcription factors plays a role for their binding and reciprocal interaction on the IFN-γ, IL-10 and Foxp-3 promoters thus dictating novel directives in gene transcription that can lead to different subsets of allergic asthma.

Acknowledgment

The author thanks Markus F. Neurath and Roman Karwot for critically reading the manuscript.

References

1 Van der Marel AP, Samsom JN, Greuter M, et al: Blockade of IDO inhibits nasal tolerance induction. J Immunol 2007; 179:894–900.

2 Baldini M, Vercelli D, Martinez FD: CD14: an example of gene by environment interaction in allergic disease. Allergy 2002;57:188–192.

3 Lauener RP, Birchler T, Adamski J, et al: Expression of CD14 and Toll-like receptor 2 in farmers' and non-farmers' children. Lancet 2002;360:465–466.

4 Holt PG, Sly PD, Martinez FD, et al: Drug development strategies for asthma: in search of a new paradigm. Nat Immunol 2004;5:695–698.

5 Stern DA, Guerra S, Halonen M, et al: Low IFN-gamma production in the first year of life as a predictor of wheeze during childhood. J Allergy Clin Immunol 2007;120:835–841.

6 Hausding M, Karwot R, Scholtes P, et al: Lung CD11c + cells from mice deficient in Epstein-Barr virus-induced gene 3 (EBI-3) prevent airway hyper-responsiveness in experimental asthma. Eur J Immunol 2007;37:1663–1677.

7 Doganci A, Neurath MF, Finotto S: The IL-6R alpha chain controls lung CD4+CD25+ Treg development and function during allergic airway inflammation in vivo. J Clin Invest 2005;115: 313–325.

8 Diveu C, Venereau E, Froger J, et al: Molecular and functional characterization of a soluble form of oncostatin M/interleukin-31 shared receptor. J Biol Chem 2006;281:36673–36682.

9 Stross C, Radtke S, Clahsen T, et al: Oncostatin M receptor-mediated signal transduction is negatively regulated by SOCS3 through a receptor tyrosine-independent mechanism. J Biol Chem 2006;281:8458–8468.

10 Doganci A, Eigenbrod T, Krug N, et al: Pathological role of IL-6 in the experimental allergic bronchial asthma in mice. Clin Rev Allergy Immunol 2005; 28:257–270.

11 Finotto S, Eigenbrod T, Karwot R, et al: Local blockade of IL-6R signaling induces lung CD4+ T cell apoptosis in a murine model of asthma via regulatory T cells. Int Immunol 2007;19:685–693.

12 Sawitzki B, Kingsley CI, Oliveira V, et al: IFN-gamma production by alloantigen-reactive regulatory T cells is important for their regulatory function in vivo. J Exp Med 2005;201:1925–1935.

13 Finotto S, Glimcher L: T cell directives for transcriptional regulation in asthma. Springer Semin Immunopathol 2004;25:281–294.

14 Finotto S, De Sanctis GT, Lehr HA, et al: Treatment of allergic airway inflammation and hyperresponsiveness by antisense-induced local blockade of GATA-3 expression. J Exp Med 2001; 193:1247–1260.

15 Lee GR, Fields PE, Flavell RA: Regulation of IL-4 gene expression by distal regulatory elements and GATA-3 at the chromatin level. Immunity 2001; 14:447–459.

16 Sel S, Wegmann M, Dicke T, et al: Effective prevention and therapy of experimental allergic asthma using a GATA-3-specific DNAzyme. J Allergy Clin Immunol 2008;121:910–916.

17 Erpenbeck, VJ, Hagenberg A, Krentel H, et al: Regulation of GATA-3, c-maf and T-bet mRNA expression in bronchoalveolar lavage cells and bronchial biopsies after segmental allergen challenge. Int Arch Allergy Immunol 2006;139:306–316.

18 Maynard CL, Harrington LE, Janowski KM, et al: Regulatory T cells expressing interleukin 10 develop from Foxp3(+) and Foxp3(−) precursor cells in the absence of interleukin 10. Nat Immunol 2007;8:931–941.

19 Doganci A*, Karwot R*, Maxeiner JH* (*contributed equally), et al: IL-2R beta Chain Signaling Controls Immunosuppressive CD4+ T Cells in the Draining Lymph Nodes and Lung during Allergic Airway Inflammation in vivo . J Immunol 2008, in press.

20 Kohl J, Wills-Karp M: Complement regulates inhalation tolerance at the dendritic cell/T cell interface. Mol Immunol 2007;44:44–56.

21 Zhou L, Ivanov II, Spolski R, et al: IL-6 programs T(H)-17 cell differentiation by promoting sequential engagement of the IL-21 and IL-23 pathways. Nat Immunol 2007;8:967–974.

22 Bettelli E, Carrier Y, Gao W, et al: Reciprocal developmental pathways for the generation of pathogenic effector TH17 and regulatory T cells. Nature 2006;441:235–238.

23 Fujiwara M, Hirose K, Kagami S, et al: T-bet inhibits both TH2 cell-mediated eosinophil recruitment and TH17 cell-mediated neutrophil recruitment into the airways. J Allergy Clin Immunol 2007;119:662–670.

24 Mehta DS, Wurster AL, Weinmann AS, et al: NFATc2 and T-bet contribute to T-helper-cell-subset-specific regulation of IL-21 expression. Proc Natl Acad Sci USA 2005;102:2016–2021.

25 Gocke AR, Cravens PD, Ben LH, et al: T-bet regulates the fate of Th1 and Th17 lymphocytes in autoimmunity. J Immunol 2007;178:1341–1348.

26 Schnyder-Candrian S, Togbe D, Couillin I, et al: Interleukin-17 is a negative regulator of established allergic asthma. J Exp Med 2006;203:715–725.

27 Karwot R, Maxeiner JH, Schmitt S, et al: Protective role of nuclear factor of activated T cells 2 in CD8+ long-lived memory T cells in an allergy model. J Allergy Clin Immunol 2008;121:992–999.

28 Liberman AC, Refojo D, Druker J, et al: The activated glucocorticoid receptor inhibits the transcription factor T-bet by direct protein-protein interaction. FASEB J 2007;21:1177–1188.

29 Tantisira KG, Hwang ES, Raby BA, et al: TBX21: a functional variant predicts improvement in asthma with the use of inhaled corticosteroids. Proc Natl Acad Sci USA 2004;28;101:18099–18104.

30 Finotto S, Neurath MF, Glickman JN, et al: Development of spontaneous airway changes consistent with human asthma in mice lacking T-bet. Science 2002;295:336–338.

31 Ivascu C, Wasserkort R, Lesche R, et al: DNA methylation profiling of transcription factor genes in normal lymphocyte development and lymphomas. Int J Biochem Cell Biol 2007;39:1523–1538.

32 Xystrakis E, Kusumakar S, Boswell S, et al: Reversing the defective induction of IL-10-secreting regulatory T cells in glucocorticoid-resistant asthma patients. J Clin Invest 2006;116:146–155.

33 Wu Y, Borde M, Heissmeyer V, et al: FOXP3 controls regulatory T cell function through cooperation with NFAT. Cell 2006;126:375–387.

Susetta Finotto, PhD
Laboratory of Cellular and Molecular Lung Immunology
First Medical Clinic, University of Mainz, Room 2:110
Obere Zahlbacher Strasse 63, DE–55131 Mainz (Germany)
Tel. +49 06131 393 3367, Fax +49 06131 393 7140, E-Mail finotto@mail.uni-mainz.de

Blaser K (ed): T Cell Regulation in Allergy, Asthma and Atopic Skin Diseases.
Chem Immunol Allergy. Basel, Karger, 2008, vol 94, pp 93–100

Immune Regulatory Mechanisms in Allergic Contact Dermatitis and Contact Sensitization

Andrea Cavani

Laboratory of Immunology, Istituto Dermopatico dell'Immacolata, IDI-IRCCS, Rome, Italy

Abstract

Contact allergy is a very common disease due to an uncontrolled immune response to chemically reactive small molecular compounds penetrating the skin. The reaction is mostly sustained by specific CD8+ and CD4+ type 1 T lymphocytes, which are recruited at the site of chemical challenge thanks to the expression of specific homing and chemokine receptors. Evidence exists that specialized subsets of T lymphocytes with regulatory function modulate immune responses to haptens by preventing the occurrence of the hypersensitivity reactions in non-allergic individuals exposed to the sensitizer. In addition, the magnitude of the inflammatory reaction in allergic individuals is also tightly regulated not only by the exhaustion/apoptosis of effector T cells at the site of chemical challenge, but also by the intervention of T-regulatory cells. Most of the T-regulatory cells involved in this process belong to the CD4+ subset, such as the IL-10-producing T cells, namely T-regulatory cells 1, and the CD4+CD25+ T-regulatory lymphocytes. In addition, reports suggest the existence of Treg activity among the CD8+ subpopulation. The currently held view is that contact allergies are the consequences of the exaggerated expansion of specific CD8+ effector T lymphocytes due to an impaired development of efficient regulatory T cells.

Copyright © 2008 S. Karger AG, Basel

The skin immune system is challenged everyday with an enormous variety of potential sensitizers which penetrate the stratum corneum and trigger the two major populations of dendritic cells (DCs) residing in the skin, the epidermal Langerhans' cells (LCs) and the dermal DCs [1]. In spite of the repeated exposure to sensitizers, only a minority of individuals will become sensitized during their life, and develop an eczematous reaction at any further exposure to the relevant chemical. Even in this case, the severity of the allergic reaction typically fluctuates in time, and, despite the persistence of the sensitizer in the skin, the inflammatory reaction which follows each hapten application is usually self-limited.

In aggregate, these observations have suggested that both sensitization to chemicals and expression of contact allergy are highly regulated events [2]. Indeed, the control of immune responses to environmental chemicals is a high priority task for the skin immune system. This task is orchestrated by skin DCs and is guaranteed by multiple mechanisms, including apoptosis of effector T lymphocytes due to activation-induced cell death, T-cell anergy, release of anti-inflammatory cytokines, and induction of specialized subsets of T lymphocytes with regulatory function (Treg) [3].

Treg cells not only prevent undesired immune responses to innocuous antigens applied onto the skin, but also promote the termination of ongoing immune responses by dampening T-cell activation at the site of hapten application in allergic subjects. Animal models of contact allergy helped to identify the mechanisms underlying immune reactions to skin sensitizers, and have been of great value in the disclosure of several subsets of Treg involved in the allergic disease.

Contact Hypersensitivity and Animal Model of Tolerance to Haptens

Much of the knowledge on the immune mechanisms of contact sensitization has derived from the mouse model of contact hypersensitivity (CHS). CHS is induced by applying the hapten onto the shaved abdomen of the mouse (sensitization phase) and is quantified by measuring the ear thickness 24 and 48 h after the ear challenge with the relevant substance (afferent phase). In this scenario, when the site of hapten sensitization is irradiated with UV-B prior to the sensitization phase, a specific immune tolerance, instead of hypersensitivity, is induced [4]. Similarly, a long-lasting tolerance to chemicals can be generated by oral feeding the animal with the sensitizer prior to skin exposure [5]. Both UV-B and oral tolerance are antigen-specific and not the consequence of a generalized immune suppression, since the animals maintain the responsiveness to unrelated antigens.

Mechanisms involved in UV-B-induced immune tolerance are multiple. UV-B irradiation strongly affects the viability and function of skin DCs [6]. UV-B irradiation causes DNA damage and apoptosis in LCs, while promoting their migration to regional lymph nodes [7]. This effect is paralleled by the reduced expression of MHC and costimulatory molecules, which results in an impaired antigen presenting capability. The release of IL-10 by resident skin cells, keratinocytes and mast cells, also contributes to dampen DC function [8, 9]. Thus, upon UV-B irradiation, immature or partially mature DCs, with poor capacity to prime for effector type 1 cells, reach the secondary lymphoid organs and may expand specific Treg populations [10]. Interestingly, UV-B-induced tolerance can be reverted by toll-like receptor agonists, such as imiquimod, which strongly activate skin DCs, and by IL-12 and IL-18 [11–13]. In particular, IL-12, other than affecting the capacity of DCs to prime for Th1/Tc1 lymphocytes, enhances DNA repair in skin LCs and reduces the immunosuppressive activity of *cis*-urocanic acid, which accumulates in the epidermis upon UV-B irradiation.

The role of Treg in UV-B-induced immunosuppression is demonstrated by the evidence that tolerance can be transferred into naive recipients with CD4+CD25+ Treg expressing high levels of CTLA-4 isolated from UV-B-irradiated syngenic animals [14]. Importantly, although tolerogenic CD4+CD25+ Treg cells can prevent induction of CH in naive animals, they fail to impede CH expression in already sensitized mice [15]. This finding depends on the homing properties of UV-B-induced Treg, which express the L-selectin for lymph node homing but not the cutaneous lymphocyte-associated antigen (CLA). Although canonic CD4+CD25+ Treg cells do not release IL-10, Tregs induced by UV-B release abundant IL-10, that, together with host-derived IL-10, contributes significantly to the immunosuppressive mechanisms.

Although conceptually similar to UV-B-induced tolerance, oral tolerance is orchestrated by the gut immune system. More than one subset of Treg cells have been found to have a role in the induction of oral tolerance: TGF-β-secreting T cells, named Th3 lymphocytes, IL-10/TGF-β-releasing T-regulatory type 1 (Tr1) lymphocytes, and, more recently, CD4+CD25+ Treg lymphocytes [16, 17]. Oral tolerance is prevented by depletion of CD4+ T lymphocytes in animals, and fails in mice lacking MHC class II molecules, in which the development of mature CD4+ T lymphocytes is greatly impaired [18]. Oral tolerance requires intact recirculation through the mesenteric lymph nodes and is impaired in CCR7-deficient mice. CCR7 is a critical chemokine receptor that targets DCs residing in the lamina propria to the mesenteric lymph nodes, where Treg cells are expanded [19]. An attractive hypothesis suggests that the expansion of Treg lymphocytes in oral tolerance depends on the presence of NK-T cells, a distinct lymphoid lineage expressing an invariant T-cell receptor (TCR) recognizing glycolipids in a CD1d-restricted fashion [20]. Indeed, oral tolerance to nickel fails in NK-T cell-deficient Ja18−/− mice. Consensus exists that cytokines, either IL-10 or TGF-β, are also involved in the mechanism of suppression. These findings demonstrated that the immune system possesses the intrinsic capacity to regulate responses to chemicals, and that tolerance can be boosted by specific experimental procedures.

T-Regulatory Cells in Contact Allergy

The hypothesis of the existence of T cells that specifically regulate immune responses towards self and allogeneic antigens has been formulated since 25 years ago [21]. However, phenotype and functional properties of Treg have been at least partially defined only in the last few years.

In the mid-1990s, the group of Roncarolo [23] and that of Sagakuchi [22] provided evidence of the existence of two distinct Treg subsets: the Tr1 cells and the CD4+CD25+ Treg lymphocytes [22, 23]. Tr1 cells are defined by the prominent IL-10 production in the absence of significant IFN-γ and/or IL-4 release. IL-5 and TGF-β can be coexpressed by certain Tr1 subpopulations. Tr1 cells suppress T-cell activation in vitro and prevent the development of experimental induced colitis when transferred in susceptible mice. Their immunomodulatory activity mostly depends on the release of IL-10, which is secreted abundantly upon TCR engagement. In vitro, IL-10 strongly inhibits the antigen presenting func-

tion of macrophages and DCs, as well as the differentiation and IL-12 release of monocyte-derived DCs [24]. IL-10 is a critical regulatory cytokine in immune responses to chemicals [25]. Administration of IL-10 prior to hapten challenge strongly impairs the effector phase of CHS in mouse. Conversely, mouse with targeted disruption of the IL-10 gene displayed enhanced cutaneous immune responses to chemicals.

The suppressive function of IL-10 in human contact allergy received only indirect confirmation. Nickel-specific Tr1 cells are enriched in peripheral blood of non-allergic individuals exposed to the metal [24]. Although to a lower frequency, nickel-specific Tr1 cells can also be isolated from ongoing contact allergy reactions to nickel in allergic individuals, indicating that they can be recruited at the site of hapten exposure where they can modulate the magnitude of the immune response. This hypothesis is confirmed by experiments showing that blocking IL-10 augments the magnitude and the duration of murine CHS reaction to haptens [25]. Of note, chemokine receptor analysis of Tr1 cells revealed the capacity of these cells to respond to a vast array of chemokines. They share with Th2 cells the expression of CCR8 and the responsiveness to CCL1 [26]. Notably, mRNA of CCL1, produced by maturing DCs, activated T cells and keratinocytes, appears late during CHS reactions, further suggesting the role of Tr1 cells in the termination of the immune response to haptens. The release of IL-10 is not limited to the Tr1 cell subset. In mouse, Th2 cells can secrete significant levels of this cytokine and could thus contribute to the regulation of CHS. In humans, both Th1 and Th2 can equally release IL-10 and their effective role in contact allergy may depend upon the ratio between these two cytokines [27]. Interestingly, effector/memory Th1 cells rendered anergic by inadequate activation have been found to release abundant IL-10 and to possess suppressive function. Although Tr1 cells have been characterized phenotypically and functionally, their origin is still debated.

Their phenotypes resemble that of a highly differentiated memory T cells with markers which belongs to both the Th1 and Th2 differentiation, such as CD30, Lag, and the IL-12Rβ2 chain [24]. However, they do not express the transcription factor Foxp3, which characterize a distinct subset of T cells with regulatory function, the CD4+CD25+ Treg lymphocytes.

CD4+CD25+ Treg lymphocytes were first identified in mouse as a distinct T-cell lineage that originates in the thymus after being positively selected by thymic epithelial cells [22]. The major function of naturally occurring CD25+ Treg is to maintain the peripheral tolerance to self antigens. Both in mouse and human the CD4+CD25+ T population represents about 5–10% of circulating CD4+ cells. Among these, Treg appears included in the CD25^{high} fraction. Additional markers for CD25+ Treg are the expression of L-selectin, which allows their recirculation through the high endothelial venules in the secondary lymphoid organs, the high levels of CTLA-4, and of the glucocorticoid-induced TNF-receptor family-related gene (GITR). CTLA-4 is a CD28 analog that binds to CD80 and CD86 and negatively regulates cell activation and IL-2 release. As mentioned, CD25+ Treg express high levels of the transcriptional factor Foxp3, which encodes a transcriptional factor named Scurfin, and has been positively correlated with both development and functions of CD25+ T cells [28]. In mouse, Foxp3 confers regulatory activity when transduced into T cells. The role of Foxp3 in the development of CD25+ Treg has been confirmed in humans: mutation of Foxp3 induces an autoimmune lymphoproliferative disorder termed subjects, termed immune dysregulation polyendocrinopathy enteropathy-X-linked (IPEX) syndrome characterized by neonatal autoimmune type 1 diabetes polyendocrinopathy, autoimmune hemolytic anemia, autoimmune enteropathy and eczema [29]. Clinical manifestations are the consequence of the uncontrolled T-cell proliferation and activation. CD25+ Treg

display a broad usage of TCR Vβ repertoire and have the characteristics of highly differentiated T cells, indicating repetitive antigen encounter and stimulation. Indeed, the CD25+ Treg population renovates continuously in vivo, but they behave as anergic cells in vitro. This characteristic limits considerably our capacity to determine their antigen specificity. Beside naturally occurring CD25+ Treg, which are responsible for the control of autoreactive T cells that escaped from thymic selection, adaptive CD25+ Treg with a broad antigenic specificity have been demonstrated to expand following encounters with exogenous antigens. Adaptive Treg regulate immune responses to environmental antigens, including bacteria, fungi, protozoa, allergenic molecules and chemicals. In human beings, it has been shown that CD4+CD25+ T cells from peripheral blood of healthy, non-allergic individuals can regulate in vitro the activation of both naive and memory nickel-specific T-cell responses [30]. In comparison, CD4+CD25+ T cells isolated from nickel-allergic subjects showed a limited or absent capacity to suppress CD4+ and CD8+ nickel-specific T cells. CD4+CD25+ Treg have a pattern of migratory behavior similar to that of Tr1 cells, both expressing high levels of CCR4 and CCR8, receptors for CCL17 and CCL1, indicating that common mechanisms govern the recruitment of distinct Treg subsets in peripheral tissues. In addition, a conspicuous fraction of circulating CD4+CD25+ T cells coexpress the CLA, and can be recruited at the site of skin inflammation. According to this hypothesis, despite the negativity of the epicutaneous reaction to nickel sulfate in non-allergic individuals, the site of nickel application displays a conspicuous T-cell infiltrate, which included CD25+ T cells. Once isolated, these infiltrating CD4+CD25+ T cells strongly suppressed in vitro nickel-specific T-cell responses. Thus, CD4+CD25+ Treg could block T-cell activation to chemicals through multiple pathways: at the site of chemical entry, by dampening the activation of chemical-reactive effector CD8+ T cells, and in secondary lymphoid organs, where they can prevent the expansion of memory-effector CD4+ and CD8+ T cells. In addition, CD4+CD25+ Treg have shown to inhibit expression of CXCR3 chemokine receptor by differentiating T cells, the latter being crucial for T-cell homing into the skin during chemical hypersensitivity reactions. Finally, it has been shown that CD25+ Treg facilitate the induction of IL-10 producing Tr1-like cells with an anergic/suppressive phenotype. Thus, development of exaggerated immune responses to chemicals may be the consequence of a defective or altered expansion and/or functional suppressive activity of specific Treg.

In vitro analyses have determined that CD25+ Treg are anergic cells, unless high IL-2 is provided. CD25+-mediated suppression requires activation via TCR, although, once activated, CD25+ Treg can regulate antigen-unrelated CD4+ and CD8+ T lymphocytes [31]. In vitro, mechanism of suppression appears independent of IL-10 and TGF-β release, and requires cell-to-cell contact between the Treg and the suppressed T cell. However, several in vivo models underlined the role of either IL-10 or TGF-β in their regulatory activity. A putative role of CTLA-4 in the suppressive activity of Treg has been suggested by many reports. In this model, CTLA-4 exposed on CD25+ Treg may interact with CD80 and CD86 expressed by activated T cells generating an outside-in signal that blocks IL-2 production. In addition, CTLA-4 interaction with CD80 and CD86 expressed by DCs induce indoleamine 2,3-dyoxigenase, an enzyme involved in tryptophan catabolism. T-cell suppression may be the consequence of tryptophan deprivation. It has been shown that CD25+ Treg express high levels of perforin and granzyme A. Induction of apoptosis of target T cells has been proposed as an additional mechanism of suppression of CD25+ Treg. The presence to redundant mechanisms involved in immunoregulation indicates that

tolerance to self as well as exogenous antigens is a critical task for the immune system. Although most of the T-regulatory cell populations described so far belong to the CD4+ T-cell subset, reports showing similar roles performed by CD8+ T cells are increasing. For example, IL-10/IL-4-releasing CD8+ T cells have been reported to expand following repeated skin administration of subimmunogenic amount of chemicals and mediate the development of low zone tolerance. CD8+ T cells with a pattern of cytokine expression similar to Tr1 lymphocytes have been shown to expand upon stimulation of naive CD8+ T cells with plasmacytoid DCs [32]. In addition, a subpopulation of CD8+CD28− T-suppressor cells have been described to regulate immune responses by inducing the expression of the inhibitory molecules immunoglobulin-like transcript (ILT)-3 and ILT-4 on DCs, which thus acquire tolerogenic activity. Their role in the regulation of chemical hypersensitivity has not been investigated, so far.

Dendritic Cells as Orchestrators of Skin Immune Responses to Haptens

Skin penetration of potential allergens can induce a protective immune response or a specific tolerance, being the latter by far the most common choice of the immune system (fig. 1). Only circumstances leading to the failure of the tolerogenic mechanisms result in uncontrolled hypersensitivity response to chemicals. DCs are the major orchestrators of the dynamic interaction between innate and adaptive immune responses, being capable of inducing either protective immune responses or unresponsiveness, depending on their functional properties [3]. LCs and dermal DCs reside in the skin in an immature status. Upon antigen encounter, skin DCs migrate to regional lymph nodes to present the antigenic determinants to naive T cells. Their maturation and mobilization is

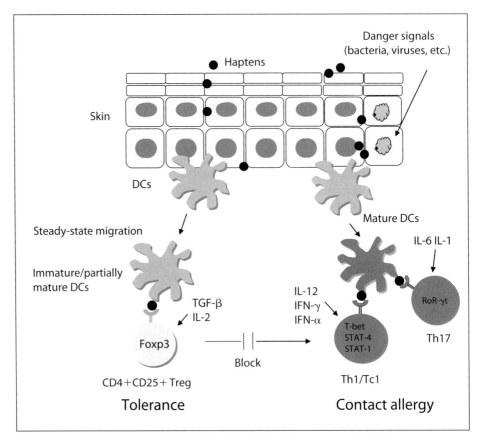

Fig. 1. Skin DCs orchestrate T-cell immune responses to haptens. Hapten penetrating the skin can induce specific tolerance or contact allergy. Tolerance is mostly mediated by the expansion of T-regulatory cells (CD4+CD25+ Treg, in particular) which are expanded in the presence of TGF-β by immature or partially mature DCs emigrating from the skin in steady-state conditions. Effector Th1 and Tc1, as well as Th17 cells, are the major protagonists of contact allergy and results from hapten presentation by fully mature DCs which emigrated from the skin in the presence of danger signals. Development of contact allergy results from the balance between regulatory and effector T cells.

strongly promoted by the exposure to a wide spectrum of agents generally named 'danger signals', which includes UVB radiation, bacteria, CpG tracts, viral products, necrotic cells, and extracellular matrix components, such as heparan sulfate. The cytokines IL-1, TNF-α and IL-18 are strongly involved in the regulation of DC migration. The relevance of the two major DC populations in contact allergy has remained undefined for years. Recently, this issue has been

evaluated in knockin mice where the human diphtheria toxin receptor was induced under the control of the CD207 gene [33]. In these mice, CHS was not affected or even augmented by intraperitoneal injection of diphtheria toxin, which determined selective apoptosis of LCs but not dermal DCs. This finding indicates that dermal DCs are the principal protagonists, whereas LCs are dispensable for the development of cutaneous responses to haptens.

DC maturation state and the cytokine milieu at the site of antigen encounter strongly affect the future properties of memory-effector T cells. Several reports demonstrated that TGF-β has a critical role in the induction of CD25+ Treg in vitro [34]. Indeed, in the presence of TGF-β, naive CD4+CD25− T cells stimulated with immature DCs or with anti-CD3 Ab rapidly convert to a CD4+CD25+ phenotype. TGF-β-induced Treg express Foxp3 and display potent immunosuppressive activity both in vitro and in vivo. In addition, modulation of DC maturation by cholera toxin, 1,25-dihydroxyvitamin D_3, mycophenolate mofetil, anti-TNF Ab, dietary anti-oxidants (α-tocopherol and vitamin C) have been reported to increase the yield of Treg upon in vitro stimulation of CD4+CD25− T cells [35]. Whether distinct DC lineages (e.g. skin LCs vs. dermal DCs) are selectively involved in the generation of Treg is a still debated attractive hypothesis.

Differentiation of effector Th1 and Tc1 cells, responsible for contact allergy, is promoted by IL-12, which is released by fully mature, but not immature DCs. In contrast, antigen presentation by immature or partially mature DCs, which have migrated in secondary lymphoid organs in steady-state conditions, often leads unresponsiveness and/or immune tolerance, due to the expansion of T cells with regulatory functions. Thus, the concomitance of danger signals during chemical exposure, such as bacteria, viruses, or the irritant property of the chemical itself, may be a relevant cofactor in breaking tolerance to skin-applied chemicals. This hypothesis is supported by recent findings demonstrating that T lymphocytes activated by toll-like receptor-triggered DCs are resistant to suppression mediated by CD25+ Treg.

Conclusions

The control of immune responses to environmental antigens penetrating the skin is a high priority task for the skin immune system. Although induction of tolerance to small molecular compounds is the most frequent consequence of chemical entry through the skin, allergy may develop in certain circumstances. A high concentration of the chemical, irritancy capacity of the sensitizer, the presence of bacteria that strongly stimulate skin DCs by triggering TLRs, are considered important factors involved in the development of uncontrolled immune responses to skin sensitizers, characterized by the expansion of effector CD8+ T cells. Studies aimed to characterize the mechanisms involved in the regulation of contact allergy have advanced since the definition of several Treg populations that dampen the activation of hapten-specific T-cell responses both in mouse and in humans. Several promising studies have shown that in vitro activation of naive T cells in the presence of cytokines (TGF-β) or drugs that modulate the antigen presenting capacity of DCs can expand antigen-specific Treg cells. These findings are critical steps for the development of innovative therapeutic approaches in contact allergy.

References

1 Kupper TS, Fuhlbrigge RC: Immune surveillance in the skin: mechanisms and clinical consequences. Nat Rev Immunol 2004;4:211–222.
2 Cavani A, Ottaviani C, Nasorri F, Sebastiani S, Girolomoni G: Immunoregulation of hapten- and drug-induced immune reactions. Curr Opin Allergy Clin Immunol 2003;3:243–247.

3 Steinman RM, Hawiger D, Nussenzweig MC: Tolerogenic dendritic cells. Annu Rev Immunol 2003;21:685–711.
4 Schwarz T: 25 years of UV-induced immunosuppression mediated by T cells – from disregarded T-suppressor cells to highly respected regulatory T cells. Photochem Photobiol 2008;84: 10–18.

5 Dubois B, Goubier A, Joubert G, Kaiserlian D: Oral tolerance and regulation of mucosal immunity. Cell Mol Life Sci 2005;62:1322–1332.
6 Tang A, Udey MC: Doses of ultraviolet radiation that modulate accessory cell activity and ICAM-1 expression are ultimately cytotoxic for murine epidermal Langerhans' cells. J Invest Dermatol 1992;99:71S–73S.

7   Schwarz A, Grabbe S, Riemann H, Aragane Y, Simon M, Manon S, Andrade S, Luger TA, Zlotnik A, Schwarz T: In vivo effects of interleukin-10 on contact hypersensitivity and delayed-type hypersensitivity reactions. J Invest Dermatol 1994;103:211–216.

8   Alard P, Kurimoto I, Niizeki H, Doherty JM, Streilein JW: Hapten-specific tolerance induced by acute, low-dose ultraviolet B radiation of skin requires mast cell degranulation. Eur J Immunol 2001;31:1736–1746.

9   Ghoreishi M, Dutz JP: Tolerance induction by transcutaneous immunization through ultraviolet-irradiated skin is transferable through CD4+CD25+ T regulatory cells and is dependent on host-derived IL-10. J Immunol 2006; 176:2635–2644.

10 Mahnke K, Qian Y, Knop J, Enk AH: Induction of CD4+/CD25+ regulatory T cells by targeting of antigens to immature dendritic cells. Blood 2003; 101:4862–4869.

11 Thatcher TH, Luzina I, Fishelevich R, Tomai MA, Miller RL, Gaspari AA: Topical imiquimod treatment prevents UV light-induced loss of contact hypersensitivity and immune tolerance. J Invest Dermatol 2006;126:821–831.

12 Schwarz A, Maeda A, Kernebeck K, van Steeg H, Beissert S, Schwarz T: Prevention of UV radiation-induced immunosuppression by IL-12 is dependent on DNA repair. J Exp Med 2005; 201:173–179.

13 Schwarz A, Maeda A, Stander S, van Steeg H, Schwarz T: IL-18 reduces ultraviolet radiation-induced DNA damage and thereby affects photoimmunosuppression. J Immunol 2006;176:2896–2901.

14 Schwarz A, Beissert S, Grosse-Heitmeyer K, Gunzer M, Bluestone JA, Grabbe S, Schwarz T: Evidence for functional relevance of CTLA-4 in ultraviolet-radiation-induced tolerance. J Immunol 2000;165:1824–1831.

15 Schwarz A, Maeda A, Schwarz T: Alteration of the migratory behavior of UV-induced regulatory T cells by tissue-specific dendritic cells. J Immunol 2007;178:877–886.

16 Faria AM, Weiner HL: Oral tolerance. Immunol Rev 2005;206:232–259.

17 Dubois B, Chapat L, Goubier A, Papiernik M, Nicolas J-F, Kaiserlian D: Innate CD4+CD25+ regulatory T cells are required for oral tolerance and inhibition of CD8+ T cells mediating skin inflammation. Blood 2003;102: 3295–3301.

18 Desvignes C, Bour H, Nicolas J-F, Kaiserlian D: Lack of oral tolerance but oral priming for contact sensitivity to dinitrofluorobenzene in major histocompatibility complex class II-deficient mice and in CD4+ T-cell-depleted mice. Eur J Immunol 1996;26:1756–1761.

19 Worbs T, Bode U, Yan S, Hoffmann MW, Hintzen G, Bernhardt G, Forster R, Pabst O: Oral tolerance originates in the intestinal immune system and relies on antigen carriage by dendritic cells. J Exp Med 2006;203:519–527.

20 Roelofs-Haarhuis K, Wu X, Gleichmann E: Oral tolerance to nickel requires CD4+ invariant NKT cells for the infectious spread of tolerance and the induction of specific regulatory T cells. J Immunol 2004;173:1043–1050.

21 Germain RN: A rose by any other name: from suppressor T cells to Tregs, approbation to unbridled enthusiasm. Immunology 2008;123:20–27.

22 Sakaguchi S: Naturally arising Foxp3-expressing CD25+CD4+ regulatory T cells in immunological tolerance to self and non-self. Nat Immunol 2005;6:345–352.

23 Groux H, O'Garra A, Bigler M, Rouleau M, Antonenko S, de Vries JE, Roncarolo MG: A CD4+ T-cell subset inhibits antigen-specific T-cell responses and prevents colitis. Nature 1997;389:737–742.

24 Cavani A, Nasorri F, Prezzi C, Sebastiani S, Albanesi C, Girolomoni G: Human CD4+ T lymphocytes with remarkable regulatory functions on dendritic cells and nickel-specific Th1 immune responses. J Invest Dermatol 2000;114:295–302.

25 Berg DJ, Leach MW, Kuhn R, Rajewsky K, Muller W, Davidson NJ, Rennick D: Interleukin-10 but not interleukin-4 is a natural suppressant of cutaneous inflammatory responses. J Exp Med 1995;182:99–108.

26 Sebastiani S, Allavena P, Albanesi C, Nasorri F, Bianchi G, Traidl C, Sozzani S, Girolomoni G, Cavani A: Chemokine receptor expression and function in CD4+ T lymphocytes with regulatory activity. J Immunol 2001;166:996–1002.

27 O'Garra A, Vieria P: TH1 cells control themselves by producing interleukin-10. Nat Rev Immunol 2007;7:425–428.

28 Zheng Y, Rudensky AY: Foxp3 in control of the regulatory T cell lineage. Nat Immunol 2007;8:457–462.

29 Le Bras S, Geha RS: IPEX and the role of Foxp3 in the development and function of human Tregs. J Clin Invest 2006;116: 1473–1475.

30 Cavani A, Nasorri F, Ottaviani C, Sebastiani S, De Pita O, Girolomoni G: Human CD25+ regulatory T cells maintain immune tolerance to nickel in healthy, nonallergic individuals. J Immunol 2003;171:5760–5768.

31 Shevach EM, DiPaolo RA, Andersson J, Zhao DM, Stephens GL, Thornton AM: The lifestyle of naturally occurring CD4+CD25+ Foxp3+ regulatory T cells. Immunol Rev 2006;212:60–73.

32 Seidel-Guyenot W, Perschon S, Dechant N, Alt R, Knop J, Steinbrink K: Low zone tolerance induced by systemic application of allergens inhibits Tc1-mediated skin inflammation. J Allergy Clin Immunol 2006;117:1170–1177.

33 Kaplan DH, Jenison MC, Saeland S, Shlomchik WD, Shlomchil MJ: Epidermal Langerhnas cells-deficient mice develop enhanced contact hypersensitivity. Immunity 2005;23:611–620.

34 Chen W, Jin W, Hardegen N, Lei KJ, Li L, Marinos N, McGrady G, Wahl SM: Conversion of peripheral CD4+CD25− naive T cells to CD4+CD25+ regulatory T cells by TGF-β induction of transcription factor Foxp3. J Exp Med 2003;198:1875–1886.

35 Adorini L, Penna G, Giarratana N, Uskokovic M: Tolerogenic dendritic cells induced by vitamin D receptor ligands enhance regulatory T cells inhibiting allograft rejection and autoimmune diseases. J Cell Biochem 2003;88:227–233.

Andrea Cavani
Laboratory of Immunology, IDI-IRCCS
via dei Monti di Creta 104, IT–00167 Rome (Italy)
Tel. +39 06 6646 4776, Fax +39 06 6646 4705
E-Mail cavani@idi.it

Blaser K (ed): T Cell Regulation in Allergy, Asthma and Atopic Skin Diseases.
Chem Immunol Allergy. Basel, Karger, 2008, vol 94, pp 101–111

Regulatory Role of T Lymphocytes in Atopic Dermatitis

Thomas Werfel · Miriam Wittmann

Department of Immunodermatology and Allergy Research,
Hannover Medical School, Hannover, Germany

Abstract

Eczema does not occur in the absence of T cells. Here we provide an overview on the regulatory impact which T cells have on the establishment and maintenance of atopic dermatitis. Particularly, we outline the role of different T-helper cell subsets (i.e. Th-1, Th-2, T-regulatory and Th-17 cells) and their distinct influence on the cutaneous inflammatory reaction at different stages of the disease. Eczema is characterized by epidermal inflammation and thus T-cell/keratinocyte interactions are of particular relevance in this condition. Alterations in innate and adaptive immunity involving T cells result in susceptibility to skin infections and in hyperreactivity reactions to environmental stimuli which in turn determine the course and severity of atopic dermatitis.

Copyright © 2008 S. Karger AG, Basel

T cells play a central role in the development and regulation of immune responses. They stimulate and suppress through mechanisms that involve direct and indirect actions on several cells, including antigen-presenting cells (APC) and tissue resident cells. Such faculty allows them to regulate the specificity, the magnitude and duration of most immune responses. Atopic dermatitis is associated with a characteristic distribution and morphology of skin lesions. The disease manifestation occurs in the upper layers of the skin. T cells enter this site from dermal vessels, interact with numerous cell types and extracellular matrix, pass the basement membrane and continue to migrate into the epidermis which is composed to over 90% of keratinocytes. Many of the T cells entering the skin seem to be allergen-specific. However, next to disease-eliciting allergens, numerous other trigger factors have been identified for atopic dermatitis over the last decades such as irritative substances and infectious microorganisms like *Staphylococcus aureus* [1, 2].

A still not completely elucidated complex interaction between susceptibility genes encoding skin barrier molecules and molecules of the inflammatory response, host environments, infectious agents and specific immunologic responses is involved in the pathophysiology of atopic dermatitis. It is probable that different patients with atopic dermatitis have a distinctive arrangement of alterations that could make them candidates for different therapies. Thus, successful management of atopic dermatitis requires a multisided approach and still is a challenge for the clinician.

Regulation of Atopic Dermatitis by T Cells – Clinical Aspects

T Lymphocytes Dominate the Cellular Infiltrate in Atopic Dermatitis

In animal models of atopic dermatitis, the eczematous rash does not occur in the absence of T cells. In humans there is a marked infiltration of mononuclear cells in eczematous skin which is predominated by CD4-positive T-helper cells. Many intralesional T cells show signs of activation and can further be distinguished by CD45RO, a marker of T-memory cells suggesting a previous contact with antigen or allergen and by the cutaneous lymphocyte-associated antigen (CLA). CLA defines the subset of skin-homing T cells that binds to E-selectin, an adhesion molecule expressed by endothelial cells in inflamed tissues during the first step of leukocyte extravasation. Most circulating CLA+ T cells display a Th-2 phenotype and are allergen-specific. Nonetheless, IL-12 appears to be a key cytokine in the regulation of CLA: it induces the rapid upregulation of $\alpha(1,3)$-fucosyltransferase VII which is involved in the expression of CLA molecules in CLA-negative Th-2 cells [3].

T cells remain present in the skin throughout the chronic phase, although in smaller numbers than seen in acute atopic dermatitis.

Clinically unaffected skin in atopic dermatitis differs from normal skin: the underlying barrier defect associated in more than 30% with filaggrin loss of function mutations first published in 2006 [4] leads to dry skin associated with a greater irritant skin response than in normal healthy skin. Microscopic studies revealed a sparse perivascular T cell infiltrate in unaffected atopic dermatitis skin that is not seen in normal healthy skin.

Role of Adaptive Immune Responses in Atopic Dermatitis Involving IgE Responses

In about 80% of adult patients with atopic dermatitis, the disease is associated with increased serum IgE levels, sensitization against aeroallergens and food allergens, and/or concomitant food allergy, allergic rhinitis and asthma. The role of T cells in eczema is indirectly indicated by the observation that primary T-cell immunodeficiency disorders frequently are associated with high serum IgE levels and eczematous skin lesions, which clear after successful bone marrow transplantation.

Th-2 cytokines are critically involved in IgE regulation and recent epidemiological data suggest a contributory role for IgE-mediated immunologic processes for the onset and course of atopic dermatitis, especially in patients with severe disease [5]. However, 20% of adult patients with eczematous skin lesions clinically and histologically indistinguishable from atopic dermatitis do not show increased serum IgE levels or specific IgE against inhalant or food allergens. Of note, this subtype of atopic dermatitis, which often manifests later in life (>20 years), still shows a marked T-cell infiltrate in the skin.

Aeroallergen-Specific T Cells Are Well-Known Initiators and Perpetuators of Eczematous Responses in Atopic Dermatitis

Pruritus and skin lesions can develop after intranasal or bronchial inhalation challenge with aeroallergens in patients with atopic dermatitis. Epicutaneous application of aeroallergens (house dust mites, weeds, animal dander and moulds) on uninvolved skin elicits eczematous reactions in a subgroup of patients with atopic dermatitis. The so-called atopy patch test has been used in recent years as a model to study T-cell-based allergen-induced pathomechanisms in the skin [6]. Importantly, the isolation of aeroallergen-specific T cells from the skin first succeeded from atopy patch test lesions. Similar techniques were applied later to isolate aeroallergen-specific T cells also from spontaneous lesional skin.

Specific immunotherapy (SIT) with aeroallergens directly addresses adaptive mechanism in hypersensitivity reactions. A meta-analysis of SIT studies revealed positive effects of subcutaneous immunotherapy on atopic dermatitis [7]. In the largest cohort study published so far, subcutaneous SIT with mite allergens was effective in moderate to severe atopic dermatitis [8]. In contrast, sublingual immunotherapy with mite allergens which has been studied in children with atopic dermatitis had beneficial effects on patients with mild eczema only [9]. As outlined below, SIT has been shown to involve regulatory mechanisms in T lymphocytes in other allergic diseases. The clinical efficacy of SIT in atopic dermatitis is therefore probably related to T-cell-mediated reactions.

Food-Specific T Cells Are Involved in Allergic Responses in Atopic Dermatitis in Children and Adults

Food allergy and atopic dermatitis may occur in the same patient. Besides typical immediate types of allergic reactions (i.e. non-eczematous reactions) which are observed in patients suffering from atopic dermatitis, foods can provoke flare-ups as shown in placebo-controlled food challenge studies [10]. The serum level of specific IgE can be predictive for the outcome of oral provocation tests in children with immediate reactions to foods. Specific T cells have been shown to be involved in the late eczematous response to food: higher proliferative responses to the allergen and specific T-cell clones can be generated from patients reacting with food-induced eczema. In addition, milk-induced eczema has also been reported to be associated in a higher rate of CLA+ lymphocytes upon in vitro stimulation with casein [10].

A murine model of food-induced atopic dermatitis confirmed the important role of specific T cells in eczema: here, C3H/HeJ mice were orally sensitized to cow's milk or peanut and thereafter exposed to the allergen. An eczematous eruption developed in approximately one third of mice after low-grade exposure to milk or peanut proteins. Histological examination of lesional skin revealed spongiosis and a cellular infiltrate mainly consisting of CD4+ lymphocytes.

Patients sensitized to pollen allergens often develop an IgE response to cross-reactive food allergens. Birch pollen-related food may lead to an exacerbation of eczema in a subpopulation of patients with atopic dermatitis and sensitization to birch pollen allergens. A birch pollen-specific T-cell response could be detected in lesional skin of these responding patients. T-cell cross-reactivity between Bet v 1 and related food allergens can occur independently of IgE cross-reactivity in vitro and in vivo. This has been shown in atopic dermatitis patients who developed late eczematous skin reactions to cooked food which was shown to elicit T-cell but not IgE-mediated responses [11].

T Cells May Contribute to the Defects in Innate Immune Response in Atopic Dermatitis

Most patients with atopic dermatitis are colonized with *S. aureus* and experience exacerbation of their skin disease after infection with this organism [2]. In patients with *S. aureus* infection, treatment with anti-staphylococcal substances can result in the reduction of skin disease. Binding of *S. aureus* to the epidermis is enhanced by atopic skin inflammation. This is supported by clinical studies demonstrating that treatment with topical corticosteroids or tacrolimus reduces *S. aureus* counts in atopic dermatitis.

Recent evidence suggests that a deficiency of the antimicrobial peptides dermcidin, cathelicidin LL-37, human β-defensin (HBD)-2 and HBD-3 contribute to the susceptibility of atopic patients to skin infections [12]. Defensins are broad-spectrum antibiotics that kill bacterial and fungal pathogens. LL-37 has been shown to display antiviral actions additional to its bactericidal and fungicidal properties. The Th-2-derived cytokines IL-4 and IL-13 have been shown to downregulate the expression of β-defensins and of LL-37 in atopic skin [2, 13]. Th-2 cells are prominent in the skin in acute eczema. Taken together, these findings may explain why atopic dermatitis patients are more prone to *S. aureus* colonization and to severe eczema herpeticatum.

Table 1. Interaction between T cells and MHC class II + cells by staphylococcal superantigens leads to numerous inflammatory reactions in the skin

---

Induction of T-cell proliferation
Induction of IL-2, IL-5, IL13, and IFN-γ production by T cells
Induction of CLA expression on T cells
Reversal of suppressive activity of Tregs
Release of cytokines (e.g. IL-12) from MHC class II + APC
Release of proinflammatory cytokines from activated
  MHC class II + keratinocytes

Microorganism Activate T Lymphocytes and Bystander Cells in the Skin in Atopic Dermatitis

An important strategy by which *S. aureus* exacerbates atopic dermatitis is by secreting exotoxins. Some of them function as superantigens, which stimulate activation of T cells and major histocompatibility (MHC) class II + APC or keratinocytes, which express MHC class II upon activation. Many effects on T lymphocytes and other cells are elicited by superantigens (table 1).

In addition, some patients with atopic dermatitis produce specific IgE antibodies directed against staphylococcal superantigens, which correlate with skin disease severity. Superantigens have been shown to penetrate into the dermis and higher doses have been shown to induce cutaneous inflammation when applied onto the skin. Low doses which do not induce visible clinical inflammation are still able to amplify aeroallergen-induced patch test responses [14].

Are T Cells Involved in Specific Immune Responses to Autoantigens in Atopic Dermatitis?

Autoimmune phenomena to human self-proteins may also contribute to the pathophysiology of atopic dermatitis. IgE against autoantigens such as Hom S1-4 have been shown to stimulate type 1 hypersensitivity reactions which in turn may contribute to the clinical cutaneous reactions in atopic dermatitis [15]. Autoallergens induce the proliferation of CLA + autoreactive T cells derived

from the blood and it is possible to generate autoreactive T-cell clones from the skin of sensitized atopic dermatitis patients [Heratizadeh et al., submitted]. Interestingly, autoallergen-specific IgE has been found early in infancy in atopic dermatitis [16]. Cross-reactivity between inhalant allergens and autoantigens may lead to autoimmunity: For example, IgE against manganese superoxide dismutase (MnSOD) from the skin-colonizing yeast *Malassezia sympodialis* cross-reacts with human MnSOD. Patients with atopic dermatitis sensitized to human MnSOD have been shown to be concurrently sensitized against the *M. sympodialis* MnSOD [17].

Cellular and Molecular Interactions of T Cells in Atopic Dermatitis

T Cells Communicate with Vascular Cells, Proinflammatory Cytokines and Chemokines in the Skin

Early events initiating atopic skin inflammation involve mechanical trauma and skin barrier disruption which may occur after scratching. This results in the rapid upregulation of proinflammatory mediators such as IL-1α, IL-1β, TNF-α and GM-CSF [18] and certainly to the release of damage-associated molecular patterns (DAMPs). Of note, some molecules also relevant to skin inflammation are classified in a subgroup of DAMPs, the 'alarmins' which are endogenous molecules that signal tissue and cell damage (e.g. HMGB1, heat-shock proteins, cathelicidins, defensins, galectins, IL-1α). These proinflammatory cytokines and molecules activate the vascular endothelium to upregulate adhesion molecules which subsequently allow infiltrating cell to transmigrate into the tissue. T-cell-endothelial cell interactions are thus crucial in acute atopic dermatitis.

Once inflammatory cells have infiltrated into the tissue, they respond to chemotactic gradients established by cytokines and chemokines, which origin from sites of injury or infection. These molecules play a central role in defining the nature of the inflammatory infiltrate in atopic dermatitis.

Do CD8+ T Cells Play a Role in Atopic Dermatitis?

Patients suffering from atopic dermatitis have increased levels of activated circulating T cells. A study revealing increased telomerase activity and shortened telomere length in atopic dermatitis indicates that T cells are chronically stimulated and have an increased cellular turnover in vivo. The high number of circulating T cells results from increased numbers of CD4+ cells whereas the absolute number of CD8+ lymphocytes is normal or even decreased in peripheral blood. However, acute psychological stress has been shown to lead to rapid, significant higher increases in the number of circulating CD8+ T lymphocytes in atopic dermatitis patients compared to healthy controls. This points to the fact that there are larger pools of this cell type close to the circulation which can be translocated into the blood during psychological stress.

The role of CD8+ T cells in atopic skin inflammation is still not well defined. It has been shown that CLA+CD8+ T cells isolated from the circulation are as potent as CLA+CD4+ T cells in the induction of IgE and enhancement of eosinophil survival. This suggests that these cells have more than bystander functions in atopic dermatitis. Recent data from a mouse model indicate that allergen-primed CD8+ T cells are required for the development of atopic dermatitis-like lesions in vivo [19].

T Cells Secrete Different Cytokines at Different Stages in Atopic Dermatitis

The onset of acute atopic dermatitis is strongly associated with the production of Th-2 cytokines, notably IL-4, IL-13 and IL-31, levels of which are significantly higher in atopic dermatitis individuals compared with control subjects [2].

Th-1 and Th-2 cytokines may contribute to the pathogenesis of local skin inflammation in atopic dermatitis with the relative contribution of each cytokine dependent on the duration of the skin lesion. In previous studies, the majority of allergen-specific T cells derived from skin lesions that had been provoked by epicutaneous application of inhalant allergens were found to produce predominantly Th-2 cytokines such as IL-4, IL-13, or IL-5. This was first considered to be a specific feature reflecting immune dysregulation in atopic dermatitis. Subsequently it was shown that the expression of IFN-γ rather than of IL-4 predominates in spontaneous or older patch test lesions. Importantly, treatment of patients that resulted in improvement of their lesions could be correlated with downregulation of IFN-γ expression, but not of IL-4, in the skin. In addition, allergen-specific T-cell clones from spontaneous atopic dermatitis lesions differed from allergen-specific T cells isolated from inhalant allergen patch test lesions by virtue of their capacity to produce IFN-γ [2].

T Lymphocytes Regulate the Cutaneous Cytokine Milieu in Atopic Dermatitis

In patients with atopic dermatitis, activated T cells with skin-homing properties, which express high levels of IFN-γ, may predominantly undergo apoptosis in the circulation, skewing the immune response to surviving Th-2 cells as a mechanism for Th-2 predominance in the circulation and in acute lesions [1]. Moreover, patients with atopic dermatitis have a genetic background of a general systemic Th-2 polarization which contributes to the higher number of circulating T cells capable of producing Th-2 cytokines.

IL-4 which is a strong inducer of a type 2 cytokine milieu itself is produced by 'early' skin-infiltrating T cells but it may also be released from mast cells, basophils or eosinophils during the acute eczematous skin reaction. Of note, the high frequency of IL-4-producing T cells in the skin is not necessarily associated with atopy since mRNA for IL-4 and T cells expressing IL-4 are found in nickel-induced patch test reactions as well.

Acute lesions show reduced expression of IL-12, a key cytokine of Th-1 polarization which was shown on the mRNA level by in situ hybridization in acute skin lesions. The reason for the relative lack in the expression of IL-12 is not completely understood yet. Skin-infiltrating CD40L+ T cells may contribute to the relative inability of IL-12 upregulation in acute eczema leading to a refractory state of constitutive APC via an intracellular ERK-dependent signaling pathway [20].

A number of factors may be involved in the switch from Th-2 towards Th-1 cytokines in older lesions. The polarization of T cells along the Th-1 lineage, resulting in IFN-γ production, is supported by IL-12, IL-23, IL-27 and by IL-18 [21]. IL-12 subunits have been found to be expressed by professional APC and by human keratinocytes. However, it is not clear whether keratinocytes are a relevant source of bioactive IL-12.

IL-23 has recently been shown to be produced by dendritic cells and by human cultured keratinocytes in healthy skin and in psoriasis – its role in atopic dermatitis has to be defined [22]. Interaction of keratinocytes with activated T cells via CD40-CD40L may enhance IL-23 production and subsequently the IFN-γ production by memory T cells [23].

IL-18 is another proinflammatory cytokine which can support Th-1 responses [24]. Keratinocytes functionally respond to IL-18 with upregulation of MHC I, reinforcement of the IFN-γ-induced MHC class II expression and production of the Th-1 attracting chemokine CXCL10 [25]. This supports the notion that IL-18 is involved in the pathogenesis of local Th-1 responses in chronic inflammatory skin diseases.

Th-2 Cytokines Have Numerous Effects on Cutaneous Cells in Atopic Dermatitis
In acute eczema, IL-4 and IL-13 induce a variety of local responses such as the induction of the adhesion molecules on endothelial cells, of chemokines or of Fc receptors on eosinophils [1]. Recent findings point to direct effects of IL-4 and

IL-13 on keratinocytes, two Th-2 cytokines which function via the same receptor in this cell type [26]. IL-13 or IL-4-stimulated keratinocytes attract CCR4+CD4+ Th-2 cells via CCL22 [27]. Moreover, IL-13 induces the expression of MMP-9 in keratinocytes [28] which may play a crucial role in atopic skin inflammation by facilitating the migration of leukocytes into the epidermis.

As mentioned above, a subgroup of patients with atopic dermatitis has a filaggrin loss-of-function mutation Recently, it was shown that filaggrin expression is reduced in atopic dermatitis even in the absence of any mutation [29]. Keratinocytes differentiated in the presence of IL-4 and IL-13 exhibited significantly reduced filaggrin gene expression and neutralization of IL-4 and IL-13 improves skin barrier integrity [30]. This indicates that Th-2 lymphocytes directly contribute to the skin barrier defect in atopic dermatitis.

A new 'Th-2'-associated cytokine is IL-31 which has been shown to be highly expressed in acute eczema (i.e. both in acute atopic and in acute allergy contact dermatitis) [31]. IL-31 is produced by T cells that express CLA and localize to the skin [32]. IL-31 appears to be a link between skin-infiltrating T cells and pruritus as has been shown in a mouse model [33]. In humans, IL-31 is significantly overexpressed in itching skin inflammation [34]. Staphylococcal superantigens induce IL-31 expression in atopic individuals. These data suggest that IL-31 may be an itch-causing mediator derived from skin-infiltrating T cells.

In chronic lichenified atopic dermatitis skin lesions, fewer IL-4 and IL-13 mRNA-expressing cells are present, but greater numbers of IL-5, GM-CSF, IL-12, and IFN-γ mRNA-expressing cells are detected. The rise in IL-5 expression during the transition from acute to chronic atopic dermatitis likely plays a role in the prolongation of eosinophil survival and function. Some of the other cytokines mentioned above support the function of macrophages and promote the Th-1-type inflammation more characteristic of chronic atopic dermatitis [35].

Do Th-17 Lymphocytes Contribute to Eczema in Atopic Dermatitis?

The range of identified effector CD4 T-cell lineages has expanded with description of Th-17 cells, which produce effector cytokines, including IL-17 (or IL-17A), IL-17F, and IL-6, and are antagonized by products of the Th-1 and Th-2 lineages. TGF-β, supported by IL-6, is necessary for initiation of Th-17 differentiation. In contrast, IL-23 signaling is not required for Th-17 commitment but instead appears to be important for amplifying and stabilizing the Th-17 phenotype.

Th-17 cells appear to be involved in protection against bacterial pathogens. In addition, Th-17 cells may also be crucial in the pathogenesis of various chronic inflammatory diseases that were formerly categorized as Th-1-mediated disorders. Whereas IL-17 may play an important role in the pathogenesis of psoriasis and contact hypersensitivity, its role in atopic dermatitis is still unclear [36]. In skin biopsy specimens recovered from acute and chronic skin lesions from patients with atopic dermatitis, IL-17 was preferentially associated with acute lesions [37].

Epicutaneous immunization with ovalbumin, which causes allergic skin inflammation with many characteristics of the skin lesions of atopic dermatitis in a mouse model was found to drive IL-17 expression in the skin. Epicutaneous, but not intraperitoneal immunization of mice with ovalbumin drove the generation of IL-17-producing T cells in draining lymph nodes and spleen and increased serum IL-17 levels. Dendritic cells trafficking from skin to lymph nodes expressed more IL-23 and induced more IL-17 secretion by naive T cells. This was inhibited by neutralizing IL-23 and by intradermal injection of anti-TGF-β neutralizing antibody in vivo. These data suggest that initial cutaneous exposure to protein antigens might selectively induce the production of IL-17 [38].

Role of Regulatory T Cells in Atopic Dermatitis

Regulatory T cells (Tregs) control the activation of autoreactive and T effector cells and are crucial for the maintenance of peripheral tolerance to self antigens. Two major groups of Tregs have been defined: natural CD4+CD25+ Tregs and adaptive Tregs, the latter being characterized by the secretion of high levels of IL-10 in combination with or without TGF-β [39]. Mutations in FoxP3, a nuclear factor expressed in natural Tregs, and a subpopulation of adaptive Tregs result in immune dysregulation polyendocrinopathy enteropathy X-linked syndrome characterized by hyper-IgE, food allergy, and eczema [40], which points to a possible role of Tregs in atopic dermatitis.

Increased numbers of peripheral blood CD4+CD25+ T cells and an overexpression of FoxP3 have been found in the blood of patients with atopic dermatitis compared to psoriasis and healthy controls [41]. Staphylococcal enterotoxin B inhibits natural Tregs in vitro [41]. Superantigens have been shown to upregulate glucocorticoid-induced TNF receptor-related protein ligand on monocytes resulting in the proliferation of natural Tregs and abrogation of their immunosuppressive activity via a cell-cell contact interaction [42].

In the skin, adaptive regulatory T lymphocytes cells but no FoxP3+ natural Tregs were detectable in atopic dermatitis in series of biopsies from 8 patients [43]. This finding was not confirmed in a study focusing on lupus erythematodes. Here, skin biopsies from patients with atopic dermatitis were used as controls and the numbers of natural Tregs were not decreased [44]. In a further recent study with 5 patients, the numbers of FoxP3+ natural Tregs were even higher in atopic dermatitis compared to healthy controls. Of note, the number of natural Tregs did not change significantly after medium dose UVA-1 radiation in that study [45].

As outlined above, SIT, which has been shown to involve adaptive and natural Tregs in respiratory allergy and insect venom allergy [46], appears to work in atopic dermatitis as well. During SIT the levels of the tolerogenic cytokine IL-10 increased in the sera of the patients with atopic dermatitis in an open study [47]. Unfortunately, no further studies are available so far on the effect of SIT on T-regulatory lymphocytes in atopic dermatitis.

T Cells Interact with Keratinocytes in Atopic Dermatitis

There is growing evidence to consider keratinocytes as active contributors to the inflammatory response in atopic dermatitis [23]. Keratinocytes play a role as immunologic sentinels in the skin as a barrier organ. As such they are equipped with receptors sensing pathogens (toll-like receptors) and danger such as tissue damage (receptors for DAMPs). They are recognized for their capacity to produce chemoattractants for leukocytes and antimicrobial peptides in response to invading microbes. Thus, this epidermal cell population plays an important role in the skin innate immunity.

Keratinocytes secrete a unique profile of chemokines and cytokines after exposure to proinflammatory cytokines. Keratinocyte-derived thymic stromal lymphopoietin (TSLP) may be of particular importance in atopic dermatitis: This protein is undetectable in normal skin or non-lesional skin in patients with atopic dermatitis, but is highly expressed in acute and chronic atopic dermatitis lesions [18]. TSLP instructs human dendritic cells to create a Th-2-permissive microenvironment by inducing the expression of OX40L which triggers the differentiation of inflammatory Th-2 cells [48].

Keratinocytes stimulated with proinflammatory cytokines have been identified as an important cellular source of chemokines which attract T cells of different subtypes [23]: CXCR3 ligands such as CXCL10 preferentially attract Th-1 cells. CCL22 and CCL17 preferentially attract Th-2 cells by binding to CCR4 [27]. CCL2 is effective on both Th-1 and Th-2 subsets. Moreover, CCL27, which is constitutively expressed by keratinocytes, binds to CCR10 expressed on most skin-homing lymphocytes.

Keratinocytes are also important cellular sources of cytokines such as the T-cell growth factor IL-15 in the skin. IL-15 has been implicated in the pathogenesis of different skin diseases by virtue of its action on the maintenance of T cells – possibly also intraepithelial T cells.

In turn, keratinocytes respond both to Th-1 and to Th-2 cytokines from T cells. Among them, IFN-γ is one of the most potent keratinocyte-activating factors. It induces surface molecules (e.g. ICAM-1, MHC class I and II, CD40, Fas), chemokines (e.g. CCL2, CCL3, CCL4, CCL5, CCL18, CCL22, CXCL10) and cytokines (e.g. IL-1, IL-6, IL-18, TGF-β) in keratinocytes. Many other molecules such as matrix metalloproteinases, growth factors, enzymes, transcription factors/pathway molecules are also upregulated [18, 23].

It has been shown that IFN-γ induces Fas on keratinocytes which renders them susceptible to apoptosis induction by infiltrating FasL+ T cells. This has been interpreted as an important event in eczema, mainly in atopic dermatitis. There is further evidence that cleavage of E-cadherin and sustained desmosomal cadherin contacts between keratinocytes that are undergoing apoptosis result in spongioform morphology in the epidermis as a hallmark of eczematous lesions. Suppression of keratinocyte activation and apoptosis thus remains a potential target for the treatment of atopic dermatitis [2].

Both CXCR3+CD4+ and CCR4+CD4+ T cells migrate in response to IFN-γ-treated human primary keratinocytes. Of note, IFN-γ also induces CCL22 production in human keratinocytes. Many IFN-γ-inducible molecules are reinforced by IL-4 or IL-13 in human keratinocytes such as CD54, CCL2, CCL5 and CXCL10 [27].

With regard to surface molecule expression of keratinocytes and their role in immunoregulation, a recent study by Loser et al. [49] showed that the member of the TNF superfamily, RANKL, is expressed on keratinocytes of inflamed human and mouse skin. In a murine system, RANKL overexpression in keratinocytes resulted in functional alterations of epidermal dendritic cells and systemic increases of regulatory CD4+CD25+ T cells. Thus, epidermal RANKL expression can change dendritic cell functions to maintain the number of peripheral CD4+CD25+ Tregs. The role of RANKL in the immunoregulation of atopic inflammation in humans remains to be elucidated.

Concluding Remarks

A complex interplay between skin-infiltrating T lymphocytes and constitutive cells or other infiltrating cells of the skin leads to up- or down-regulation of inflammatory reactions and polarization of cytokine pattern in the skin into the Th-2 or Th-1 direction in atopic dermatitis. T lymphocytes are the major cell population among the cell populations infiltrating the skin and probably have the key role in the regulation of the pathologic skin reaction. They therefore are the major target cells of therapeutical approaches both with traditional anti-inflammatory substances and with newer approaches addressing Tregs in a more direct way.

References

1 Leung DY, Boguniewicz M, Howell MD, Nomura I, Hamid QA: New insights into atopic dermatitis. J Clin Invest 2004;113:651–657.

2 Akdis CA, Akdis M, Bieber T, Bindslev-Jensen C, Boguniewicz M, Eigenmann P, Hamid Q, Kapp A, Leung DY, Lipozencic J, Luger TA, Muraro A, Novak N, Platts-Mills TA, Rosenwasser L, Scheynius A, Simons FE, Spergel J, Turjanmaa K, Wahn U, Weidinger S, Werfel T, Zuberbier T: Diagnosis and treatment of atopic dermatitis in children and adults: European Academy of Allergology and Clinical Immunology/American Academy of Allergy, Asthma and Immunology/PRACTALL Consensus Report. Allergy 2006;61:969–987.

3 Biedermann T, Lametschwandtner G, Tangemann K, Kund J, Hinteregger S, Carballido-Perrig N, Rot A, Schwarzler C, Carballido JM: IL-12 instructs skin homing of human Th2 cells. J Immunol 2006;177:3763–3770.

4 Palmer CN, Irvine AD, Terron-Kwiatkowski A, Zhao Y, Liao H, Lee SP, Goudie DR, Sandilands A, Campbell LE, Smith FJ, O'Regan GM, Watson RM, Cecil JE, Bale SJ, Compton JG, DiGiovanna JJ, Fleckman P, Lewis-Jones S, Arseculeratne G, Sergeant A, Munro CS, El Houate B, McElreavey K, Halkjaer LB, Bisgaard H, Mukhopadhyay S, McLean WH: Common loss-of-function variants of the epidermal barrier protein filaggrin are a major predisposing factor for atopic dermatitis. Nat Genet 2006;38:441–446.

5 Williams H, Flohr C: How epidemiology has challenged three prevailing concepts about atopic dermatitis. J Allergy Clin Immunol 2006;118:209–213.

6 Turjanmaa K, Darsow U, Niggemann B, Rance F, Vanto T, Werfel T: EAACI/GA2LEN position paper: present status of the atopy patch test. Allergy 2006;61:1377–1384.

7 Bussmann C, Bockenhoff A, Henke H, Werfel T, Novak N: Does allergen-specific immunotherapy represent a therapeutic option for patients with atopic dermatitis? J Allergy Clin Immunol 2006;118:1292–1298.

8 Werfel T, Breuer K, Rueff F, Przybilla B, Worm M, Grewe M, Ruzicka T, Brehler R, Wolf H, Schnitker J, Kapp A: Usefulness of specific immunotherapy in patients with atopic dermatitis and allergic sensitization to house dust mites: a multicentre, randomized, dose-response study. Allergy 2006;61:202–205.

9 Pajno GB, Caminiti L, Vita D, Barberio G, Salzano G, Lombardo F, Canonica GW, Passalacqua G: Sublingual immunotherapy in mite-sensitized children with atopic dermatitis: a randomized, double-blind, placebo-controlled study. J Allergy Clin Immunol 2007;120:164–170.

10 Werfel T, Breuer K: Role of food allergy in atopic dermatitis. Curr Opin Allergy Clin Immunol 2004;4:379–385.

11 Bohle B, Zwolfer B, Heratizadeh A, Jahn-Schmid B, Antonia YD, Alter M, Keller W, Zuidmeer L, van Ree R, Werfel T, Ebner C: Cooking birch pollen-related food: divergent consequences for IgE- and T cell-mediated reactivity in vitro and in vivo. J Allergy Clin Immunol 2006;118:242–249.

12 McGirt LY, Beck LA: Innate immune defects in atopic dermatitis. J Allergy Clin Immunol 2006;118:202–208.

13 Howell MD, Boguniewicz M, Pastore S, Novak N, Bieber T, Girolomoni G, Leung DY: Mechanism of HBD-3 deficiency in atopic dermatitis. Clin Immunol 2006;121:332–338.

14 Langer K, Breuer K, Kapp A, Werfel T: *Staphylococcus aureus*-derived enterotoxins enhance house dust mite-induced patch test reactions in atopic dermatitis. Exp Dermatol 2007;16:124–129.

15 Mittermann I, Aichberger KJ, Bunder R, Mothes N, Renz H, Valenta R: Autoimmunity and atopic dermatitis. Curr Opin Allergy Clin Immunol 2004;4:367–371.

16 Mothes N, Niggemann B, Jenneck C, Hagemann T, Weidinger S, Bieber T, Valenta R, Novak N: The cradle of IgE autoreactivity in atopic eczema lies in early infancy. J Allergy Clin Immunol 2005;116:706–709.

17 Schmid-Grendelmeier P, Fluckiger S, Disch R, Trautmann A, Wuthrich B, Blaser K, Scheynius A, Crameri R: IgE-mediated and T cell-mediated autoimmunity against manganese superoxide dismutase in atopic dermatitis. J Allergy Clin Immunol 2005;115:1068–1075.

18 Homey B, Steinhoff M, Ruzicka T, Leung DY: Cytokines and chemokines orchestrate atopic skin inflammation. J Allergy Clin Immunol 2006;118: 178–189.

19 Hennino A, Vocanson M, Toussaint Y, Rodet K, Benetiere J, Schmitt AM, Aries MF, Berard F, Rozieres A, Nicolas JF: Skin-infiltrating CD8+ T cells initiate atopic dermatitis lesions. J Immunol 2007;178:5571–5577.

20 Wittmann M, Alter M, Stunkel T, Kapp A, Werfel T: Cell-to-cell contact between activated CD4+ T lymphocytes and unprimed monocytes interferes with a TH1 response. J Allergy Clin Immunol 2004;114:965–973.

21 Hunter CA: New IL-12-family members: IL-23 and IL-27, cytokines with divergent functions. Nat Rev Immunol 2005;5:521–531.

22 Piskin G, Sylva-Steenland RM, Bos JD, Teunissen MB: In vitro and in situ expression of IL-23 by keratinocytes in healthy skin and psoriasis lesions: enhanced expression in psoriatic skin. J Immunol 2006;176:1908–1915.

23 Wittmann M, Werfel T: Interaction of keratinocytes with infiltrating lymphocytes in allergic eczematous skin diseases. Curr Opin Allergy Clin Immunol 2006;6:329–334.

24 Dinarello CA: Interleukin-18 and the pathogenesis of inflammatory diseases. Semin Nephrol 2007;27:98–114.

25 Wittmann M, Purwar R, Hartmann C, Gutzmer R, Werfel T: Human keratinocytes respond to interleukin-18: implication for the course of chronic inflammatory skin diseases. J Invest Dermatol 2005;124:1225–1233.

26 Purwar R, Werfel T, Wittmann M: Regulation of IL-13 receptors in human keratinocytes. J Invest Dermatol 2007;127:1271–1274.

27 Purwar R, Werfel T, Wittmann M: IL-13-stimulated human keratinocytes preferentially attract CD4+CCR4+ T cells: possible role in atopic dermatitis. J Invest Dermatol 2006;126:1043–1051.

28 Purwar R, Kraus M, Werfel T, Wittmann M: Modulation of keratinocyte-derived MMP-9 by IL-13: a possible role for the pathogenesis of epidermal inflammation. J Invest Dermatol 2008;128: 59–66.

29 Howell MD: The role of human β defensins and cathelicidins in atopic dermatitis. Curr Opin Allergy Clin Immunol 2007;7:413–417.

30 Howell MD, Kim BE, Gao P, Grant AV, Boguniewicz M, Debenedetto A, Schneider L, Beck LA, Barnes KC, Leung DY: Cytokine modulation of atopic dermatitis filaggrin skin expression. J Allergy Clin Immunol 2007; 120:150–155.

31 Neis MM, Peters B, Dreuw A, Wenzel J, Bieber T, Mauch C, Krieg T, Stanzel S, Heinrich PC, Merk HF, Bosio A, Baron JM, Hermanns HM: Enhanced expression levels of IL-31 correlate with IL-4 and IL-13 in atopic and allergic contact dermatitis. J Allergy Clin Immunol 2006;118:930–937.

32 Bilsborough J, Leung DY, Maurer M, Howell M, Boguniewicz M, Yao L, Storey H, LeCiel C, Harder B, Gross JA: IL-31 is associated with cutaneous lymphocyte antigen-positive skin homing T cells in patients with atopic dermatitis. J Allergy Clin Immunol 2006; 117:418–425.

33 Takaoka A, Arai I, Sugimoto M, Honma Y, Futaki N, Nakamura A, Nakaike S: Involvement of IL-31 on scratching behavior in NC/Nga mice with atopic-like dermatitis. Exp Dermatol 2006;15:161–167.

34 Sonkoly E, Muller A, Lauerma AI, Pivarcsi A, Soto H, Kemeny L, Alenius H, Dieu-Nosjean MC, Meller S, Rieker J, Steinhoff M, Hoffmann TK, Ruzicka T, Zlotnik A, Homey B: IL-31: a new link between T cells and pruritus in atopic skin inflammation. J Allergy Clin Immunol 2006;117:411–417.

35 Fiset PO, Leung DY, Hamid Q: Immunopathology of atopic dermatitis. J Allergy Clin Immunol 2006;118: 287–290.

36 Van Beelen AJ, Teunissen MB, Kapsenberg ML, de Jong EC: Interleukin-17 in inflammatory skin disorders. Curr Opin Allergy Clin Immunol 2007;7: 374–381.

37 Toda M, Leung DY, Molet S, Boguniewicz M, Taha R, Christodoulopoulos P, Fukuda T, Elias JA, Hamid QA: Polarized in vivo expression of IL-11 and IL-17 between acute and chronic skin lesions. J Allergy Clin Immunol 2003;111:875–881.

38 He R, Oyoshi MK, Jin H, Geha RS: Epicutaneous antigen exposure induces a Th17 response that drives airway inflammation after inhalation challenge. Proc Natl Acad Sci USA 2007;104:15817–15822.

39 Akdis M, Blaser K, Akdis CA: T regulatory cells in allergy: novel concepts in the pathogenesis, prevention, and treatment of allergic diseases. J Allergy Clin Immunol 2005;116:961–968.

40 Torgerson TR, Ochs HD: Immune dysregulation, polyendocrinopathy, enteropathy, X-linked: forkhead box protein 3 mutations and lack of regulatory T cells. J Allergy Clin Immunol 2007;120:744–750.

41 Ou LS, Goleva E, Hall C, Leung DY: T regulatory cells in atopic dermatitis and subversion of their activity by superantigens. J Allergy Clin Immunol 2004;113:756–763.

42 Cardona ID, Goleva E, Ou LS, Leung DY: Staphylococcal enterotoxin B inhibits regulatory T cells by inducing glucocorticoid-induced TNF receptor-related protein ligand on monocytes. J Allergy Clin Immunol 2006;117: 688–695.

43 Verhagen J, Akdis M, Traidl-Hoffmann C, Schmid-Grendelmeier P, Hijnen D, Knol EF, Behrendt H, Blaser K, Akdis CA: Absence of T-regulatory cell expression and function in atopic dermatitis skin. J Allergy Clin Immunol 2006;117:176–183.

44 Franz B, Fritzsching B, Riehl A, Obekrle N, Klemke CD, Sykora J, Quick S, Stumpf C, Hartmann M, Enk A, Ruzicka T, Krammer PH, Suri-Payer E, Kuhn A: Low number of regulatory T cells in skin lesions of patients with cutaneous lupus erythematosus. Arthritis Rheum 2007;56:1910–1920.

45 Schnopp C, Rad R, Weidinger A, Weidinger S, Ring J, Eberlein B, Ollert M, Mempel M: Fox-P3-positive regulatory T cells are present in the skin of generalized atopic eczema patients and are not particularly affected by medium-dose UVA1 therapy. Photodermatol Photoimmunol Photomed 2007;23:81–85.

46 Verhagen J, Taylor A, Akdis M, Akdis CA: Targets in allergy-directed immunotherapy. Expert Opin Ther Targets 2005;9:217–224.

47 Bussmann C, Maintz L, Hart J, Allam JP, Vrtala S, Chen KW, Bieber T, Thomas WR, Valenta R, Zuberbier T, Sager A, Novak N: Clinical improvement and immunological changes in atopic dermatitis patients undergoing subcutaneous immunotherapy with a house dust mite allergoid: a pilot study. Clin Exp Allergy 2007;37:1277–1285.

48 Ito T, Wang YH, Duramad O, Hori T, Delespesse GJ, Watanabe N, Qin FX, Yao Z, Cao W, Liu YJ: TSLP-activated dendritic cells induce an inflammatory T-helper type 2 cell response through OX40 ligand. J Exp Med 2005;202:1213–1223.

49 Loser K, Mehling A, Loeser S, Apelt J, Kuhn A, Grabbe S, Schwarz T, Penninger JM, Beissert S: Epidermal RANKL controls regulatory T-cell numbers via activation of dendritic cells. Nat Med 2006;12:1372–1379.

Thomas Werfel
Department of Immunodermatology and Allergy Research, Hannover Medical School
DE–30449 Hannover (Germany)
Tel. +49 511 924 6450, Fax +49 511 924 6440
E-Mail Werfel.thomas@mh-hannover.de

Blaser K (ed): T Cell Regulation in Allergy, Asthma and Atopic Skin Diseases.
Chem Immunol Allergy. Basel, Karger, 2008, vol 94, pp 112–123

T-Cell Regulation in Helminth Parasite Infections: Implications for Inflammatory Diseases

Rick M. Maizels[a] · Maria Yazdanbakhsh[b]

[a]Institute of Immunology and Infection Research, University of Edinburgh, Edinburgh, UK, and [b]Leiden University Medical Center, Leiden, The Netherlands

Abstract

The field of infectious disease immunology is at an exciting intersection with new concepts in immune regulation meeting with the dynamics of infectious diseases. We discuss how the identification of regulatory mechanisms has already helped develop new models to understand helminth infections, which remain among the most prevalent chronic diseases in the world today. The epidemiological imbalance between helminth infections in developing countries, and intensifying allergies and autoimmune pathologies in the industrialised nations, seems to reflect a fundamental shift in regulation of immune responsiveness. Experimental studies have verified that helminths can downmodulate a range of immunopathological conditions, with the regulatory T cell being one of the most common mechanisms in play. We discuss further the context of host genetic predisposition, together with the impact of infection on the evolution of the human immune system, and suggest future strategies to harness our new understanding of helminth organisms in order to control both infectious and non-infectious immunological disorders.

Infections with helminth parasites remain extraordinarily prevalent in many developing countries, with >25% of the human population currently infected. Helminth diseases are also amongst the most neglected communicable diseases in the world today [1]. Current options for intervention are limited. Pharmacological treatments rely on a few, long-standing compounds which are compromised by rapid re-infection, variable compliance, and emerging resistance, while trial vaccines have rarely succeeded in evoking strong resistance [2]. A major challenge for immunology is to develop a new paradigm to explain the persistence of helminths, as a platform for new intervention strategies.

One likely reason for the prevalence of helminths is their undoubted ability to downregulate the host immune system at both the antigen-specific and polyclonal levels [3]. In many chronic diseases, such as schistosomiasis and lymphatic filariasis, peripheral blood T cells show dramatically impaired parasite antigen-specific responsiveness [4], as discussed in more detail below. Moreover, from early reports of immunosuppression in animal models of infection, to studies in Africa linking vaccine failure to heavy helminth infection, there is clear evidence that infections can diminish reactivity to bystander antigens, particularly with increasing intensity of

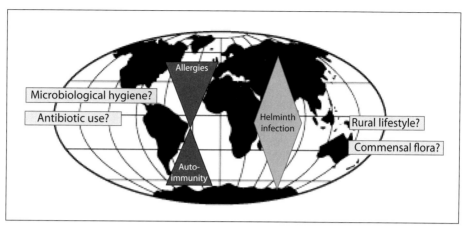

Fig. 1. Gradient of helminth infections and immunopathologies worldwide. The diagram illustrates the inverse prevalence of allergies and autoimmune disease (hourglass) compared to helminth parasitic infections (diamond). Many other environmental and microbiological factors are likely to influence the incidence of immunopathologies; it has been suggested that the reduced level of bacterial exposure in industrialised countries and/or use of antibiotics in infancy (left-hand boxes) may increase propensity to allergies; conversely, a rural lifestyle and certain commensal bacterial species (right-hand boxes) have been associated with protection from allergy. Global image is reproduced with thanks from http://www.graphicmaps.com/clipart.htm.

the worm burden. Intriguingly, many carriers of infection are both asymptomatic and hyporesponsive, suggesting that a state of immune tolerance or anergy has been established which protects the host from pathology as well as the parasite from elimination [5].

At the population level, there is also evidence that exposure to helminths is associated with lower frequencies of allergic and autoimmune disorders [6], and the inverse correlation between infections and immunopathologies is evident at the global scale (fig. 1). This relationship can be summarised in the hygiene hypothesis, which posits that with declining intensity and prevalence of infectious agents, the immune system becomes over-reactive to innocuous substances such as allergens and autoantigens [6–11]. Critical to a new interpretation of this hypothesis have been signal publications identifying the regulatory T cell (Treg) population as major immunological

controllers of human immunopathologies, including atopic dermatitis and other allergic disorders [12–14] as well as type 1 diabetes and other autoimmune diseases [15]. With the appreciation that Tregs play an important role in a significant range of infectious diseases [16], it is timely for us to summarise below the epidemiological and experimental evidence for helminth modulation of host T-cell populations and T-cell-mediated diseases in the context of allergy and autoimmunity.

Epidemiology of Helminth Infections, Allergies and Autoimmune Pathologies

Parasitic helminths, such as *Ascaris lumbricoides*, *Trichuris trichiura*, hookworms, schistosomes and filarial nematodes are highly prevalent in tropical and subtropical areas of the world [1]. These infections often overlap and affect more than 1 billion people, primarily in rural areas of the world but also among urban dwellers living in poverty. Helminth infections disproportionally affect younger people and show a strongly overdispersed intensity pattern with a few 'wormy people' carrying the highest burden of infection and acting as a reservoir for transmission. Re-infection after chemotherapy is the rule rather than the exception. With increasing economic development, sanitation and access to medical treatment, the prevalence of these infections is now declining in urban areas of the tropics. The disappearance of geohelminth infections in Western Europe occurred in the last century for similar reasons. However as recently as 1936, it was reported that 50% of schoolchildren on Terschelling, one of the Northern Islands in the Netherlands, were infected with *Ascaris* and *Trichuris*. Since that time, concerns in Western Europe have re-focussed on the alarming increase in inflammatory diseases such as allergies.

The ISAAC Study (http://isaac.auckland.ac.nz) examined the international prevalence patterns of asthma, allergic rhinoconjunctivitis and eczema in children aged from 6 to 8 years and from 12 to 14 years. Phase I of the study was conducted in 156 centres in 56 countries, including 6 in Africa, 18 in Asia (including the Middle East) and 9 in Latin America. The results indicated that the highest prevalence of symptoms of asthma (wheeze in past 12 months) were in countries such as the UK (18.4%), New Zealand (29.7%), Ireland (33%) or USA (22.9%) and lowest among others in Indonesia (2.1%), Albania (2.6%) or China (average of 5%) [17]. On the whole, developing countries tended to have a lower prevalence of symptoms of allergic disorders compared with countries with full economic development.

Since then, numerous studies have documented that the prevalence of asthma, rhinitis and eczema has been increasing not only in industrialised developed countries [18], but also among affluent people in developing countries [19]. In both environments, it appears that a rural lifestyle confers protection against allergic disorders whereas urbanisation appears to be an important disease risk factor. For example, among traditional rural farmers in Germany and Eastern Europe, there is little allergy compared to major urban centres. Further analysis of ISAAC data indicated that in addition to affluence and dietary factors, infections [20] might play a role in the variations recorded in prevalence of allergic disorders. In 1989, Strachan [21] suggested that frequent exchange of childhood infections among siblings in large and less affluent families was responsible for the lower incidence of allergic diseases.

This proposition stimulated key studies that related either indirect or direct measurements of infection to the presence of allergies in human subjects. As markers of past exposure to pathogens, antibodies to hepatitis A, to *Toxoplasma gondii* or to *Helicobacter pylori* [22] as well as cellular responses to mycobacterial antigens [23], were shown to be inversely associated with prevalence of asthma or skin prick test positivity. When relating active infections to allergic disorders, respiratory viral infections appear to exacerbate asthma [24], while parasitic helminth infections are often negatively associated with allergic disorders [reviewed in 6]. Given the overall pattern of complementary epidemiological distribution of parasitic helminth infections and allergies, and their inverse trends over time, it is tempting to speculate that there may be an important relationship between helminth infections and allergic diseases. However, human studies do not all provide a statistically significant link between helminth infection and mitigated allergic reactivity. Indeed, reports indicate increased risk of allergic sensitization, atopy and symptoms in the context of some helminth infections [e.g. 25].

In a recent meta-analysis of published data on the relationship between intestinal helminth infections (*Ascaris, Trichuris* and hookworms) and allergies, no consistent role for these infections in preventing allergic asthma was found, although hookworm infections did seem to show some protective effect [26]. It is important to note that this analysis combined studies from areas where prevalence of infection varied from very low to very high. The intensity and chronicity of helminth infections, however, has previously been suggested to be a crucial factor in the impact of parasitism on allergies, with allergic responses quite possibly exacerbated at very low or infrequent levels of infection [27]. Thus, there may be a threshold effect, in which a certain minimum intensity of infection must be reached before systemic reduction of bystander responses would be observed, and/or a certain stage of the infection that must be established [28]. Moreover, the ability of different species of helminths to modulate allergic reactivity is likely to differ widely. *Ascaris* and *Trichuris* infections have largely an intestinal passage and residence; hookworms have an interstitial migratory phase, while both filarial nematodes and schistosomal trematodes cause systemic infections. As each species enters into a different interaction with the host, the influence of infection on the immune system and allergic reactivities will very likely vary. In this respect, where multiple studies have examined the same helminth infection, as in schistosomiasis, a consistent relationship has emerged, showing that in each case this infection exerts a suppressive effect on allergic disorders [29–31].

Epidemiological data linking helminth infections with prevalence of autoimmune diseases are almost non-existent. However, recently, Fleming and Cook [32] have charted multiple sclerosis (MS) prevalence against *T. trichiura* prevalence for 35 different developed and developing countries, showing a dichotomous relationship with only a few instances (e.g. Argentina) where intermediate levels of both conditions were observed. Interestingly, it was reported that in Argentina, MS patients who acquired helminth infections subsequent to diagnosis of autoimmune disease

suffered far lower relapse rates and clinical deterioration compared to uninfected, matched patients [33]. Moreover, in the latter study, the authors were able to show higher Treg-associated activity in helminth-infected patients, as discussed further below.

Immune Regulation in Human Helminth Infections

A key characteristic of chronic helminth infections is the antigen-specific T-cell hyporesponsiveness, which is alleviated after drug treatment, indicating that current helminth infections exert a modifiable regulatory effect on the immune system. In humans, schistosomiasis and filarial infections (lymphatic filariasis and onchocerciasis) have long been associated with IL-10 and TGF-β, the neutralisation of which leads to recovery of antigen-specific cellular responses [34] Such suppressive cytokines are associated with pivotal cells of the immune system: antigen presenting cells and Tregs (fig. 2). Direct evidence for the presence of Tregs during chronic helminth infections was obtained when regulatory phenotype T-cell clones were isolated from onchocerciasis patients [35]. More recently, further evidence on the activity of Tregs, and the anergisation of effector cells, during chronic helminth infections has been reported. In lymphatic filariasis, infected patients show higher levels of CTLA-4 expression in peripheral blood T cells than do uninfected, and in vitro IL-5 responses (associated with protection) are significantly enhanced in the presence of anti-CTLA-4 antibody [36]. In vitro studies have indicated that live filarial parasites, but not worm extracts, induce upregulation of genes associated with T-cell anergy in peripheral blood mononuclear cells of infected subjects, together with upregulation of Foxp3 mRNA among natural Tregs [37]. Analysis of patients with *Schistosoma mansoni* infections in Kenya has documented high levels of CD4+ CD25++ cells in 40% of

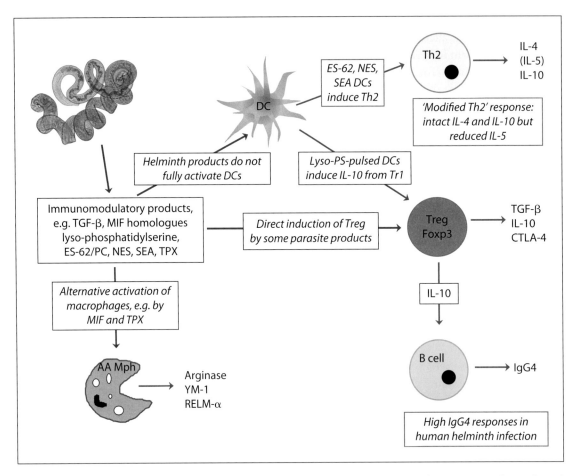

Fig. 2. Potential mechanisms for expansion of immunoregulatory cell activity by helminth parasites. Products released from live helminths have been shown to induce a state of partial activation in DCs, which disposes them strongly towards Th2 induction or even (in the case of DCs pulsed with *S. mansoni* lyso-phosphatidylserine, lyso-PS), towards IL-10 producing Tr1 cells. Where Th2 responses predominate in human helminth infection, they are frequently of a 'modified' phenotype, in which IL-5, eosinophliia and IgE are all downregulated. Some parasite products appear able to directly induce Foxp3 expression in naive T cells, converting them to Treg function. IL-10 of either Th2 or Treg origin may act on B cells to enhance switching to IgG4 and block IgE production. Finally, additional parasite products can influence the differentiation of macrophages towards the 'type 2' phenotype of alternative activation and release of arginase, the chitinase-like product Ym-1 and the resistin-like molecule RELM-α. TGF-β = Transforming growth factor-β; MIF = macrophage migration inhibitory factor; ES-62/PC = the phosphorylcholine-conjugated 62-kDa excretory-secretory product of adult *Acanthocheilonema viteae* filarial worms; NES = *Nippostrongylus brasiliensis* excretory-secretory antigens; SEA = schistosome egg antigen; TPX = thioredoxin peroxidase.

infected subjects, and showed that these levels decreased after treatment with Praziquantel, indicating that active infection leads to the expansion of CD4+ CD25++ cells [38]. However, as studies to date have not examined the functional activity of these cells, the dynamic development and resolution of Tregs during human infections is still awaiting clarification.

A further striking feature of chronic helminth infections is an extreme isotype bias towards IgG4

[39]. This non-complement-fixing antibody sub-class is generally <5% of total serum antibody, yet dominates the antifilarial antibody response. A recent study by Satoguina et al. [40] has helped us to integrate the cytokine and isotype observations, as IL-10 was shown to drive B-cell production of IgG4. High IgG4, known to be indicative of active filarial infection [41], may indeed reflect the level of immunoregulatory cell activity in the patient, a supposition supported by the accelerated loss of IgG4 in patients following curative drug therapy [42]. Both the cytokine profile (high IL-4, IL-10, low IL-5) and the isotype balance (high IgG4 and low IgE) in asymptomatic helminth infections are highly reminiscent of the 'modified Th2 response' observed in desensitised patients treated for allergic disorders [43].

Exploiting the knowledge that has recently developed on the induction of regulatory immune pathways by helminths, clinical trials were and are being initiated to study the effect of these parasites on inflammatory diseases. Currently, *Trichuris suis* is being used to treat patients with ulcerative colitis and Crohn's disease, with promising initial results [44]. Future studies are planned to examine the effect of hookworms on allergic airway diseases [45] and of *T. suis* on MS [11].

Experimental Evidence for Immune Regulation in Animal Models

The first indications of immune downregulation in animal models of helminth infection were found in the 1970s, in the modulation of liver granulomas over time in chronic schistosome infection [46]. Subsequently, many other reports described suppression of T-cell bystander antigen and mitogen responses during infections with filarial parasites in rodents [47] as well as in larger animals. The link to immune system pathologies was then made, e.g. *S. mansoni* infection of mice protects them from diabetes [48].

With the emergence of the Th1/Th2 paradigm, it was soon clear that helminth infections elicited a remarkably polarised Th2 response [49], which readily spilled over into bystander antigens [50]. High levels of IL-4 induction, from basophils and eosinophils as well as T cells [51], as well as suppression of dendritic cell IL-12 required for Th1 differentiation [52, 53], result in an overwhelming type-2 environment, which also promotes the development of alternatively activated macrophages [3]. The same bias can be achieved with secreted products from helminths [54, 55], and indeed Schramm [56] has identified a single component of schistosome egg antigen (SEA) which directly induces IL-4 production leading to the selective induction of Th2 responses. The anti-helminth Th2 response also engenders a high level of IL-10, and Th2 IL-10 production is dependent upon initial IL-4 [57]. Hence, it is important to appreciate that immune regulation by IL-10 in helminth infections may result from either (or both) Th2 and Tr1 production of this cytokine.

Most recently it has become clear that many helminth parasites stimulate Treg populations. Expression of Foxp3 among CD4+ T cells rises soon after infection with *Heligmosomoides polygyrus* [58] and in a model of a chronic filarial parasite infection (*Litomosoides sigmodontis*). In schistosomiasis, control of inflammatory liver disease has been most clearly associated with Tregs, as CD4+CD25+ [59] or Foxp3-transduced [60] T cells. A key issue, highlighted in the human but experimentally tractable in the mouse, is whether the high IL-10 environment can be attributed to Th2, Tr1-Foxp3−, or 'natural' Foxp3+ Treg cells. In fact, all may play a part, although the majority of IL-10 in murine helminth infections now appears to be produced by CD25− Th2 effector populations [61, 62]. While effector populations may produce IL-10, in other respects they may be functionally anergised. Thus, in vitro proliferation in response to antigen challenge is ablated, in a manner reminiscent of the human setting, and CD25− effectors are found to express high levels of GITR and CTLA-4 [63].

The likelihood that helminth-induced Treg populations also act to protect parasites from clearance is supported by experiments in which antibodies to Treg surface markers (GITR and CD25) result in clearance of in mice [63]. Thus, for the first time it has been demonstrated that nullifying Treg activity can 'cure' chronic helminth parasite infection by allowing the immune system to operate at full potential. Equally, antibodies to CD25 and CTLA induce mice to kill the majority of *Litomosoides* filarial parasites. These results support the proposal that during chronic infection, the host immune system fully recognises parasite antigens, but is hampered from reacting to them effectively by the activity of parasite-specific suppressor/regulatory mechanisms. Thus, immunity (whether naturally evoked or vaccine-elicited) requires the removal of suppressive cells if it is to be expressed to its full potential. In both mouse models and human studies on lymphatic filariasis [36], this expression of immunity is thought to depend on IL-5, known to be a key cytokine for eosinophil-mediated killing of parasites which is upregulated following depletion of the Treg population.

Models of Allergies and Autoimmunity – Helminths Acting Through T Cells?

In a broad range of model systems, helminth infections have proven to abrogate immunopathologies of both allergic and autoimmune aetiology. Interestingly, while each helminth tested has been strongly Th2-inducing, their suppressive effects are found on both Th1 (autoimmune) and Th2 (allergic) diseases. In allergy models, among the first reports was of mice infected with *Strongyloides stercoralis*, in which airway responses to ovalbumin were suppressed relative to uninfected controls [64]. Similarly, airway allergy is suppressed by infection with *Nippostrongylus brasiliensis* [65] and *H. polygyrus* [62]. In a different model of anaphylaxis, schistosome infection has been found to be protective in mice [66]. In the *H. polygyrus* model, suppression of allergy could be achieved by transfer of CD4+CD25+ Tregs from infected allergen-naive mice to sensitized, uninfected recipients. This experiment demonstrated that inhibition of pathology was not simply due to antigenic competition (particularly where parasites like *N. brasiliensis* traverse the airways), and identified helminth-induced Tregs as a likely mediator of the allergic suppression (fig. 2).

Suppression of allergy by a transferred T-cell population also argues against protection mediated by high IgE levels, which are a common feature of all helminth models. The proposition, in humans, that high polyclonal (or parasite-specific) IgE blocks allergen-specific IgE reactions is widely held, although not supported by evidence that cell FcεR density is extremely plastic, so that blocking by parasite-specific IgE is unlikely to be effective [67].

H. polygyrus also protects mice from food allergy [68] and from colitis in the gut [69]. These reports underline the broad-spectrum activity of parasite-induced regulation, and argue that regulatory cells (perhaps not only Tregs) driven by infection in one site (such as the gut), disseminate throughout the body. Hence, the efficacy of regulation may depend as much on the migratory capacity of these cells (facilitated perhaps by CD103 [70]), as on their arithmetic number or origin as 'natural' or 'adaptive' types.

In autoimmunity models, similar interactions occur. Thus, mice exposed to *S. mansoni* ova are protected from two different autoimmune diseases, type 1 diabetes [71] and experimental allergic encephalomyelitis [72, 73]. In these instances, a Th2 immune deviation might equally explain the amelioration of Th1 pathology, and experimental testing of this possibility remains to be undertaken.

Helminths and the Innate Immune System

With their wide variety of habitats and lifestyles, helminth parasites necessarily interact with the full range of innate immune system components including dendritic cells (DCs), macrophages and granulocytes as well as vascular endothelial cells, and the gastrointestinal epithelium. From the viewpoint of T-cell regulation, perhaps the most significant of these is the helminth-DC interface (fig. 2). Helminth antigens, in vitro, induce a 'muted' response from immature DCs, which is related to the propensity to induce Th2, rather than Th1, responsiveness [52, 53, 74].

In humans, most studies of DCs have been based on the exposure of monocyte-derived DCs (moDCs) [75] to helmith-derived products. On their own, helminth-derived extracts with Th2-inducing capacity do not lead to strong moDC [76] or Langerhans' cell [77] maturation but exert inhibitory effects on different costimulatory molecules expressed on DCs. For example, Langerhans' cells exposed to filarial larvae downregulate HLA class I and II [77], while moDCs exposed to microfilariae downregulate DC-SIGN, but not HLA molecules [78]. Whether the downregulation of such molecules is involved in the lower capacity of such antigen presenting cells to support T-cell proliferation [76, 77] is as yet unknown. Moreover, it is interesting to note the effect that helminth-derived molecules have on activation of DCs. Exposure of human moDCs to *S. mansoni* extracts seems to allow expression of CD83, a maturation marker, in response to TLR ligands [79], yet these cells have impaired CD86 expression [van Riet, unpubl. data]. Studies of excretory/secretory products released from *N. brasiliensis* (NES) and *H. poly-gyrus* (HP-ES) on murine bone marrow-derived dendritic cells (BMDC) showed that responses to TLR ligation are impaired in BMDCs exposed to helminth products [52, 80]. Similarly, the activation of DCs induced in vivo [81] or in vitro [80] via OVA exposure was suppressed when helminth-derived molecules were used. Taken together it is clear that helminth-derived molecules are able to affect DC function in such a way that their ability to activate T cells is significantly hampered.

Interestingly, there is also evidence that specific molecules, such as lysophosphatidylserine (PS), stimulate DCs to induce Tregs rather than effector T-cell responses [79], as represented in figure 2. The question of the extent to which the ability of helminths to induce a Th2 response overlaps with their induction of a regulatory response, remains an important one to address. Is the inhibition of 'classic' TLR or non-TLR mediated activation important for Th2 rather than regulatory responses? To what extent is the 'non-classic' activation of TLRs involved? With respect to this, it is of great interest that molecules expressed by helminths such as LNFPIII [82], Lyso-PS [79] or ES-62 [83] have TLR-activating capacities with downstream effects that are distinct from 'classic' pro-inflammatory TLR ligands, raising the question whether other co-receptors are involved in switching 'classic' to 'non-classic' TLR activity. It is clear that the delineation of molecular events that determine DC involvement in the effector/regulatory switchpoint in T-cell responsiveness is very relevant not only to helminth infections but also to inflammatory diseases.

With respect to allergies, the role that innate receptors, such as TLRs, play in the development and progression of this disease has largely been extrapolated from genetic studies. Polymorphisms in the TLR-2 and TLR-4 genes, in certain populations, have been associated with susceptibility to asthma. In animal models of allergies, the influence of TLR ligation in most settings is considered to stimulate or amplify reactivity [84]. However, it is also known that in the specific context of TLR2−/− mice, there is a reduction in Treg function, and aggravated schistosome pathology [85].

Given the possibility of 'non-classic' TLR activation, the different outcomes of TLR-knockout experiments might be very context-dependent. The expression levels of TLRs and the association with allergic diseases may support this. Microbial exposure seems to increase TLR expression, more specifically TLR-2, in European farmers, a population in whom prevalence of allergies is significantly lower than in non-farmers [86]. However, the finding that human helminth infection may reduce TLR expression [87] would appear to contradict the findings in European farmers, as helminth infections tend to protect against allergic diseases. The question remains whether the nature of infections present in the different populations accounts for the up- or downregulation of TLR expression, despite both populations being protected from the development of allergic disorders and the data clearly indicate a complex relationship that has still to be unravelled.

Learning from Helminths to Treat Allergy and Autoimmunity

Recent developments in immunology now offer a conceptual framework to understand the link between helminth infection and immunomodulation. Parasites induce Treg populations which suppress antiparasite effector cells, as part of the parasites' own strategy for survival in the host. At the same time, they can dampen bystander responses to allergens and autoantigens. Can we develop new interventions based on products from the helminths? In principle, yes, but we have yet to analyse how their expansion of Tregs can be focussed in an antigen-specific manner, as a further broad-spectrum immunosuppressive agent will not necessarily prove useful in selectively ablating allergy or autoimmunity.

Our perspective is thus one of general significance to chronic infection, as well as one that will provide specific pathways to novel treatments of human schistosomiasis, and lymphatic filariasis. These two diseases represent a massive public health problem with 300 million people infected in the world today. Intervention by ablating parasite-specific Tregs in these patients will solve the specific problems of schistosomiasis and filarial diseases, while at the same time proving a principle which will be applicable to chronic infections in general.

Acknowledgements

R.M.M. is supported by grants from The Wellcome Trust, The Medical Research Council and The European Commission; M.Y. is supported by grants from The European Commission.

References

1 Hotez PJ, Molyneux DH, Fenwick A, et al: Control of neglected tropical diseases. N Engl J Med 2007;357:1018–1027.

2 Maizels RM, Holland M, Falcone FH, Zang XX, Yazdanbakhsh M: Vaccination against helminth parasites: the ultimate challenge for immunologists? Immunol Rev 1999;171:125–148.

3 Maizels RM, Balic A, Gomez-Escobar N, Nair M, Taylor M, Allen JE: Helminth parasites: masters of regulation. Immunol Rev 2004;201:89–116.

4 Yazdanbakhsh M, Paxton WA, Kruize YCM, et al: T-cell responsiveness correlates differentially with antibody isotype levels in clinical and asymptomatic filariasis. J Infect Dis 1993;167:925–931.

5 Maizels RM, Yazdanbakhsh M: Regulation of the immune response by helminth parasites: cellular and molecular mechanisms. Nat Rev Immunol 2003;3:733–743.

6 Yazdanbakhsh M, Kremsner PG, van Ree R: Allergy, parasites, and the hygiene hypothesis. Science 2002;296:490–494.

7 Bach J-F: Regulatory T cells under scrutiny. Nat Rev Immunol 2003;3:189–198.

8 Kamradt T, Göggel R, Erb KJ: Induction, exacerbation and inhibition of allergic and autoimmune diseases by infection. Trends Immunol 2005;26:260–267.

9 Maizels RM: Infections and allergy – helminths, hygiene and host immune regulation. Curr Opin Immunol 2005;17:656–661.

10 Schaub B, Lauener R, von Mutius E: The many faces of the hygiene hypothesis. J Allergy Clin Immunol 2006;117:969–978.

11 Fleming J, Fabry Z: The hygiene hypothesis and multiple sclerosis. Ann Neurol 2007;61:85–89.

12 Akdis M, Blaser K, Akdis CA: T regulatory cells in allergy: novel concepts in the pathogenesis, prevention, and treatment of allergic diseases. J Allergy Clin Immunol 2005;116:961–969.

13 Strickland DH, Stumbles PA, Zosky GR, et al: Reversal of airway hyperresponsiveness by induction of airway mucosal CD4+CD25+ regulatory T cells. J Exp Med 2006.

14 Umetsu DT, Dekruyff RH: The regulation of allergy and asthma. Immunol Rev 2006;212:238–255.

15 Arif S, Tree TI, Astill TP, et al: Autoreactive T cell responses show proinflammatory polarization in diabetes but a regulatory phenotype in health. J Clin Invest 2004;113:451–463.

16 Belkaid Y: Regulatory T cells and infection: a dangerous necessity. Nat Rev Immunol 2007;7:875–999.

17 International Study of Asthma and Allergies in Childhood (ISAAC) Steering Committee: Worldwide variation in prevalence of symptoms of asthma, allergic rhinoconjunctivitis, and atopic eczema. Lancet 1998;351:1225–1232.

18 Eder W, Ege MJ, von Mutius E: The asthma epidemic. N Engl J Med 2006;355:2226–2235.

19 Von Hertzen LC, Haahtela T: Asthma and atopy – the price of affluence? Allergy 2004;59:124–137.

20 Von Mutius E, Pearce N, Beasley R, et al: International patterns of tuberculosis and the prevalence of symptoms of asthma, rhinitis, and eczema. Thorax 2000;55:449–453.

21 Strachan DP: Hay fever, hygiene, and household size. BMJ 1989;299:1259–1260.

22 Matricardi PM, Rosmini F, Ferrigno L, et al: Cross-sectional retrospective study of prevalence of atopy among Italian military students with antibodies against hepatitis A virus. BMJ 1997;314:999–1003.

23 Shirakawa T, Enomoto T, Shimazu S, Hopkin JM: The inverse association between tuberculin responses and atopic disorder. Science 1997;275:77–79.

24 Mallia P, Johnston SL: How viral infections cause exacerbation of airway diseases. Chest 2006;130:1203–1210.

25 Palmer LJ, Celedon JC, Weiss ST, Wang B, Fang Z, Xu X: *Ascaris lumbricoides* infection is associated with increased risk of childhood asthma and atopy in rural China. Am J Respir Crit Care Med 2002;165:1489–1493.

26 Leonardi-Bee J, Pritchard D, Britton J: Asthma and current intestinal parasite infection: systematic review and meta-analysis. Am J Respir Crit Care Med 2006;174:514–523.

27 Yazdanbakhsh M, van den Biggelaar A, Maizels RM: Th2 responses without atopy: immunoregulation in chronic helminth infections and reduced allergic disease. Trend Immunol 2001;22:372–377.

28 Smits HH, Hammad H, van Nimwegen M, et al: The protective effect of *Schistosoma mansoni* infection on allergic asthma depends on intensity and chronicity of infection. J Allergy Clin Immunol 2007;120:932–940.

29 Araujo MI, Lopes AA, Medeiros M, et al: Inverse association between skin response to aeroallergen and *Schistosoma mansoni* infection. Int Arch Allergy Immunol 2000;123:145–148.

30 Van den Biggelaar A, van Ree R, Roderigues LC, et al: Decreased atopy in children infected with *Schistosoma haematobium*: a role for parasite-induced interleukin-10. Lancet 2000;356:1723–1727.

31 Medeiros M Jr, Figueiredo JP, Almeida MC, et al: *Schistosoma mansoni* infection is associated with a reduced course of asthma. J Allergy Clin Immunol 2003;111:947–951.

32 Fleming JO, Cook TD: Multiple sclerosis and the hygiene hypothesis. Neurology 2006;67:2085–2086.

33 Correale J, Farez M: Association between parasite infection and immune responses in multiple sclerosis. Ann Neurol 2007;61:97–108.

34 King CL, Mahanty S, Kumaraswami V, et al: Cytokine control of parasite-specific anergy in human lymphatic filariasis. Preferential induction of a regulatory T-helper type 2 lymphocyte subset. J Clin Invest 1993;92:1667–1673.

35 Satoguina J, Mempel M, Larbi J, et al: Antigen-specific T regulatory-1 cells are associated with immunosuppression in a chronic helminth infection (onchocerciasis). Microbes Infect 2002;4:1291–1300.

36 Steel C, Nutman TB: CTLA-4 in filarial infections: implications for a role in diminished T-cell reactivity. J Immunol 2003;170:1930–1938.

37 Babu S, Blauvelt CP, Kumaraswami V, Nutman TB: Regulatory networks induced by live parasites impair both Th1 and Th2 pathways in patent lymphatic filariasis: implications for parasite persistence. J Immunol 2006;176:3248–3256.

38 Watanabe K, Mwinzi PN, Black CL, et al: T regulatory cell levels decrease in people infected with *Schistosoma mansoni* on effective treatment. Am J Trop Med Hyg 2007;77:676–682.

39 Ottesen EA, Skvaril F, Tripathy SR, Poindexter RW, Hussain R: Prominence of IgG4 in the IgG antibody response to human filariasis. J Immunol 1985;134:2707–2712.

40 Satoguina JS, Weyand E, Larbi J, Hoerauf A: T regulatory-1 cells induce IgG4 production by B cells: role of IL-10. J Immunol 2005;174:4718–4726.

41 Kwan-Lim G-E, Forsyth KP, Maizels RM: Filarial-specific IgG4 response correlates with active *Wuchereria bancrofti* infection. J Immunol 1990;145:4298–4305.

42 Atmadja AK, Atkinson R, Sartono E, Partono F, Yazdanbakhsh M, Maizels RM: Differential decline in filarial-specific IgG1, IgG4 and IgE antibodies following diethylcarbamazine chemotherapy of *Brugia malayi* infected patients. J Infect Dis 1995;172:1567–1572.

43 Platts-Mills T, Vaughan J, Squillace S, Woodfolk J, Sporik R: Sensitisation, asthma, and a modified Th2 response in children exposed to cat allergen: a population-based cross-sectional study. Lancet 2001;357:752–756.

44 Summers RW, Elliott DE, Urban JF Jr, Thompson RA, Weinstock JV: *Trichuris suis* therapy for active ulcerative colitis: a randomized controlled trial. Gastroenterology 2005;128:825–832.

45 Mortimer K, Brown A, Feary J, et al: Dose-ranging study for trials of therapeutic infection with *Necator americanus* in humans. Am J Trop Med Hyg 2006;75:914–920.

46 Boros DL, Pelley RP, Warren KS: Spontaneous modulation of granulomatous hypersensitivity in *Schistosoma mansoni*. J Immunol 1975;114:1437–1441.

47 Lammie PJ, Katz SP: Immunoregulation in experimental filariasis. II. Responses to parasite and nonparasite antigens in jirds with *Brugia pahangi*. J Immunol 1983;130:1386–1389.

48 Cooke A, Tonks P, Jones FM, et al: Infection with *Schistosoma mansoni* prevents insulin-dependent diabetes mellitus in non-obese diabetic mice. Parasite Immunol 1999;21:169–176.

49 Pearce EJ, Caspar P, Grzych J-M, Lewis FA, Sher A: Downregulation of Th1 cytokine production accompanies induction of Th2 responses by a parasitic helminth, *Schistosoma mansoni*. J Exp Med 1991;173:159–166.

50 Kullberg MC, Pearce EJ, Hieny SE, Sher A, Berzofsky JA: Infection with *Schistosoma mansoni* alters Th1/Th2 cytokine responses to a non-parasite antigen. J Immunol 1992;148: 3264–3270.

51 Voehringer D, Shinkai K, Locksley RM: Type 2 immunity reflects orchestrated recruitment of cells committed to IL-4 production. Immunity 2004;20:267–277.

52 Balic A, Harcus Y, Holland MJ, Maizels RM: Selective maturation of dendritic cells by *Nippostrongylus brasiliensis* secreted proteins drives T-helper type 2 immune responses. Eur J Immunol 2004;34:3047–3059.

53 Cervi L, MacDonald AS, Kane C, Dzierszinski F, Pearce EJ: Dendritic cells copulsed with microbial and helminth antigens undergo modified maturation, segregate the antigens to distinct intracellular compartments, and concurrently induce microbe-specific Th1 and helminth-specific Th2 responses. J Immunol 2004;172:2016–2020.

54 Holland MJ, Harcus YM, Riches PL, Maizels RM: Proteins secreted by the parasitic nematode *Nippostrongylus brasiliensis* act as adjuvants for Th2 responses. Eur J Immunol 2000;30: 1977–1987.

55 Pearce EJ, Kane C, Sun J, J JT, McKee AS, Cervi L: Th2 response polarization during infection with the helminth parasite *Schistosoma mansoni*. Immunol Rev 2004;201:117–126.

56 Schramm G, Mohrs K, Wodrich M, et al: IPSE/α1, a glycoprotein from *Schistosoma mansoni* eggs, induces IgE-dependent, antigen-independent IL-4 production by murine basophils in vivo. J Immunol 2007;178:6023–6027.

57 Balic A, Harcus YM, Taylor MD, Brombacher F, Maizels RM: IL-4R signaling is required to induce IL-10 for the establishment of Th2 dominance. Int Immunol 2006;18:1421–1431.

58 Finney CA, Taylor MD, Wilson MS, Maizels RM: Expansion and activation of CD4+CD25+ regulatory T cells in *Heligmosomoides polygyrus* infection. Eur J Immunol 2007;37:1874–1886.

59 Hesse M, Piccirillo CA, Belkaid Y, et al: The pathogenesis of schistosomiasis is controlled by cooperating IL-10-producing innate effector and regulatory T cells. J Immunol 2004;172:3157–3166.

60 Singh KP, Gerard HC, Hudson AP, Reddy TR, Boros DL: Retroviral Foxp3 gene transfer ameliorates liver granuloma pathology in *Schistosoma mansoni*-infected mice. Immunology 2005; 114:410–417.

61 McKee AS, Pearce EJ: CD25+CD4+ cells contribute to Th2 polarization during helminth infection by suppressing Th1 response development. J Immunol 2004;173:1224–1231.

62 Wilson MS, Taylor M, Balic A, Finney CAM, Lamb JR, Maizels RM: Suppression of allergic airway inflammation by helminth-induced regulatory T cells. J Exp Med 2005;202:1199–1212.

63 Taylor M, Le Goff L, Harris A, Malone E, Allen JE, Maizels RM: Removal of regulatory T cell activity reverses hyporesponsiveness and leads to filarial parasite clearance in vivo. J Immunol 2005;174:4924–4933.

64 Wang CC, Nolan TJ, Schad GA, Abraham D: Infection of mice with the helminth *Strongyloides stercoralis* suppresses pulmonary allergic responses to ovalbumin. Clin Exp Allergy 2001; 31:495–503.

65 Wohlleben G, Trujillo C, Muller J, et al: Helminth infection modulates the development of allergen-induced airway inflammation. Int Immunol 2004; 16:585–596.

66 Mangan NE, Fallon RE, Smith P, van Rooijen N, McKenzie AN, Fallon PG: Helminth infection protects mice from anaphylaxis via IL-10-producing B cells. J Immunol 2004;173:6346–6356.

67 Mitre E, Norwood S, Nutman TB: Saturation of immunoglobulin E (IgE) binding sites by polyclonal IgE does not explain the protective effect of helminth infections against atopy. Infect Immun 2005;73:4106–4111.

68 Bashir ME, Andersen P, Fuss IJ, Shi HN, Nagler-Anderson C: An enteric helminth infection protects against an allergic response to dietary antigen. J Immunol 2002;169:3284–3292.

69 Elliott DE, Setiawan T, Metwali A, Blum A, Urban JF Jr, Weinstock JV: *Heligmosomoides polygyrus* inhibits established colitis in IL-10-deficient mice. Eur J Immunol 2004;34: 2690–2698.

70 Suffia I, Reckling SK, Salay G, Belkaid Y: A role for CD103 in the retention of CD4+CD25+ Treg and control of *Leishmania major* infection. J Immunol 2005;174:5444–5455.

71 Cooke A, Tonks P, Jones FM, et al: Infection with *Schistosoma mansoni* prevents insulin-dependent diabetes mellitus in non-obese diabetic mice. Parasite Immunol 1999;21:169–176.

72 La Flamme AC, Ruddenklau K, Backstrom BT: Schistosomiasis decreases central nervous system inflammation and alters the progression of experimental autoimmune encephalomyelitis. Infect Immun 2003; 71:4996–5004.

73 Sewell D, Qing Z, Reinke E, et al: Immunomodulation of experimental autoimmune encephalomyelitis by helminth ova immunization. Int Immunol 2003;15:59–69.

74 MacDonald AS, Straw AD, Dalton NM, Pearce EJ: Th2 response induction by dendritic cells: a role for CD40. J Immunol 2002;168:537–540.

75 Kapsenberg ML: Dendritic-cell control of pathogen-driven T-cell polarization. Nat Rev Immunol 2003;3:984–993.

76 Semnani RT, Liu AY, Sabzevari H, et al: *Brugia malayi* microfilariae induce cell death in human dendritic cells, inhibit their ability to make IL-12 and IL-10, and reduce their capacity to activate CD4+ T cells. J Immunol 2003;171: 1950–1960.

77 Semnani RT, Law M, Kubofcik J, Nutman TB: Filaria-induced immune evasion: suppression by the infective stage of *Brugia malayi* at the earliest host-parasite interface. J Immunol 2004;172:6229–6238.

78 Talaat KR, Bonawitz RE, Domenech P, Nutman TB: Preexposure to live *Brugia malayi* microfilariae alters the innate response of human dendritic cells to *Mycobacterium tuberculosis*. J Infect Dis 2006;193:196–204.

79 Van der Kleij D, Latz E, Brouwers JFHM, et al: A novel host-parasite lipid crosstalk: schistosomal lysophosphatidylserine activates toll-like receptor 2 and affects immune polarization. J Biol Chem 2002;277:48122–48129.

80 Segura M, Su Z, Piccirillo C, Stevenson MM: Impairment of dendritic cell function by excretory-secretory products: a potential mechanism for nematode-induced immunosuppression. Eur J Immunol 2007;37:1887–1904.

81 Silva SR, Jacysyn JF, Macedo MS, Faquim-Mauro EL: Immunosuppressive components of *Ascaris suum* down-regulate expression of costimulatory molecules and function of antigen-presenting cells via an IL-10-mediated mechanism. Eur J Immunol 2006;36:3227–3237.

82 Thomas PG, Carter MR, Atochina O, et al: Maturation of dendritic cell 2 phenotype by a helminth glycan uses a toll-like receptor 4-dependent mechanism. J Immunol 2003;171:5837–5841.

83 Goodridge HS, Marshall FA, Else KJ, et al: Immunomodulation via novel use of TLR4 by the filarial nematode phosphorylcholine-containing secreted product, ES-62. J Immunol 2005;174:284–293.

84 Horner AA, Raz E: Do microbes influence the pathogenesis of allergic diseases? Building the case for toll-like receptor ligands. Curr Opin Immunol 2003;15:614–619.

85 Layland LE, Rad R, Wagner H, da Costa CU: Immunopathology in schistosomiasis is controlled by antigen-specific regulatory T cells primed in the presence of TLR2. Eur J Immunol 2007;37:2174–2184.

86 Lauener RP, Birchler T, Adamski J, et al: Expression of CD14 and toll-like receptor 2 in farmers' and non-farmers' children. Lancet 2002;360:465–466.

87 Babu S, Blauvelt CP, Kumaraswami V, Nutman TB: Diminished T cell TLR expression and function modulates the immune response in human filarial infection. J Immunol 2006;176: 3885–3889.

Rick M. Maizels
Institute of Immunology and Infection Research
University of Edinburgh
West Mains Road, Edinburgh EH9 3JT (UK)
Tel. +44 131 650 5511, Fax +44 131 650 5450, E-Mail address.rick.maizels@ed.ac.uk

Blaser K (ed): T Cell Regulation in Allergy, Asthma and Atopic Skin Diseases.
Chem Immunol Allergy. Basel, Karger, 2008, vol 94, pp 124–137

Immune Regulation and Tolerance to Fungi in the Lungs and Skin

Luigina Romani · Paolo Puccetti

Department of Experimental Medicine and Biochemical Sciences,
University of Perugia, Perugia, Italy

Abstract

The balance of pro- and anti-inflammatory signaling is a pre-requisite for successful host/fungal interactions and requires the coordinate actions of both innate and adaptive immune systems. Although inflammation is an essential component of the protective response to fungi, its dysregulation may significantly worsen fungal diseases and limit protective antifungal immune responses. The newly described Th17 developmental pathway may play an inflammatory role previously attributed to uncontrolled Th1 responses and serve to accommodate the seemingly paradoxical association of chronic inflammatory responses with fungal persistence in the face of an ongoing inflammation. In this scenario, unrestricted fungal growth could result from the activation of not only pathogenic Th17 cells, but also Th2 cells whose activation is strictly dependent on fungal burden. The capacity of regulatory T cells (Tregs) to inhibit aspects of innate and adaptive antifungal immunity is required for protective tolerance to fungi. Indoleamine 2,3-dioxygenase (IDO) and tryptophan catabolites contribute to such a homeostatic condition by providing the host with immune defense mechanisms adequate for protection, without necessarily eliminating fungal pathogens – which would impair immune memory – or causing an unacceptable level of tissue damage. IDO and tryptophan metabolites may prove to be potent regulators capable of taming overzealous or heightened inflammatory host responses.   Copyright © 2008 S. Karger AG, Basel

Fungi belonging to the *Ascomycota* as well as to the *Basidiomycota* are capable of causing a wide spectrum of infections and diseases. According to the site of infection, mycoses are designated as superficial, cutaneous, subcutaneous, and systemic or deep. These clinical classifications blend into each other, for example, a deep mycosis, such as coccidioidomycosis, may begin with cutaneous lesions, and a subcutaneous mycosis, such as sporotrichosis, may disseminate to become a systemic disease. Opportunistic fungal infections occur in patients with defective immunity. *Candida* species remain the fourth most important cause of hospital-acquired bloodstream infections. Invasive aspergillosis, mostly by *Aspergillus fumigatus* and *Aspergillus terreus*, and other mold infections are a leading cause of infection-related death in hematopoietic stem cell transplant recipients. Despite marked reductions in the rates of AIDS-associated fungal infections, such as cryptococcosis in developed countries, the burden of these diseases in those countries is large and increasing.

Fungal Diseases

Fungal diseases include type I hypersensitivity, the most prevalent disease caused by molds, and a large number of other illnesses, including allergic

Table 1. Allergic fungal diseases

Fungus	Diseases	Ref.
Aspergillus spp.	ABPA	4
Alternaria, Aspergillus, Cladosporium, Penicillium	Allergic sinusitis, Allergic rhinitis, Hypersensitivity pneumonitis	2
Molds	Asthma	3
Malassezia spp.	Atopic dermatitis	6, 11
Dermatophytes	Allergy	23
Candida albicans	CMC	7

ABPA = Allergic bronchopulmonary aspergillosis; CMC = chronic mucocutaneus candidiasis.

bronchopulmonary mycoses, allergic chronic sinusitis, hypersensitivity pneumonitis and atopic eczema/dermatitis syndrome (AEDS – formerly atopic dermatitis) [1, 2] (table 1). Many airborne fungi are involved, including species of *Alternaria, Aspergillus, Cladosporium* and *Penicillium*, and exposure may be indoors, outdoors or both. Hypersensitivity may occur in association with the state of colonization observed with a fungus ball that forms in an ectatic bronchus, and even in the nasal sinuses. In contrast to pollen-derived allergies, fungal allergies are frequently linked with allergic asthma and associated with asthma severity [3]. Sensitization to molds has been reported in asthmatic patients and in chronic rhinosinusitis [2]. In addition, allergic bronchopulmonary aspergillosis (ABPA) is frequent in patients with asthma and cystic fibrosis [4]. However, the prevalence of fungal sensitization is not known mainly due to the lack of standardized fungal extracts and to an overwhelming number of fungal species able to elicit IgE-mediated reactions [1]. Recent work based on high-throughput cloning of fungal allergens revealed that fungi are able to produce extremely complex repertoires of cross-reactive allergens. There is evidence that fungal sensitization also contributes to autoreactivity against self antigens due to shared epitopes with homologous fungal allergens [5].

The skin can be a portal of entry for fungal infections when the epithelial barrier is breached or it can be a site for disseminated, systemic fungal disease. Fungal infections of the skin range from generally benign conditions, such as congenital candidiasis, to potentially fatal infections with opportunistic pathogens, including *Aspergillus* and the Zygomycetes. The two most common cutaneous fungal infections are caused by one or more of the fungal species in the keratinophilic genera *Microsporum, Trichophyton*, or *Epidermophyton* and *Malassezia* spp. Although *Malassezia* yeasts are a part of the normal microflora, they have been associated with a number of diseases affecting the human skin, such as pityriasis versicolor, folliculitis, seborrheic dermatitis and dandruff, AEDS, psoriasis, and – less commonly – with other dermatologic disorders such as confluent and reticulated papillomatosis, onychomycosis, and transient acantholytic dermatosis [6]. Recent studies of the interaction of *Malassezia* spp. with innate cells have highlighted the potential of the fungus to modulate the immune response directed against it [6]. In the normal skin, the fungus may downregulate the inflammatory response, through the production of immunosuppressive transforming growth factor (TGF)-β_1 and interleukin (IL)-10, allowing it to live as a commensal. In contrast, in AEDS and psoriasis, both chronic inflammatory skin diseases, the skin barrier may provide an environment that can enhance the release of allergens as well as the ability of the fungus to upregulate the production of molecules involved in hyperproliferation and cell migration thus exacerbating psoriatic lesions. Therefore, an inflammatory cycle seems to be at work, the manipulation of which may offer strategies to control or prevent exacerbations of these diseases. A similar vicious circle may be at work in chronic mucocutaneous candidiasis

(CMC), a primary immune deficiency presenting as an inability to clear yeasts, mostly *Candida albicans*, that consequently persist and recur in infections of the skin, nails and mucous membranes [7]. Most CMC patients also develop accompanying endocrine and inflammatory disorders that suggest an underlying deregulation of the inflammatory and immune responses [7].

Features of Fungal Diseases

Phylogenetically conserved allergen structures are known to play a role as cross-reactive allergens in fungal allergy [5]. As a result of molecular mimicry and cross-reactivity with structurally related human proteins, perpetration of the inflammatory reactions and tissue damage releasing intracellular self antigens occurred in both skin diseases and ABPA [5]. These findings highlight two major features of mucosal fungal diseases, namely molecular mimicry as a basic mechanism involved in mediating chronic allergic diseases and the deleterious effect of a deregulated inflammation, to which both the host and the fungus contribute. Both features underline the existence of complex and unusual relationships of fungi with the vertebrate immune system, partly due to some prominent features. Among these, the ability to reversibly switch from one form to the other in infection which may have resulted in an expanded repertoire of cross-regulatory and overlapping antifungal host responses at different body sites, and, for commensals, the highly effective strategies of immune evasion they must have evolved to survive in the host environment. However, because fungal diseases are rare, a stable host-parasite interaction is a likely condition for most fungi. This condition requires that the elicited immune response be strong enough to allow host survival with or without pathogen elimination and to establish commensalism/persistency without excessive pro-inflammatory pathology. Therefore, the balance of pro- and anti-inflammatory signaling is a prerequisite for successful host/fungal interactions and requires the coordinate actions of both innate and adaptive immune systems [8].

Immunity to Fungi: Connecting the Innate to the Adaptive Immune System through DCs

Innate Immunity

Protective immunity against fungal pathogens is achieved by the integration of two distinct arms of the immune system, the innate and adaptive (or antigen-specific) responses. The two systems are distinguished by whether the antigen receptors are encoded in the germ line (innate immunity) or generated somatically by gene rearrangement or hypermutation (adaptive immunity). Most of the innate mechanisms are inducible upon infection and their activation requires specific recognition of conserved molecular structures of fungi by pattern recognition receptors (PRRs), including toll-like receptors (TLRs) and C-type lectin receptors [9]. A number of cell wall components of fungi may act through several distinct PRRs, each activating specific antifungal programs on phagocytes and dendritic cells (DCs). The inflammatory response is initially mediated by cells of the innate immune system followed by a later adaptive immune response, which responds to the signals originated by the innate immune system. However, another emerging function of innate immunity is that it also has a role in sterile inflammation, that is, inflammation and the ensuing tissue damage, caused by endogenous TLR ligands. In this regard, TLR activation itself is a double-edged sword and is involved in the pathogenesis of autoimmune, chronic inflammatory disorders such as asthma, rheumatoid arthritis, and infectious diseases.

A number of innate immune deficits mediate susceptibility to cutaneous infections [10]. There is considerable evidence that patients with AEDS have an unusual propensity for colonization by certain microbes (including *Malassezia* and

Candida) that is associated, among others, to defects in antimicrobial peptides, such as defensins, cathelicidins and dermcidin, key players of cutaneous immunity. Altered expression of extracellular (TLR) and intracellular (Nod/CARD; nucleotide-binding oligomerization domain/ caspase recruitment domain containing protein) family members is found in patients with dermatological diseases [11]. AEDS patients carrying the TLR-2 (Arg753Gln) or TLR-4 (Thr399Ile) single nucleotide polymorphisms had increased disease severity characterized by markedly elevated IgE antibodies to allergens. Moreover, in the lungs, most of the inhaled fungal spores are eliminated by exclusion mechanisms, which include physical barriers, such as mucus, and cilia as well as a variety of innate mediators of the collectin family, such as lung surfactant proteins, mannose-binding lectins and pentraxin 3 [12].

In vertebrates, antigen-independent recognition of fungi by the innate immune system leads to the immediate mobilization of immune effector and regulatory mechanisms that provide the host with the generation of antigen-specific T-helper (Th) effector cells that are endowed with the ability to release a distinct panel of cytokines, capable of activating and deactivating signals to effector phagocytes. To limit the pathologic consequences of excessive inflammatory cell-mediated immune reactions, the immune system also resorts to a number of protective mechanisms, including the generation of regulatory T cells (Tregs). The T-cell compartment of innate and adaptive immunity provides vertebrates with the potential to survey for and respond specifically to an incredible diversity of antigens.

Dendritic Cells
DCs are uniquely adept at decoding the fungus-associated information and translating it in qualitatively different adaptive Th responses [13]. Both human and murine DCs recognize and internalize a number of fungi, including *A. fumigatus*, *C. albicans*, and *Malassezia furfur* and are

affected by fungi and their products. Different PRRs determine the functional plasticity of DCs in response to fungi and contribute to the discriminative recognition of the different fungal morphotypes [13]. The uptake of the different fungal elements occurs through different receptors and forms of phagocytosis and implicates a lectin-like pathway for unicellular forms and opsono-dependent pathways for filamentous forms. The engagement of distinct PRRs by distinct fungal morphotypes also translates into downstream signaling events, ultimately regulating cytokine production and costimulation, an event greatly influenced by fungal opsonins and antibodies [13]. Natural killer cells, abundantly present in AEDS patients [14], also influence the activation program of DCs in response to *Malassezia* [15], eventually leading to pro-inflammatory cytokine production and maintenance of inflammation in AEDS lesions. A role for inflammatory epidermal DCs in the pathogenesis of inflammation seen in AEDS lesions has recently been described [16]. A remarkable and important feature of DCs is their capacity to produce IL-10 in response to fungi. These IL-10–producing DCs activate CD4+ CD25+ Tregs that are essential components of antifungal resistance (see below).

Overall, the ability of a given DC subset to respond with flexible activating programs to the different stimuli as well as the ability of different subsets to convert into each other confer unexpected plasticity to the DC system [13]. In this regard, as further discussed below, through their ability to produce type I IFNs, plasmacytoid DCs (pDCs) indisputably drive protective antiviral inflammation but have also been implicated in the induction and exacerbation of the inflammatory process associated with autoimmunity and allergy [17]. The bipolar functions of pDCs, and of the associated type I IFN response, appear to be an intrinsic ability of the immune system to co-activate cytostatic mechanisms, induce the death of pathogenic T cells and polarize T cells towards a Treg-cell phenotype. Tryptophan catabolism may, in principle, fulfill all the requirements to effect these functions [18, 19].

By subverting the morphotype-specific program of activation of DCs, innate environmental factors qualitatively affect DC functioning and Th/Treg selection in vivo, ultimately impacting on fungal virulence. In this scenario, the qualitative development of Th-cell responses to fungi may not primarily depend on the nature of the fungal form being phagocytosed and presented, but rather on the type of cell signaling initiated by the ligand-receptor interaction in DCs. For commensals, the paradigm would predict that specific forms of the fungus cannot be regarded as absolutely indicative of saprophytism or infection at a given site. The selective exploitation of receptor-mediated entry of fungi into DCs could explain the full range of host immune-parasite relationships, including saprophytism and infection. Importantly, as hyphae – more than yeasts – activate DCs for the local induction of Tregs [8], it appears that in addition to the induction of phase-specific products enhancing fungal survival within the host, transition to the hyphal phase of the fungus could implicate the induction of immunoregulatory events that allow for fungal persistence in the absence of the pathological consequences of an exaggerated immunity and possible autoimmunity, this condition representing the very essence of fungal commensalism [8].

Adaptive Th Immunity
Serological and skin reactivity surveys indicate the occurrence of acquired immunity to fungi. Lymphocytes from healthy subjects show proliferative responses after stimulation with fungal antigens and produce a number of different cytokines. Due to their action on circulating leukocytes, the cytokines produced by fungus-specific T cells are instrumental in mobilizing and activating antifungal effectors, thus providing prompt and effective control of infectivity once the fungus has established itself in tissues or spread to internal organs [20]. Generation of a dominant Th1 response dri-

ven by IL-12 is essentially required for the expression of protective immunity to fungi. Through the production of the signature cytokine IFN-γ and help for opsonizing antibodies, the activation of Th1 cells is instrumental in the optimal activation of phagocytes at sites of infection. Therefore, the failure to deliver activating signals to effector phagocytes may predispose patients to chronic infections, limit the therapeutic efficacy of antifungals and antibodies and favor persistency and/or commensalism. The clinical circumstances in which fungal infections occur definitely suggest an association with impaired cell-mediated immunity. Patients with CMC have documented altered patterns of cytokine production in response to *Candida* spp. with decreased production of type 1 cytokines and increased levels of IL-10 [21]. Cell-mediated immunity is the major defense mechanism in dermatophyte infection and is stimulated by glycopeptide fungal antigens and downregulated by fungal keratinases [10]. Similar to dermatophytes, the ability of *C. albicans* to persist in host tissues may involve primarily the immunosuppressive property of its major cell wall glycoprotein, mannan [20].

The inflammatory allergic manifestations that follow the contact or inhalation of fungi all constitute compelling evidence of the pathogenic role of T-cell dysreactivity in fungal diseases. In patients with defective IL-12/IFN-γ pathway, such as those with hyperimmunoglobulinemia E syndrome, fungal infections and allergy are both observed [20]. Allergy is an overzealous Th2 response to environmental allergens, both airborne and ingested. Allergic asthma is characterized by chronic inflammation followed by airway remodeling. IL-4-dependent Th2 cells, that dampen protective Th1 responses and favor fungal allergy, are present in patients with fungal allergy and are associated with elevated levels of antifungal IgE, IgA, and IgG [1, 2]. Moreover, and consistent with the inflammatory state, patients with pulmonary aspergillosis are genetically low producers of both TGF-β and IL-10 [22]. AEDS is characterized by increased systemic Th2 responses and a combination of Th2 and Th1 responses in the skin lesions [23]. Around 30–80% of patients with AEDS have specific serum IgE and/or positive skin-prick test and atopy patch test reactions to *Malassezia* spp. [6]. Several allergens of *Malassezia* have been defined the distribution of which varies, with some specific to a particular species of *Malassezia* and others common to several species. It is intriguing that Th2 cytokines inhibit the release of antimicrobial peptides in the skin [24].

A recent, intriguing study has highlighted the role of chitin, a polymerized sugar and fundamental component of arthropods and fungi, in allergic reactions [25]. Although chitin itself does not occur in humans, chitinases are present in the human genome and chitinase expression is markedly increased in human asthma [26]. It has been suggested that the ability of a host to produce chitinases would be an important determinant in an individual's propensity toward atopy and/or asthma in response to fungi. Recent insights regarding the development of allergic diseases have also suggested a role for 'inflammatory T cells' or Th17 cells, producing IL-17, as a link between T-cell inflammation and granulocytic influx as observed in allergic airway [27] and dermal [28] inflammation (see below).

There is evidence that fungal sensitization also contributes to autoreactivity against self antigens due to shared epitopes between fungal and human proteins [29]. The underlying mechanism seems to be molecular mimicry perpetuating severe chronic allergic diseases. Cross-reactivity between fungal and human proteins has been demonstrated for MnSOD, cyclophilin, acid ribosomal protein P2 and thioredoxin [1, 5, 30]. In AEDS patients with *Malassezia sympodialis* colonization of the skin, specific IgE antibodies against human MnSOD were detected while the application of human recombinant MnSOD on healthy skin elicited an eczematous reaction [31]. Similarly in ABPA, the release of intracellular self antigens as a consequence of inflammation

processes causing tissue damage has been proposed [29]. In skin tests, a humoral autoimmune response to the human P2 protein was seen in patients with ABPA or with severe AEDS [30].

Driving Inflammation: Contribution of the Th17 Pathway

The inflammatory response to fungi may serve to limit infection but an overzealous or heightened inflammatory response may contribute to pathogenicity, as documented by the occurrence of severe fungal infections in patients with immunoreconstitution disease [32]. For *Candida*, the failure to resolve inflammation associated with defective fungal clearance characterizes CMC [7]. For *Aspergillus,* the association of persistent inflammation with the fungus is common in patients with allergy [3].

IL-12, by initiating and maintaining Th1 responses, was thought to be responsible for overreacting immune and autoimmune disorders. This was also the case in fungal infections where immunoregulation proved to be essential in fine-tuning inflammation and uncontrolled Th1/Th2 antifungal reactivity [20]. Recent studies have suggested a greater diversification of the CD4+ T-cell effector repertoire than that encompassed by the Th1/Th2 paradigm [33]. Th17 cells are now thought to be a separate lineage of effector Th cells contributing to immune pathogenesis previously attributed to the Th1 lineage. The presence of TGF-β together with IL-6 and other inflammatory mediators favors the Th17 pathway, leading to the emergence of Th17 cells that are stabilized by DC-derived IL-23. IL-12 and IL-23 are members of a family of pro-inflammatory heterodimeric cytokines that share a common p40 subunit linked to the IL-12p35 chain or the IL-23p19 chain. Th17 cells, which produce IL-17 preferentially, promote neutrophil-mediated inflammation and although linked to resistance to several bacterial and parasitic infections, correlate with disease severity and immunopathology in diverse infections. With growing understanding of the contribution of the IL-23 and Th17 axis to various organ-related autoimmune and inflammatory diseases, there has been an interest in targeting many aspects of this pathway for therapeutic interventions.

Recent results showed that Th17 cells are induced in response to *C. albicans* and *A. fumigatus*, through innate signaling via Dectin-1/CARD9 [34] and TLR/MyD88 [35] and inhibited through negative regulators of TLRs [unpubl. observation] and TRIF [36]. Although IL-17 contributed to neutrophil mobilization in disseminated candidiasis [37], the Th17 pathway – and not the uncontrolled Th1 response – is associated with defective pathogen clearance and failure to resolve inflammation and to initiate protective immune responses against both fungi [35, 36]. Both IL-23 and IL-17 impaired the antifungal effector activities of neutrophils and activated the inflammatory program of neutrophils by counteracting the IFN-γ-dependent activation of indoleamine 2,3-dioxygenase (IDO), known to limit the inflammatory status of neutrophils against fungi [38, 39] (see below). This accounted for the high inflammatory pathology and tissue destruction associated with Th17 cell activation, as IL-17 neutralization increased fungal clearance, ameliorated inflammatory pathology and restored protective Th1 antifungal resistance [35]. The finding that IL-23 and IL-17 promote inflammation, while subverting protective antifungal immunity, may serve to accommodate the seemingly paradoxical association of chronic inflammatory responses with fungal persistence in the face of an ongoing inflammation. In this scenario, the unrestricted fungal growth will result from the activation of not only pathogenic Th17 cells but also Th2 cells, whose activation is strictly dependent on fungal burden. However, because both IL-17A and IL-17F may contribute to the expression of airway inflammation and pulmonary hyperreactivity, free soluble IL-17A is increased in asthma [40] and allergic cellular and humoral responses are suppressed in IL-17-deficient mice [41], these findings indicate that the Th17 pathway may be directly involved in fungal-associated allergic lung diseases.

The above considerations may help to accommodate fungi, either commensals or ubiquitous, within immune homeostasis and its dysregulation. If the ability to subvert the inflammatory program through the IL-23 and Th17 may eventually lead to immune dysregulation, their ability to activate Tregs (see below), that are integral and essential components of protective immunity to fungi [8], may represent a mechanism whereby dysregulated immunity is prevented (fig. 1). These new findings provide a molecular connection between the failure to resolve inflammation and lack of antifungal immune resistance and point to strategies for immune therapy that attempt to limit inflammation to stimulate an effective immune response.

Dampening Inflammation and Allergy to Fungi: The Role of Treg Subsets

The control of the immune response is pivotal for preventing damage. In addition to efficient control of pathogens, tight regulatory mechanisms are required in order to balance protective immunity and immunopathology both in allergic asthma [42] and skin diseases [43]. Prolonged inflammation is a hallmark of a wide range of chronic diseases and autoimmunity. Chronic infection and inflammation are considered two of the most important epigenetic and environmental factors contributing to those diseases. To limit the pathologic consequences of an excessive inflammatory cell-mediated reaction, the immune system resorts to a number of protective mechanisms. CD4+ T cells making immunoregulatory cytokines such as IL-10, TGF-β and IL-4 have long been known and discussed in terms of immune deviation or class regulation [44]. More

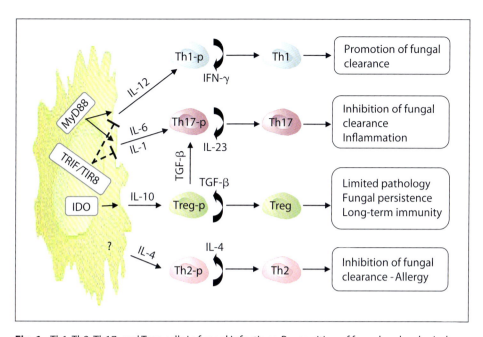

Fig. 1. Th1, Th2, Th17, and Treg cells in fungal infections. Recognition of fungal molecules induces distinct activating programs in DCs, leading to antifungal immunity in vivo. Those include activation of an immunogenic, MyD88-dependent program in DCs culminating in the production of IL-12 – and eventually leading to protective Th1 cells, producing IFN-γ – or of IL-6/IL-1/IL-23, which activate pathogenic Th17 cells (promoting inflammation and dampening Th1 responses). By as yet unknown receptors and downstream cellular events, the production of IL-4 leads to activation of Th2 responses opposing antifungal function in effector cells and promoting allergic manifestations. The activation of a tolerogenic program in DCs results in induction of IDO and subsequent IL-10 production, which is causally linked to activation of Tregs, suppressing both Th1 and Th2 antifungal immunity, and antagonizing Th17 cell development, in such a way that sufficient immunity remains for controlling fungal growth but preventing undesirable immunopathology. This results in the generation of long-term immunity in the face of fungal persistence. Solid and dotted lines – positive and negative signals, respectively.

recently, Tregs, capable of fine-tuning protective antimicrobial immunity in order to minimize harmful immune pathology, have become an integral component of the immune response. Tregs serve to restrain exuberant immune reactivity, which in many chronic infections benefits the host by limiting tissue damage. However, the Treg responses may handicap the efficacy of protective immunity.

Besides ensuring self-tolerance, different types of Tregs actively participate in immune responses.

Naturally occurring CD4+CD25+ Tregs (nTregs), expressing the Treg-lineage specification factor, forkhead box P3 – Foxp3 – originate in the thymus and survive in the periphery as natural regulators, whereas inducible (or adaptive) Tregs (iTregs) cells develop from naive CD4+ T cells in the periphery. Peripheral development of Foxp3+ Tregs represents a mechanism that helps broaden the Treg repertoire in specialized anatomical sites. In this regard, specialized intestinal DCs promote Foxp3 expression via a

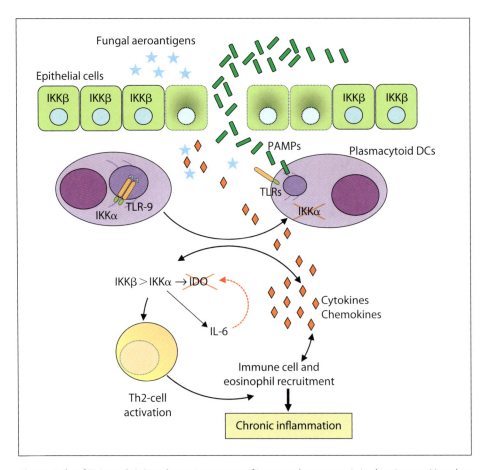

Fig. 2. Role of TLRs and IDO in the maintenance of immune homeostasis in the airways. Harmless aeroantigen is prevented from initiating airway inflammation by the integrity and antimicrobial defense of the epithelium. TLR-9-driven induction of IDO and consequent inhibition of Th2 cells likely contrast the onset of allergic inflammation [for details, see 49]. Several cell types in bronchial and pulmonary tissues mediate this effect, including epithelial and endothelial cells, as well as lung plasmacytoid DCs. Some degree of activation of the canonical NF-κB signaling pathway (IKKβ) contributes to maintenance of epithelial barrier integrity, yet noncanonical NF-κB signaling (IKKα) provides IDO-dependent regulatory effects to mucosal homeostasis. Under conditions of unopposed Th2 cell activation, allergic inflammation will develop, resulting in an epithelial defect. Persistent activation of the canonical NF-κB pathway occurs in response to different PAMPs (pathogen-associated molecular patterns, recognized by TLRs). This, in turn, promotes production of IDO-inhibitory IL-6 and favors Th2-cell expansion and sustains the pathogenetic triad of airway hyperresponsiveness, eosinophilia, and IgE production.

mechanism that is dependent on local TGF-β and retinoic acid, a vitamin A metabolite [45]. Recent studies have also revealed a reciprocal relationship between the development of Foxp3+ Tregs and effector T cells, so that naive CD4+ T cells differentiate into Foxp3+ Tregs in the presence of TGF-β or into Th17 cells in the presence of TGF-β and IL-6. Thus T-cell activation in the presence of innate stimuli diverts iTreg generation to Th17 generation [46].

Tregs with tolerogenic activity have been described in fungal infections [8]. Treg induction is defective in patients with CMC [47]. CD4+ CD25+Foxp3+ nTregs operating in the respiratory or the gastrointestinal mucosa accounted for the lack of pathology associated with fungal clearance and/or persistence in mice with fungal pneumonia or mucosal candidiasis [8, 48]. Fungal growth, inflammatory immunity, and tolerance to *C. albicans* and *A. fumigatus* were all controlled by the coordinate activation of nTregs – limiting early inflammation at the sites of infection – and pathogen-induced iTregs, which regulated the expression of adaptive Th immunity in secondary lymphoid organs. Early in infection, inflammation was controlled by the expansion, activation and local recruitment of nTregs suppressing neutrophils through the combined actions of IL-10 and cytotoxic T lymphocyte antigen (CTLA)-4 acting on IDO (see below). Late in infection, the inflammatory immunity was modulated by iTregs, which acted through activation of IDO in DCs and prevented Th17 cell development [36]. In fungal allergy, tolerogenic iTregs inhibited Th2 cells and prevented allergy to the fungus [39]. Collectively, these observations suggest that the capacity of Tregs to inhibit aspects of innate and adaptive immunity is pivotal in their regulatory function and further support the concept of 'protective tolerance' to fungi, implying that a host's immune defense may be adequate for protection without necessarily eliminating fungal pathogens – which would impair immune memory – or causing an unacceptable level of tissue damage [8].

Tryptophan Catabolism and Allergy: Fungi Are Next in Line

There is an increasing appreciation of the unifying role that the immunosuppressive pathway of tryptophan catabolism mediated by the enzyme IDO may have in promoting tolerance under a variety of physiopathologic conditions [18, 19, 49]. Modulation of tryptophan catabolism represents a general mechanism of action of Tregs expressing surface CTLA-4 [50], and different cell types respond to CTLA-4 engagement of CD80 receptor molecules with the activation of IDO, including conventional and pDCs, CD4+ T cells, and polymorphonuclear leukocytes involved in *Candida*-specific immunity [8, 49]. The bulk of these studies suggests that IDO-expressing pDCs may have a general and important role in regulating T-cell homeostasis and preventing immunopathogenesis, including that associated with infection [8, 49].

Paradigm of Reverse and Noncanonical in Fungal Infections

Thanks to primary ligands having evolved into ancillary receptors, a mechanism of intercellular communication has emerged during evolution ('reverse signaling') that enables a ligand-bearing cell to receive an immediate feedback upon activation of the cognate receptor on adjacent cells. The term reverse signaling was introduced in immunology to indicate a two-way communication between cells or cell types via a single pair of transducing molecules – acting reciprocally as ligands and receptors ('coreceptors') – whereby information actually flows in both directions, but one direction ('forward') is of greater or longer-standing importance [49]. More recently, reverse and noncanonical signaling (R&N) has been used to indicate Treg conditioning of DCs via costimulatory ligands that, expressed by DCs, transduce intracellular signals back into the DCs where they activate the noncanonical pathway of the transcription factor NF-κB [51]. R&N involves Tregs expressing CTLA-4 and GITR (glucocorticoid-induced tumor necrosis factor receptor), is mediated by at least two coreceptor pairs – CTLA-4 and CD80; GITR and GITR ligand (GITRL) – and results in transcriptional activation of type I IFN genes (in pDCs) and *Indo* (in conventional and pDCs). R&N is an effector mechanism of Treg function, a means of self-propagation by Tregs, and participates in the pharmacologic induction of Tregs [51]. In fungal infections, R&N cooperates with TLR signaling, mediating protective responses, optimally balanced between inflammation and tolerance. As a matter of fact, most of the information regarding the interface between TLR signaling and R&N in microbial immunity has been gathered in experimental models of candidiasis and aspergillosis [8, 49].

R&N in Fungal Infections Is Not Toll-Free and Is Exploited by Corticosteroids

Experimental models of ABPA have been used to demonstrate a pivotal role for Treg cells, pDCs and tryptophan catabolism in protecting mice from allergic airway inflammation [39]. A recent study has shown the IDO-dependent effects of dexamethasone on the hypersensitivity response to *Aspergillus* antigens in the murine lung [51]. Consistent with the responsiveness of ABPA to corticosteroid treatment [52], the Th2- allergic phenotype was greatly attenuated by dexamethasone, which enhanced production of IL-10 and enhanced *Foxp3* transcripts, both markers of protective Treg activity in *Aspergillus* allergy. The data demonstrate that dexamethasone downregulates exacerbating Th2 responses in ABPA by inhibiting the expansion and activation of Th2 cells and upregulates the expression of *Foxp3* via mechanisms that require R&N-dependent tryptophan catabolism [51].

It is intriguing that fungi have exploited IDO manipulation as a mean to induce or subvert the tolerogenic program of pDCs [8]. Regulation of IDO activity in pDCs occurred in a morphotype-dependent manner and, interestingly, in an opposite manner for *Candida* and *Aspergillus*. IDO activity was promoted by *Candida* hyphae and by *Aspergillus* resting conidia and inhibited by *Aspergillus* swollen conidia or hyphae. The implication is that *Candida* hyphae, by promoting tolerance, contribute to commensalism and eventually to immunoevasion while swollen *Aspergillus* conidia promote host inflammatory response by subverting tolerance.

Can IDO Help in the Fight Against Fungal Allergy?

Traditionally recognized for its role in infection, pregnancy, transplantation, autoimmunity and neoplasia, the IDO mechanism has revealed an unexpected potential in the control of inflammation, allergy, and allergic airway inflammation, all conditions in which the pDCs could have a protective function. As predicted by the 'hygiene hypothesis' – that is, an early reduction in microbial burden may predispose to allergy [53] and autoimmunity [54] – epidemiological and experimental data suggest now that certain microorganisms induce a state of protective tolerance in the gut to which TLRs [55], inhibition of canonical NF-κB [56] and IDO [57] jointly contribute. In the airways, experimental eosinophilia and hyperresponsiveness were inhibited by soluble CTLA-4 [58], a TLR-9 ligand [59] and by IKKα-dependent induction of IDO through reverse signaling [51]. These data suggest that IDO modulation by noncanonical NF-κB – the latter in balance with its canonical counterpart – is essential for the maintenance of TLR-driven immune homeostasis in the airways. It is conceivable that fungal aeroantigen is prevented from initiating airway inflammation by the integrity and antimicrobial defense of the epithelium, in an environment in which TLR9-driven induction of IDO and consequent inhibition of Th2 cells will contrast the onset of allergic inflammation. Asymptomatic atopy associated with increased IDO activity and IL-10 production in seasonal allergen exposure has been described [60]. Clinical trials of TLR-9-based immunotherapy are presently ongoing, suggesting that 'TLR-9 ligands may revolutionize the treatment of allergic diseases' [61].

Conclusion: Targeting R&N-Mediated Immune Homeostasis in Fungal Allergy

While some degree of activation of the NF-κB signaling pathway likely contributes to maintenance of epithelial barrier integrity, noncanonical NF-κB signaling could contribute IDO-dependent regulatory effects to the overall local immune homeostasis. Persistent activation of the canonical NF-κB pathway through the TLR-MyD88 pathway favors Th2 cell expansion and promotes allergic inflammation [62]. Plasmacytoid DCs and noncanonical NF-κB, activated by TLR-9 signaling, may oppose pathogenesis by polarizing T cells towards an IL-10-producing Treg phenotype. Accumulating Tregs – expressing surface cytotoxic T CTLA-4 and GITR – could further expand their own population through R&N in pDCs, after engagement of CD80 and GITRL, respectively. The combined effects of tryptophan starvation and production of kynurenines (immunoactive tryptophan catabolites), resulting from the sustained activation of IDO, will act as a major stimulus for the local Treg-cell generation and other regulatory effects. Glucocorticoids and TLR-9 ligands or modulators could greatly help restore local homeostasis, by directly inhibiting the canonical NF-κB (as is the case for glucocorticoids) or by promoting GITRL- and TLR-9-dependent activation of the noncanonical NF-κB pathway.

In summary, regulation through tryptophan catabolism appears to be an essential component of host responses to fungi such that its manipulation may allow fungi to either evade or promote immune activation.

As the effects of treatments with antifungal agents on symptoms and clinical findings in patients with allergic fungal diseases are controversial [52], targeting R&N-mediated immune homeostasis in fungal diseases is a promising option.

Acknowledgements

We thank Dr. Cristina Massi Benedetti for editorial assistance. This study was supported by the Specific Targeted Research Project 'EURAPS' (LSHM-CT-2005), contract No. 005223 (FP6) and 'MANASP' (LSHE-CT-2006), contract No. 037899 (FP6).

References

1 Crameri R, Weichel M, Fluckiger S, Glaser AG, Rhyner C: Fungal allergies: a yet unsolved problem. Chem Immunol Allergy 2006;91:121–133.
2 Simon-Nobbe B, Denk U, Poll V, Rid R, Breitenbach M: The spectrum of fungal allergy. Int Arch Allergy Immunol 2007;145:58–86.
3 Denning DW, O'Driscoll BR, Hugaboam CM, Bowyer P, Niven RM: The link between fungi and severe asthma: a summary of the evidence. Eur Respir J 2006;27:615–626.
4 Virnig C, Bush RK: Allergic bronchopulmonary aspergillosis: a US perspective. Curr Opin Pulm Med 2007;13:67–71.
5 Zeller S, Glaser AG, Vilhelmsson M, Rhyner C, Crameri R: Immunoglobulin-E-mediated reactivity to self antigens: a controversial issue. Int Arch Allergy Immunol 2007;145:87–93.
6 Ashbee HR: Recent developments in the immunology and biology of *Malassezia* species. FEMS Immunol Med Microbiol 2006;47:14–23.
7 Lilic D: New perspectives on the immunology of chronic mucocutaneous candidiasis. Curr Opin Infect Dis 2002;15:143–147.
8 Romani L, Puccetti P: Protective tolerance to fungi: the role of IL-10 and tryptophan catabolism. Trends Microbiol 2006;14:183–189.
9 Brown, GD: Dectin-1: a signalling non-TLR pattern-recognition receptor. Nat Rev Immunol 2006;6:33–43.
10 McGirt LY, Beck LA: Innate immune defects in atopic dermatitis. J Allergy Clin Immunol 2006;118:202–208.
11 Baker BS: The role of microorganisms in atopic dermatitis. Clin Exp Immunol 2006;144:1–9.
12 Montagnoli C, Bozza S, Gaziano R, Zelante T, Bonifazi P, Moretti S, Bellocchio S, Pitzurra L, Romani L: Immunity and tolerance to *Aspergillus fumigatus*. Novartis Found Symp 2006; 279:66–77.
13 Romani L, Bistoni F, Puccetti P: Fungi, dendritic cells and receptors: a host perspective of fungal virulence. Trends Microbiol 2002;10:508–514.
14 Buentke E, D'Amato M, Scheynius A: *Malassezia* enhances natural killer cell-induced dendritic cell maturation. Scand J Immunol 2004;59:511–516.

15 Buentke E, Scheynius A: Dendritic cells and fungi. APMIS 2003;111:789–796.

16 Guttman-Yassky E, Lowes MA, Fuentes-Duculan J, Whynot J, Novitskaya I, Cardinale I, Haider A, Khatcherian A, Carucci JA, Bergman R, Krueger JG: Major differences in inflammatory dendritic cells and their products distinguish atopic dermatitis from psoriasis. J Allergy Clin Immunol 2007;119:1210–1217.

17 Colonna M, Trinchieri G, Liu YJ: Plasmacytoid dendritic cells in immunity. Nat Immunol 2004;5:1219–1226.

18 Grohmann U, Fallarino F, Puccetti P: Tolerance, DCs and tryptophan: much ado about IDO. Trends Immunol 2003;24:242–248.

19 Mellor AL, Munn DH: IDO expression by dendritic cells: tolerance and tryptophan catabolism. Nat Rev Immunol 2004;4:762–774.

20 Romani L: Immunity to fungal infections. Nat Rev Immunol 2004;4:1–23.

21 Lilic D, Gravenor I, Robson N, Lammas DA, Drysdale P, Calvert JE, Cant AJ, Abinun M: Deregulated production of protective cytokines in response to Candida albicans infection in patients with chronic mucocutaneous candidiasis. Infect Immun 2003;71:5690–5699.

22 Sambatakou H, Pravica V, Hutchinson IV, Denning DW: Cytokine profiling of pulmonary aspergillosis. Int J Immunogenet 2006;33:297–302.

23 Woodfolk JA: Allergy and dermatophytes. Clin Microbiol Rev 2005;18:30–43.

24 Rieg S, Steffen H, Seeber S, Humeny A, Kalbacher H, Dietz K, Garbe C, Schittek B: Deficiency of dermcidin-derived antimicrobial peptides in sweat of patients with atopic dermatitis correlates with an impaired innate defense of human skin in vivo. J Immunol 2005;174:8003–8010.

25 Burton OT, Zaccone P: The potential role of chitin in allergic reactions. Trends Immunol 2007.

26 Zhu Z, Zheng T, Homer RJ, Kim YK, Chen NY, Cohn L, Hamid Q, Elias JA: Acidic mammalian chitinase in asthmatic Th2 inflammation and IL-13 pathway activation. Science 2004;304:1678–1682.

27 Bullens DM: Measuring T-cell cytokines in allergic upper and lower airway inflammation: can we move to the clinic? Inflamm Allergy Drug Targets 2007;6:81–90.

28 Zheng Y, Danilenko DM, Valdez P, Kasman I, Eastham-Anderson J, Wu J, Ouyang W: Interleukin-22, a Th17 cytokine, mediates IL-23-induced dermal inflammation and acanthosis. Nature 2007;445:648–651.

29 Crameri R, Faith A, Hemmann S, Jaussi R, Ismail C, Menz G, Blaser K: Humoral and cell-mediated autoimmunity in allergy to Aspergillus fumigatus. J Exp Med 1996;18:265–270.

30 Mayer C, Appenzeller U, Seelbach H, Achatz G, Oberkofler H, Breitenbach M, Blaser K, Crameri R: Humoral and cell-mediated autoimmune reactions to human acidic ribosomal P2 protein in individuals sensitized to Aspergillus fumigatus P2 protein. J Exp Med 1999;189:1507–1512.

31 Schmid-Grendelmeier P, Fluckiger S, Disch R, Trautmann A, Wuthrich B, Blaser K, Scheynius A, Crameri R: IgE-mediated and T cell-mediated autoimmunity against manganese superoxide dismutase in atopic dermatitis. J Allergy Clin Immunol 2005;115:1068–1075.

32 Singh N, Perfect JR: Immune reconstitution syndrome associated with opportunistic mycoses. Lancet Infect Dis 2007;7:395–401.

33 Dong C: Diversification of T-helper-cell lineages: finding the family root of IL-17-producing cells. Nat Rev Immunol 2006;6:329–333.

34 Leibundgut-Landmann S, Gross O, Robinson MJ, Osorio F, Slack EC, Tsoni SV, Schweighoffer E, Tybulewicz V, Brown GD, Ruland J, Reis ESC: Syk- and CARD9-dependent coupling of innate immunity to the induction of T-helper cells that produce interleukin-17. Nat Immunol 2007;8:630–638.

35 Zelante T, De Luca A, Bonifazi P, Montagnoli C, Bozza S, Moretti S, Belladonna ML, Vacca C, Conte C, Bistoni F, Puccetti P, Kastelein RA, Kopf M, Romani L: The Th17 pathway promote inflammation and impairs antifungal immune resistance. Eur J Immunol 37:2695–2706.

36 De Luca A, Montagnoli C, Zelante T, Bonifazi P, Bozza S, Moretti S, D'Angelo C, Vacca C, Boon L, Bistoni F, Puccetti P, Fallarino F, Romani L: Functional yet balanced reactivity to Candida albicans requires both TRIF and MyD88 and IDO-dependent inhibition of Rorc. J Immunol 2007;179:5999–6008.

37 Huang W, Na L, Fidel PL, Schwarzenberger P: Requirement of interleukin-17A for systemic anti-Candida albicans host defense in mice. J Infect Dis 2004;190:624–631.

38 Bozza S, Fallarino F, Pitzurra L, Zelante T, Montagnoli C, Bellocchio S, Mosci P, Vacca C, Puccetti P, Romani L: A crucial role for tryptophan catabolism at the host/Candida albicans Interface. J Immunol 2005;174:2910–2918.

39 Montagnoli C, Fallarino F, Gaziano R, Bozza S, Bellocchio S, Zelante T, Kurup WP, Pitzurra L, Puccetti P, Romani L: Immunity and tolerance to Aspergillus involve functionally distinct regulatory T cells and tryptophan catabolism. J Immunol 2006;176:1712–1723.

40 Linden A, Laan M, Anderson GP: Neutrophils, interleukin-17A and lung disease. Eur Respir J 2005;25:159–172.

41 Nakae S, Komiyama Y, Nambu A, Sudo K, Iwase M, Homma I, Sekikawa K, Asano M, Iwakura Y: Antigen-specific T cell sensitization is impaired in IL-17-deficient mice, causing suppression of allergic cellular and humoral responses. Immunity 2002;17:375–387.

42 Herrick CA, Bottomly K: To respond or not to respond: T cells in allergic asthma. Nat Rev Immunol 2003;3:405–412.

43 Lima HC: Role of regulatory T cells in the development of skin diseases. An Bras Dermatol 2006;81:269–281.

44 O'Garra A, Vieira P: Regulatory T cells and mechanisms of immune system control. Nat Med 2004;10:801–805.

45 Mucida D, Park Y, Kim G, Turovskaya O, Scott I, Kronenberg M, Cheroutre H: Reciprocal TH17 and regulatory T cell differentiation mediated by retinoic acid. Science 2007;317:256–260.

46 Bettelli E, Oukka M, Kuchroo VK: Th-17 cells in the circle of immunity and autoimmunity. Nat Immunol 2007;8:345–350.

47 Ryan KR, Lawson CA, Lorenzi AR, Arkwright PD, Isaacs JD, Lilic D: CD4+CD25+ T-regulatory cells are decreased in patients with autoimmune polyendocrinopathy candidiasis ectodermal dystrophy. J Allergy Clin Immunol 2005;116:1158–1159.

48 Montagnoli C, Bacci A, Bozza S, Gaziano R, Mosci P, Sharpe AH, Romani L: B7/CD28-dependent CD4+CD25+ regulatory T cells are essential components of the memory-protective immunity to *Candida albicans*. J Immunol 2002;169:6298–6308.

49 Puccetti P, Grohmann U: IDO and regulatory T cells: a role for reverse signaling and non-canonical NF-κB activation. Nat Rev Immunol 2007;7: 817–823.

50 Fallarino F, Grohmann U, Hwang KW, Orabona C, Vacca C, Bianchi R, Belladonna ML, Fioretti MC, Alegre ML, Puccetti P: Modulation of tryptophan catabolism by regulatory T cells. Nat Immunol 2003;4:1206–1212.

51 Grohmann U, Volpi C, Fallarino F, Bozza S, Bianchi R, Vacca C, Orabona C, Belladonna ML, Ayroldi E, Nocentini G, Boon L, Bistoni F, Fioretti MC, Romani L, Riccardi C, Puccetti P: Reverse signaling through GITR ligand enables dexamethasone to activate IDO in allergy. Nat Med 2007;13:579–586.

52 Judson MA, Stevens DA: Current pharmacotherapy of allergic bronchopulmonary aspergillosis. Expert Opin Pharmacother 2001;2:1065–1071.

53 Wills-Karp M, Santeliz J, Karp CL: The germless theory of allergic disease: revisiting the hygiene hypothesis. Nat Rev Immunol 2001;1:69–75.

54 Bach JF: The effect of infections on susceptibility to autoimmune and allergic diseases. N Engl J Med 2002; 347:911–920.

55 Rakoff-Nahoum S, Paglino J, Eslami-Varzaneh F, Edberg S, Medzhitov R: Recognition of commensal microflora by toll-like receptors is required for intestinal homeostasis. Cell 2004;118: 229–241.

56 Neish AS, Gewirtz AT, Zeng H, Young AN, Hobert ME, Karmali V, Rao AS, Madara JL: Prokaryotic regulation of epithelial responses by inhibition of IκB-α ubiquitination. Science 2000; 289:1560–1563.

57 Gurtner GJ, Newberry RD, Schloemann SR, McDonald KG, Stenson WF: Inhibition of indoleamine 2,3-dioxygenase augments trinitrobenzene sulfonic acid colitis in mice. Gastroenterology 2003;125:1762–1773.

58 Padrid PA, Mathur M, Li X, Herrmann K, Qin Y, Cattamanchi A, Weinstock J, Elliott D, Sperling AI, Bluestone JA: CTLA4Ig inhibits airway eosinophilia and hyperresponsiveness by regulating the development of Th1/Th2 subsets in a murine model of asthma. Am J Respir Cell Mol Biol 1998;18:453–462.

59 Hayashi T, Beck L, Rossetto C, Gong X, Takikawa O, Takabayashi K, Broide DH, Carson DA, Raz E: Inhibition of experimental asthma by indoleamine 2,3-dioxygenase. J Clin Invest 2004; 114:270–279.

60 Von Bubnoff D, Fimmers R, Bogdanow M, Matz H, Koch S, Bieber T: Asymptomatic atopy is associated with increased indoleamine 2,3-dioxygenase activity and interleukin-10 production during seasonal allergen exposure. Clin Exp Allergy 2004;34: 1056–1063.

61 Hessel EM, Chu M, Lizcano JO, Chang B, Herman N, Kell SA, Wills-Karp M, Coffman RL: Immunostimulatory oligonucleotides block allergic airway inflammation by inhibiting Th2 cell activation and IgE-mediated cytokine induction. J Exp Med 2005;202: 1563–1573.

62 Zaph C, Troy AE, Taylor BC, Berman-Booty LD, Guild KJ, Du Y, Yost EA, Gruber AD, May MJ, Greten FR, Eckmann L, Karin M, Artis D: Epithelial-cell-intrinsic IKK-β expression regulates intestinal immune homeostasis. Nature 2007;446:552–556.

Luigina Romani, MD, PhD
Department of Experimental Medicine and Biochemical Sciences
University of Perugia
Via del Giochetto, IT–06122 Perugia (Italy)
Tel./Fax +39 075 585 3411, E-Mail lromani@unipg.it

Blaser K (ed): T Cell Regulation in Allergy, Asthma and Atopic Skin Diseases.
Chem Immunol Allergy. Basel, Karger, 2008, vol 94, pp 138–149

Control of Delayed-Type Hypersensitivity by Ocular-Induced CD8+ Regulatory T Cells

Robert E. Cone · Subhasis Chattopadhyay · James O'Rourke

Department of Immunology and the Connecticut Lions Vascular Vision Center,
University of Connecticut Health Center, Farmington, Conn., USA

Abstract

The immunoregulatory pathway from the eye to the peripheral immune system is comprised of the iris, ciliary body, circulation, thymus and spleen, and is influenced by the sympathetic nervous system. At the splenic end of this pathway are antigen-specific CD8+ regulatory T cells (Tregs) that mediate directly the suppression of T cells that effect delayed-type hypersensitivity (DTH). Here we review investigations that demonstrate: (i) the injection of antigen into the anterior chamber (AC) attracts circulating monocytic cells to the iris/ciliary body that recirculate to the thymus and spleen. In the thymus, ocular-influenced monocytic cells activate natural killer T (NKT) cells that migrate to the spleen where, in concert with the ocular-influenced monocytic emigrants, they (ii) activate CD4+ and CD8+ immunoregulatory T cells. (iii) The generation of the CD8+ Tregs is dependent on NKT cells in the thymus and the periphery that are influenced by the sympathetic nervous system. (iv) The suppression of DTH by the AC-induced CD8+ Tregs is dependent on the cytokines transforming growth factor-β and interferon-γ and is restricted by the expression of major histocompatibility complex-associated Qa-1^b antigens. In aggregate, this oculo-thymic-splenic pathway is a well-controlled response to ocular injury that utilizes a systemic response to antigen that may protect ocular tissue and systemic tissue.

'What's past is prologue'
William Shakespeare, The Tempest

Almost 40 years ago, in the heady days of the birth of T-cell immunobiology, as immunologists intensely investigated T-cell interactions with B cells and antigen presenting cells that *promoted* an immune response, Gershon and his colleagues [1, 2] presented an observation and (courageous) proposal that T cells also *downregulated* an immune response in an antigen-specific manner. The paradigm that developed from the information generated by many laboratories was that 'helper T cells' (Lyt-1, today's CD4+ cell) induced the activation of Lyt-2 (today's CD8+ T cell) 'suppressor' T cells that performed the suppression of the activation and/or activity of effector T cells. These complex interactions were antigen-specific and replete with 'feedback' mechanisms. The CD8+ suppressor T cells that were demonstrated suppressed the induction of antibody formation, the delayed-type hypersensitivity (DTH) response and the generation of cytotoxic T cells. The suppressor T cells were defined as: (1) antigen-specific; (2) inducible by antigen, and (3) CD8+.

Suppressor T cells were also shown to express a major histocompatibility complex (MHC) class II marker, I-J. However, because I-J was never cloned and its presence in the MHC never shown formally, there was considerable doubt as to the significance of I-J [reviewed in 3, 4].

Almost coincident with Gershon's untimely passing, doubts were raised about the concept of cell-mediated immunoregulation. However, after a long interregnum, cell-mediated immunoregulation was revived with the description of naturally occurring, thymus-derived CD4+, CD25+, FoxP3+ regulatory T cells (Tregs) that exert a non-(antigen)-specific regulation of the activation of T or B cells [5, 6]. In general, Tregs have been shown to regulate antigen-induced proliferation in vitro and/or the induction or manifestations of autoimmunity in vivo. Presently, in addition to Treg, other CD4+ T cells and T cells expressing the NK1.1 marker (NKT) expressed by natural killer cells perform a significant immunoregulatory function [reviewed in 3, 7]. These T cells, as first demonstrated earlier, also participate in the induction of CD8+ suppressor T cells (see below). Presently, there is renewed attention on cell-mediated immune regulation and a growing list of Tregs, B cells and antigen presenting cells [7]. Significantly, CD8+ suppressor T cells mediate the antigen-specific suppression of T-cell effector activity as well as the induction of effector T cells. This suppressor T-cell population may be comprised of several phenotypically distinct CD8+ T cells [8]. Ironically, these cells are sometimes referred to as a 'new' Treg. To be consistent with current usage we will use the terminology CD8+ Treg (rather than suppressor T cell) for cells that mediate directly the suppression of effector T cells. Despite the description of CD8+ Tregs years ago, there are still questions concerning: (1) the mechanism(s) of the activation of CD8+ suppressor T cells; (2) the nature of the specificity of CD8+ suppressor T cells, and (3) the mechanisms of the suppression of effector cells by CD8+ suppressor T cells.

Because the CD8+ Treg is specific for the inducing antigen [1–4, 7], the isolation and/or investigation of these cells is limited by their clonal distribution. Moreover, CD8+ Tregs are generated during a Th1-biased immune response [7, 9]. Therefore, unraveling the mechanisms of activation of these cells is difficult because of the many immune-related events that induce their generation.

Suppression of Cell-Mediated Immunity by CD8+ Regulatory T Cells

Suppressor T Cells Redux

Although early work with CD8+ suppressor T cells centered on the suppression of antibody responses in vitro [1, 2], more recent investigations demonstrate a profound CD8+ T-cell-mediated regulation of cell-mediated in vivo immune responses (table 1) including the induction of experimental autoimmune encephalomyelitis (EAE). Moreover, CD8+ Treg-mediated suppression may be directed towards epitopes expressed by TCR variable regions [3, 14]. If these Tregs are 'anti-TCR idiotypic', the generation of these cells is likely dependent on an immune response. In that regard, CD8+ Tregs are usually detected *later* in an immune response [3]. Most of the reports of CD8+ T-cell regulation of autoimmunity do not discriminate between the suppression of the induction of the autoimmune disease and suppression of the effector T cells. Preliminary work by our laboratory has shown that splenic CD8+ cells generated by the injection of myelin basic protein into the ocular anterior chamber (AC) suppress the antigen-induced production of interferon (IFN)-γ by a CD4+ encephalitogenic T-cell clone and the induction of EAE by that clone but do not suppress the proliferation of that clone induced by antigen. However, this may be due to an artifact because the activity of CD8+

Table 1. Suppression of cell-mediated immunity by CD8+ suppressor T cells

Response	In vitro	In vivo	IV	ID	Induction	Effector	Ref.[1]
DTH		+	–	+	–	+	
Protein		+	–	+	–	+	3, 7, 9–13,
Peptide		+	–	+	–	+	16
Hapten (CS)		+	–	+	–	+	
EAE		+	+	nt	+	+	3, 7, 10, 15
Antigen-induced proliferation	±	–					17
Antigen-induced cytokine production	+				nt	+	17

CS = Contact sensitivity; EAE = experimental autoimmune encephalomyelitis; nt = not tested.
[1]Not comprehensive.

Tregs diminishes with time [R.E. Cone and A.T. Vella, unpubl. observations].

Suppression of the DTH Response

The induction and regulation of CD8+ Tregs in vivo is complex and dependent on several cell types [2, 3]. In vivo, the induction of CD8+ suppressor T cells required Lyt-1+ (CD4) 'suppressor-inducer T cells that did not *directly* suppress DTH. The mechanism of this induction was not clear but appeared to be mediated by antigen-specific, soluble molecules produced by the 'suppressor-inducer' T cells [18]. Additionally, the in vivo induction of CD8+ suppressor T cells requires cells sensitive to the cytotoxic effects of cyclophosphamide [19, 20].

The suppression of DTH (in vivo) by CD8+ Tregs affords a direct demonstration of the suppressive effects of these cells on effector T cells because adoptive transfer assays demonstrate a suppressive effect on the DTH response within 24 h of the introduction of CD8+ Tregs into the challenge site for DTH *at the time of challenge with the antigen*. The ability of CD8+ suppressor T cells to suppress directly DTH in vivo has been measured by the local adoptive transfer assay (LAT) that transfers DTH to naive recipients by

the transfer of Tregs with immune T cells and challenge with antigen [21] or by the local transfer of suppression (LTS); an injection of Tregs into immunized animals at the site challenged with antigen [12]. In the LAT a suppressive population of cells inhibits the DTH reaction elicited by the transferred immune cells that occurs within 24 h of challenge with antigen. The LTS [12], like the LAT, selectively measures the direct suppressive activity of CD8+ suppressor cells on effector T cells in DTH. However, CD4+ T cells (that would include CD4+, CD25+, FoxP3+ Tregs) do not suppress the contact sensitivity *reaction*. Moreover, the suppression of contact sensitivity by spleen cells recovered from mice that received an injection of trinitrophenylated bovine serum albumin into the AC (AC-SPL cells, i.e. spleen cells from donors that received an injection of antigen into the AC) is specific for the antigen that induced the CD8+ AC-SPL Tregs [12, 17]. The LTS is sufficiently sensitive such that as few as 1,500 cells containing suppressor T cells suppress DTH [R.E. Cone and R. Sharafieh, unpubl. observations]. Since as little as one effector cell can mediate a DTH reaction [22], it is not surprising that very few suppressor

T cells could suppress the in vivo response. Moreover, immunization of the donors of suppressor T cells increases the number of splenic CD8+ suppressor T cells that suppress specifically DTH in the LTS [R.E. Cone, Y. Lemire, and R. Sharafieh, unpubl. observations]. These observations are consistent with those demonstrating that antigen-specific CD8+ suppressor T cells are amplified by immunization [3].

Induction of Splenic CD8+ Suppressor T Cells via the Eye's Anterior Chamber

CD8+ suppressor T cells have been induced by 'tolerogenic protocols' such as the intravenous injection of antigen (without adjuvant), ingestion of antigen [reviewed in 3] and the injection of antigen into the AC of the eye. The injection of antigen into the AC induces the antigen-specific suppression of DTH (and other forms of cell-mediated immunity) as well as the suppression of IgG2 antibodies specific for the antigen injected into the AC [reviewed in 10]. This model of anterior chamber-associated immune deviation (ACAID) has provided insight into the complex cellular pathways that induce and/or regulate the systemic production of CD8+ suppressor T cells that mediate the suppression of DTH (fig. 1). ACAID can be transferred to naive or immunized mice by monocytic cells expressing the macrophage marker F4/80 [23–27]. It is believed that circulating monocytic cells from donors that received an injection of antigen into the AC (intracameral injection) are derived from the AC of the eye, probably the iris and ciliary body. The ability of resident monocytic iris cells to migrate from the iris has been questioned [28, 29]. However, ACAID can be transferred or splenic CD8+ Tregs induced by less than 100 ACAID-inducing monocytic cells [10] suggesting that the number of cells leaving the iris could be very small. Additionally, the injection of antigen into the AC, indeed, injection only, induces the influx of circulating monocytic cells [30] that probably interact with iris dendritic cells and transforming growth factor (TGF)-β in aqueous humor that could induce a suppressive phenotype in the F4/80+ cells. Exposure of F4/80+ peritoneal exudate cells ex vivo to TGF-β and antigen or monocytic iris cells from a donor that received an intercameral injection of antigen 'converts' these cells to a suppressive phenotype similar to that of circulating monocytic cells found after the intracameral injection of antigen [24, 26, 31]. The F4/80+ cells that entered the eye migrate from the eye to the thymus and spleen [30] and in the spleen, CD8+ T cells and the F4/80+ cells interact with Qa-1+ B lymphocytes [32], NKT cells [33] and recent thymic NKT cell emigrants (Thy$_{reg}$ activated by ocular-derived F4/80+ cells that migrated to the thymus) [12]. The induction of splenic CD8+ Tregs after the injection of antigen into the AC is highly specific to the antigen injected into the AC [10, 12]. Because the induction and cellular transfer of the suppression of DTH is antigen-specific, either the antigen-specific Thy$_{reg}$ are a subpopulation of NKT cells or an additional population of antigen-specific (or antigen-bearing) cells in the thymocyte population is transferred. Moreover, the CD4–, CD8–, NK1.1+ recent thymic emigrants do not become peripheral CD4+ NKT cells or the CD8+ Tregs that activate or mediate (respectively) the suppression of DTH [12]. The mechanism of participation of the recent thymic emigrants and/or the peripheral CD4+ T cells in the induction of the generation or activity of the CD8+ Tregs is not known. However, preliminary results from our laboratory suggest that the CD4+ T cells may provide the IFN-γ that facilitates the DTH-suppressive activity of the CD8+ Tregs [34, and see below]

Afferent and Efferent Mechanisms for Ocular-Induced CD8+ Regulatory T Cells

The peripheral immune system is highly innervated by sympathetic neurons that exert potent

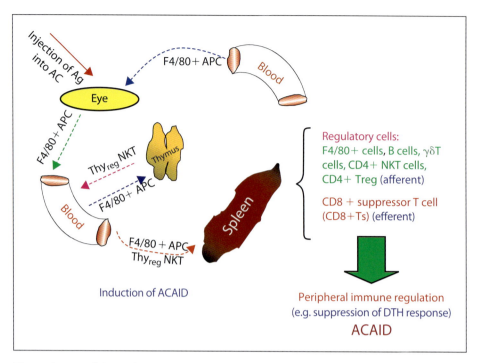

Fig. 1. Organ/cellular pathways in the induction of CD8+ suppressor T cells by the injection of antigen into the anterior chamber (AC). The injection of antigen into the AC induces a recruitment of F4/80+ monocytic cells to the iris. Interactions with iris monocytic cells, antigen and TGF-β in aqueous humor induces an immunosuppressive phenotype in the recruited cells. These cells then recirculate from the AC to the thymus and the spleen. In the spleen, F4/80+ cells interact with B cells, peripheral NKT cells, recent thymic NKT emigrants and CD8+ T cells with the generation of CD8+ suppressor T cells that effect the suppression of a DTH reaction.

regulation of an immune response [35–38]. For example, DTH-induced swelling (but not the production of IFN-γ) is not induced in mice whose sympathetic nervous system (SNS) has been ablated chemically by the injection of the SNS-neurotoxic 6-hydroxydopamine (OHDA) although immunized, 6-OHDA-treated mice make more IgM and IgG1 and antibodies in response to the injected antigen than untreated mice [37]. This apparent immune deviation in chemically sympathectomized mice is also reflected in mice that do not express receptors for SNS-derived neuropeptide Y (NPY) [38].

6-OHDA-treated mice do not produce splenic CD8+ Tregs detected in the LTS after the injection

of antigen into the AC [38]. However, peripheral blood monocytes that transfer the induction of the suppression of DTH after the injection of antigen into the AC are not affected by 6-OHDA. Functional regulatory thymic NKT cells are not recovered from mice receiving 6-OHDA and the number of liver NKT cells required for the induction of DTH [39] is diminished in 6-OHDA-treated mice [36]. Since the production of splenic suppressor T cells is restored in 6-OHDA-treated mice by functional regulatory thymocytes from AC-injected donors, it is likely 6-OHDA affects thymic and liver NKT cells but not the precursors of suppressor T cells. Although thymic NKT cells are required for the induction of the suppressor-

Cone · Chattopadhyay · O'Rourke

effector cells, the role of liver NKT cells for the *induction* of splenic CD8+ Tregs is not known. Additionally, the role of the SNS in the activation/activity of splenic CD8+ Tregs raises significant issues concerning the effects of stress on the generation and/or maintenance of immune regulation that impacts on immune defense and the regulation of autoimmune disease. In this regard, chemical sympathectomy potentiates the induction of EAE [40]. This may be due in part to a loss in the induction of CD8+ Tregs in chemically sympathectomized mice.

The mechanisms of the influence of the SNS on the induction of CD8+ Tregs are likely directed towards both the activation and function of these cells (fig. 2). Sympathetic neurons are a source of (i) norepinephrine that has strong immunoregulatory effects [35] including the proliferation of liver NKT cells necessary for the initiation of contact sensitivity reactions; (ii) immunomodulatory NPY [38] that may promote the production of IFN-γ necessary for the function of CD8+ suppressor T cells (see below), and (iii) tissue plasminogen activator (t-PA) [41] that converts plasminogen to plasmin that in turn is an activator of immunosuppressive TGF-β [42].

Antigen Specificity of the Suppression of DTH by CD8+ Regulatory T Cells

CD8+ Tregs with varying (cell surface) phenotypes have been described [reviewed in 8]. It is not known whether these varied phenotypes represent distinct lineages or various states of activation. Nevertheless, because at least eight distinct CD8+ Treg phenotypes have been described, the suppressive mechanisms of these cells may differ.

As discussed above, the LTS facilitates investigations of the mechanisms that enable the suppression of DTH by CD8+ Tregs because the assay is complete within 24 h. In other words, to probe the mechanisms and antigen specificity of suppression, manipulations can be made that only influence the suppression of the DTH response after the immunized mice are challenged.

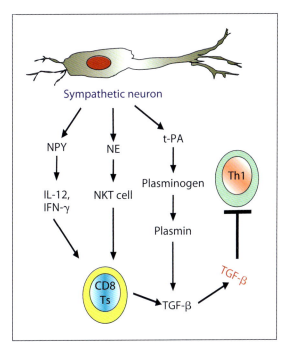

Fig. 2. Sympathetic neurons influence the development or activity of CD8+ suppressor T cells. Sympathetic neurons are a source of neuropeptide Y (NPY), norepinehprine (NE) or tissue plasminogen activator (t-PA) that respectively, (i) activate IL-12, IFN-γ necessary for the activity of suppressor T cells, (ii) NKT cells required to generate CD8+ suppressor T cells after the injection of antigen into the AC, (iii) the conversion of plasminogen to plasmin that activates immunosuppressive TGF-β produced by the CD8+ suppressor T cells.

Because the induction of splenic CD8+ Tregs via the intracameral injection of antigen is specific to the antigen injected into the AC [10], antigen presenting cells must present the cognate antigen to inducer T cells and to the precursors of splenic CD8+ Tregs. The antigen is likely presented to the suppressor T cells in the spleen by B lymphocytes that obtained the antigen from the (migrating) F4/80+ monocytic cells [32]. The specificity of the CD8+ Tregs may be directed towards T-cell receptor (TCR) V-region epitopes [3, 43, 44]. Evidence suggests that the antigen for CD8+

Tregs is a TCR V-region peptide, but direct demonstration that CD8+ Tregs are stimulated by and bind TCR peptides is presently lacking.

Qa-1[b] Restriction of CD8+ Suppressor T-Cell-Mediated Suppression

MHC-associated Qa-1 protein antigens have been implicated as integral and restrictive for the suppressive activity of CD8+ Tregs [3, 7, 14, 32, 43–45]. It has been proposed that CD94/NKG2A receptors for Qa-1:Qa-1[b] interaction-mediated immune regulation may restrict TGF-β-mediated suppression of an immune response [30, 43–45]. Conceivably, the inhibitory arm of CD94/NKG2 becomes effective via NKG2A signaling through the active immunoreceptor tyrosine-based inhibitory motif (ITIM) as compared to its immunoreceptor tyrosine-based activating motif (ITAM) by NKG2C/E [46, 47]. In addition, if the TCR of CD8+ Treg is restricted by Qa-1, suppression may require ligation of Qa-1: peptide complexes on the effector cells. To investigate further an association between the expression of Qa-1[b] antigens and the suppressive activity of CD8+ Tregs derived from donors that received an intracameral injection of antigen (AC-SPL cells), we determined the ability of AC-SPL cells mismatched with immunized recipient mice for MHC class I H2 or Qa-1[b] antigens to suppress recipient DTH in the LTS. AC-SPL cells do not suppress DTH in H-2-matched recipients but suppress contact sensitivity in H-2 mismatched mice that share the Qa-1[b] haplotype with the AC-SPL spleen Tregs [48]. Collectively these data demonstrate that suppression of DTH is not restricted by MHC class I H2 antigens but appears to be associated with the Qa-1[b] haplotype of the recipient of AC-SPL CD8+ Tregs (fig. 3).

Antibodies to CD94 and NKG2A receptors for Qa-1[b] and to Qa-1[b] inhibit the in vivo suppression of DTH by AC-SPL cells when the antibodies are included in the inoculum of AC-SPL cells injected into a DTH challenge site [49]. Moreover, splenic CD8+ suppressor T cells can-

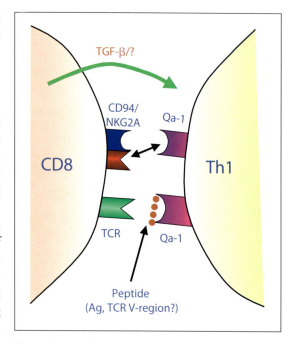

Fig. 3. Proposed suppressive mechanism of CD8+ suppressor T cells. The TCR of suppressor T cells engages Qa-1/peptide (TCR V-region?) on a T effector cells or antigen presenting cells. CD94/NKG2A also engages Qa-1. Engagement of the entire complex triggers the secretion of TGF-β by the suppressor T cell that suppresses the effector T cell that induces the DTH reaction.

not be induced in DBA/2J mice deficient in the expression of Qa-1[b] antigens and CD94/NKG2A receptors for Qa-1[b] by the injection of antigen into the AC [49]. These results, taken together with the results of others, suggest that the CD8+ suppressor T cells induced by intracameral antigen may be specific for TCR V-region peptides presented by Qa-1[b] proteins on Th1 effector cells and/or antigen presenting cells. Here, CD94 would function as a co-receptor by binding to Qa-1[b]. This scheme is analogous to that of CD8 on cytotoxic T cells ligating MHC class I H2 antigens during cell-mediated cytotoxicity. When the TCR/CD94/NKG2A 'connects' to this 'synapse', a signal is transduced to the suppressor T cell to express and/or secrete TGF-β (and/or other

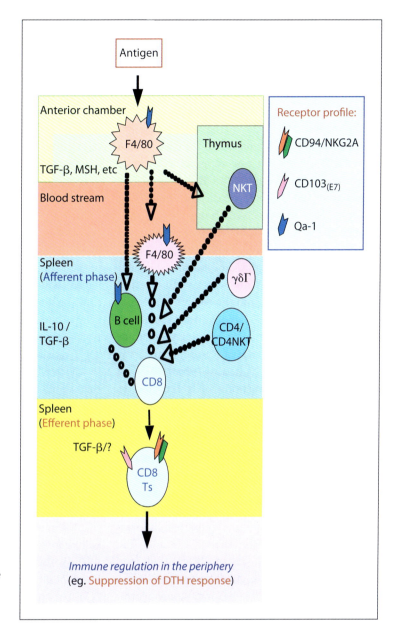

Fig. 4. Cell interactions, cell surface determinants and cytokines in the ACAID pathway to CD8 suppressor T cells.

immunosuppressive cytokines?) that specifically suppress the Th1 'target' cell (fig. 4). The mechanism of CD94/NKG2A-mediated immune regulation on DTH effector cells (Th1 cells) is not known.

IFN-γ Facilitates the Suppression of DTH by Splenic CD8+ Suppressor T Cells

IFN-γ, a major cytokine in cell-mediated immunity, has been shown to also exert strong downregulatory effects on cell-mediated autoimmunity

[50–53]. Because the induction of CD8+ Tregs by intracameral injection of antigen was diminished or absent when mice were immunized to promote a Th1 response, we reasoned that CD8+ Tregs may be dependent on IFN-γ. However, the suppression of contact sensitivity by intracamerally-induced splenic CD8+ Tregs is independent of perforin or Fas ligand [53], indicating that these CD8+ Tregs do not suppress effector T cells by cytotoxicity. Although CD8+ suppressor T cells were not detected readily by the LTS in IFN-γ–/– mice that received an injection of antigen into the AC, the spleen cells from these mice suppressed contact sensitivity if treated with IFN-γ [53]. Moreover, peripheral blood mononuclear cells recovered from IFN-γ–/– mice that received an injection of antigen into the AC are capable of transferring the suppression of contact sensitivity when injected intravenously into recipient mice [R.E. Cone and R. Sharafieh, unpubl. observations] indicating that the lack of IFN-γ does not affect the antigen presenting cells required to induce the splenic CD8+ Tregs. Additionally, IFN-γ does not restore the ability of spleen cells from mice that received an injection of antigen into the AC but lack a receptor for IFN-γ to suppress contact sensitivity. The removal of spleen cells expressing a receptor for IFN-γ from spleen cells recovered from mice receiving intracameral antigen removes all CD8+ T cells that suppress contact sensitivity in the LTS [X. Li and R.E. Cone, unpubl. results]. These observations and the enhancement of contact sensitivity when IFN-γ is injected into the challenge site concomitant with the challenge with antigen indicates that IFN-γ is not directly suppressive in the LTS. Collectively, these observations demonstrated that CD8+ Tregs are generated in the absence of stimulation with IFN-γ but require IFN-γ to perform a suppressive function. This *immediate* effect of IFN-γ on the ability of the CD8+ Tregs to suppress contact sensitivity suggests that IFN-γ may affect the expression of cell surface molecules on the CD8+ regulatory cells required for

suppression, for example CD94/NKG2A receptors for Qa-1, or CD103 [54] and/or the suppressive mechanism itself.

TGF-β Is a Mechanism of CD8+ Treg-Mediated Suppression of DTH

Among the many roles for TGF-β in development and homeostasis, this cytokine plays a major role in the induction and mediation of immunoregulation [55]. TGF-β may be instrumental in the immunoregulatory properties of CD4+ Tregs, but the evidence is indirect. The injection of antibodies to t-PA (an activator of plasmin) that activates TGF-β [56] or antibodies to TGF-β into a site of immunized mice challenged with antigen enhances contact sensitivity [57]. It is notable here that t-PA is produced by sympathetic neurons that influence the generation and possibly the activity of CD8+ suppressor T cells [41, and see below].

CD8+ Tregs produce TGF-β [16, 50, 57, 58] that could be an extracellular and/or cellular mechanism to suppress effector T cells. We have investigated this issue by determining the susceptibility of effector T cells insensitive to TGF-β to the DTH-suppressive mechanisms of T cells induced by the injection of antigen into the AC. The DTH response in the LTS is not suppressed by CD8+ regulatory (spleen) cells stimulated by an injection of antigen into the AC in mice [59] that transgenically express the dominant negative receptor for TGF-β, dnTGF-bRII in all T cells and TGF-β-resistant mice lacking the E3 ubiquitin ligase Cbl-b (Cbl-b–/– mice [60]. Moreover, the inclusion of anti-TGF-β antibodies with the AC-induced suppressor T cells in the LTS blocks the suppression of DTH [R.E. Cone and S. Chattopadhyay, unpubl. results]. Taken together, these results strongly suggest that the suppression of DTH by intracamerally-induced CD8+ Tregs is mediated by TGF-β (fig. 3). Recently, Kapp et al. [61] reported that CD8+ Tregs induced in vitro by TGF-β suppress the rejection of a transplanted heart by TGF-β-independent mechanisms. Since multiple CD8+

Treg phenotypes have been described (see below), it is probable that the mechanisms behind CD8-mediated suppression of a transplanted heart and contact sensitivity differ.

Conclusion

'Those that cannot remember the past are condemned to relive it'

George Santayana

Most of the CD8+ suppressor T cells are distinct from the canonical CD4+, CD25+, FoxP3+ Tregs, although it has been reported that some CD8+ suppressor T cells activated by exogenous TGF-β express the transcription factor FoxP3 [61]. The systemic induction of splenic suppressor T cells via the AC involves interactions between several cell types and the expression of cell surface proteins central to the induction and/or performance of suppression (fig. 4). The in vivo generation of CD8+ suppressor T cells is clearly antigen-driven. Thus, the production of these antigen (TCR V-region?)-specific cells is an immune response that can be measured.

The generation of CD8+ Tregs occurs by special activation during an immune response. Therefore, the means to expand these cells and utilize them therapeutically can be determined so that 'nascent' CD8+ Tregs could be activated by the injection of antigen into the AC or by cytokines (TGF-β?) used to activate antigen presenting cells that in turn participate in ocular pathways that activate CD8+ Tregs.

Acknowledgements

Work in the authors' laboratories is supported by grant EY017289, EY 017537 National Eye Institute, USPHS and the Connecticut Lions Eye Research Foundation.

References

1 Gershon RK, Kondo K: Infectious immunological tolerance. Immunology 1971; 21:903–914.
2 Green D, Flood PM, Gershon RK: Immunoregulatory T cell pathways. Annu Rev Immunol 1983;1:439–463.
3 Jiang H, Chess L: The specific regulation of immune responses by CD8+ T cells restricted by the MHC class IB molecule, Qa-1. Annu Rev Immunol 2000;18:185–216.
4 Dorf ME, Kuchroo VK, Collins M: Suppressor T cells: some answers but more questions. Immunol Today 1992;13: 241–243.
5 Shevach EM: From vanilla to 28 flavors: multiple varieties of T regulatory cells. Immunity 2006;25:195–201.
6 Sakaguchi S, Fukuma K, Kuribayashi K, Masuda T: Organ-specific autoimmune diseases induced in mice by elimination of T cell subset. I. Evidence for the active participation of T cells in natural self-tolerance; deficit of a T cell subset as a possible cause of autoimmune disease. J Exp Med 1985;161:72–85.
7 Jiang H, Chess L: An integrated model of immunoregulation mediated by regulatory T cell subsets. Adv Immunol 2004;83:253–288.
8 Tang XL, Smith R, Kumar V: Specific control of immunity by regulatory CD8 T cells. Cell Mol Immunol 2006;2:1–9.
9 Li X, Taylor S, Zegarelli B, Shen S, O'Rourke J, Cone RE: The induction of splenic suppressor T cells through an immune-privileged site requires an intact sympathetic nervous system. J Neuroimmunol 2004;153:40–49.
10 Niederkorn JY: Regulatory T cells and the eye. Chem Immunol Allergy 2007; 92:131–139.
11 Kosiewicz MM, Streilein JW: Intraocular injection of class II-restricted peptide induces an unexpected population of CD8 regulatory cells. J Immunol 1996;157:1905–1912.
12 Li X, Wang Y, Urso D, O'Rourke J, Cone RE: Thymocytes induced by antigen injection into the anterior chamber activate splenic CD8 suppressor cells and enhance the production of IgG1 antibodies. Immunology 2004;113:44–56.
13 Ptak W, Gershon RK: Immunological agnosis: a state that derives from T suppressor cell inhibition of antigen-presenting cells Proc Natl Acad Sci USA 1982;79:2645–2648.
14 Jiang H, Ware R, Stall A, Flaherty L, Chess L, Pernis B: CD8+ T cells that specifically delete autologous CD4+ T cells expressing Vβ8 TCR: role of the Qa-1 molecule. Immunity 1995;2: 185–194.
15 Faunce DE, Terajewicz A, Stein-Streilein J: In vitro generated tolerogenic APC induce CD8+ T regulatory cells that can suppress ongoing experimental autoimmune encephalomyelitis. J Immunol 2004;172:1991–1998.

16 Szczepanik M, Bryniarski K, Tutaj M, Ptak M, Skrzeczynska J, Askenase PW, Ptak W: Epicutaneous immunization induces αβ T-cell receptor CD4 CD8 double-positive non-specific suppressor T cells that inhibit contact sensitivity via transforming growth factor-β. Immunology 2005;115:42–54.

17 Wang Y, Ghali Wa-el, Pingle P, Traboulsi A, Dalal T, O'Rourke J, Cone RE: Splenic T cells from mice receiving intracameral antigen suppress in-vitro antigen-induced proliferation and interferon-γ production by sensitized lymph node cells. Ocular Immunol Inflamm 2003;11:39–52.

18 Cone RE: Soluble extracellular antigen-specific T cell immunoproteins. J Leuk Biol 1996;59:605–612.

19 Marcinkiewicz J, Bryniarski K, Ptak W: Cyclophosphamide uncovers two separate macrophage subpopulations with opposite immunogenic potential and different patterns of monokine production. Cytokine 1994;6:472–477.

20 Waldrep JC, Kaplan HJ: Anterior chamber-associated immune deviation induced by TNP-splenocytes (TNP-ACAID). II. Suppressor T-cell networks. Invest Ophthalmol Vis Sci 1983; 24:1339–1345.

21 Niederkorn JY, Streilein JW: Characterization of the suppressor cell(s) responsible for anterior chamber-associated immune deviation (ACAID)-induced in BALB/c mice by P815 cells. J Immunol 1985;134:1381–1387.

22 Marchal G, Seman M, Milon G, Truffa-Bachi P, Zilberfarb V: Local adoptive transfer of skin delayed-type hypersensitivity initiated by a single T lymphocyte. J Immunol 1982;129:954–958.

23 Wilbanks GA, Streilein JW: Macrophages capable of inducing anterior chamber-associated immune deviation demonstrate spleen-seeking migratory properties. Reg Immunol 1991;4:130–137.

24 Wilbanks GA, Mammolenti M, Streilein JW: Studies on the induction of anterior chamber-associated immune deviation (ACAID). II. Eye-derived cells participate in generating blood-borne signals that induce ACAID. J Immunol 1991;146:3018–3924.

25 Wang Y, Goldschneider I, O'Rourke J, Cone RE: Blood mononuclear cells induce regulatory NK thymocytes in anterior chamber-associated immune deviation. J Leukoc Biol 2001;69:741–746.

26 Li X, Shen S, Urso D, Kalique S, Park SH, Sharafieh S, O'Rourke J, Cone RE: Phenotypic and immunoregulatory characteristics of monocytic iris cells. Immunology 2006;117:566–575.

27 Lin HH, Faunce DE, Stacey M, Terajewicz A, Nakamura T, Zhang-Hoover J, Kerley M, Mucenski ML, Gordon S, Stein-Streilein J: The macrophage F4/80 receptor is required for the induction of antigen-specific efferent regulatory T cells in peripheral tolerance. J Exp Med 2005;201: 1615–1625.

28 Camelo S, Voon ASP, Blunt S, McMenamin PG: Local retention of soluble antigen by potential antigen presenting cells in the anterior segment of the eye. Invest Ophthalmol Vis Sci 2003;44:5315–5320.

29 Dulforce PA, Garman KL, Seitz GW, Fleischmann RI, Crespo SM, Planck SR, Parker DC, Rosenbaum JT: APCs in the anterior uveal tract do not migrate to draining lymph nodes. J Immunol 2004;172:6701–6708.

30 Cone RE, Chattopadhyay S, Sharafieh R, Li JC, O'Rourke J, Goldschneider I: Intracameral injection of antigen attracts circulating monocytic cells associated with anterior chamber-associated immune deviation to iris, blood and thymus. Association for Research in Vision and Ophthalmology, Annual Meeting, Fort Lauderdale, 2007, Abstr No 5208.

31 Hara Y, Caspi RR, Wiggert B, Dorf M, Streilein JW: Analysis of an in vitro-generated signal that induces systemic immune deviation similar to that elicited by antigen injected into the anterior chamber of the eye. J Immunol 1992;149:1531–1538.

32 D'Orazio TJ, Mayhew E, Niederkorn JY: Ocular immune privilege promoted by the presentation of peptide on tolergenic B cells in the spleen. II. Evidence for presentation by Qa-1. J Immunol 2001;166:26–32.

33 Faunce DE, Sonoda K-H, Stein-Streilein J: MIP-2 mediated recruitment of NKT cells to the spleen during tolerance induction. J Immunol 2001; 166:313–321.

34 Cone RE, Li X, Sharafieh R, O'Rourke J, Vella AT: The suppression of delayed-type hypersensitivity by CD8+ regulatory T cells requires interferon-γ. Immunology 2007;120: 112–119.

35 Elenkov IJ, Wilder RL, Chrousos GP, Vizi SS: The sympathetic nerve – an integrative interface between two supersystems: the brain and the immune system. Pharmacol Rev 2000; 52:595–628.

36 Li X, Taylor S, Zegarelli B, Shen S, O'Rourke J, Cone RE: The induction of splenic suppressor T cells through an immune-privileged site requires an intact sympathetic nervous system. J Neuroimmunol 2004;153:40–49.

37 Madden KS, Felten SY, Felten DF, Sundaresan PR, Livnat S: Sympathetic neural modulation of the immune system. Brain Behav Immun 1989;3:72–83.

38 Wheway J, Mackay CR, Newton RA, Sainsbury A, Boey D, Herzog H, Mackay FA: fundamental bimodal role for neuropeptide Y1 receptor in the immune system. J Exp Med 2005;202: 1527–1538.

39 Campos RA, Szczepanik M, Lisbonne M, Itakura A, Leite-de-Moraes M, Askenase PW, Cone RE: Invariant NKT cells rapidly activated via immunization with diverse contact antigens collaborate in vitro with B-1 cells to initiate contact sensitivity. J Immunol 2006; 177:3686–3694.

40 Pal E, Tabira T: Autonomic regulation of experimental autoimmune encephalomyelitis: the role of interferon-γ. Neuroimmunomodulation 2002;10:80–84.

41 Jiang X, Wang Y, Hand AR, Gillies C, Cone RE, Kirk J, O'Rourke J: Storage and release of tissue plasminogen activator by sympathetic axons in resistance vessel walls. Microvasc Res 2002; 64:438–447.

42 Gomez-Duran A, Mulero-Navarro S, Chang X, Fernandez-Salguero PM: LTBP-1 blockade in dioxin receptor-null mouse embryo fibroblasts decreases TGF-β activity: role of extracellular proteases plasmin and elastase. J Cell Biochem 2006;97:380–392.

43 Jiang H, Curran S, Ruiz-Vazquez E, Liang B, Winchester R, Chess L: Regulatory CD8+ T cells fine-tune the myelin basic protein-reactive T cell receptor Vβ repertoire during experimental autoimmune encephalomyelitis. Proc Natl Acad Sci USA 2003;100:8378–8383.

44 Tang X, Maricic I, Purohit N, Bakamjian B, Reed-Loisel LM, Beeston T, Jensen P, Kumar V: Regulation of immunity by a novel population of Qa-1-restricted CD8αα+TCRαβ+>+T cells. J Immunol 2006;177:7645–7655.

45 Noble A, Zhao ZS, Cantor H: Suppression of immune responses by CD8 cells. II. Qa-1 on activated B cells stimulates CD8 cell suppression of T-helper 2 responses. J Immunol 1998; 160:566–571.

46 Bertone S, Schiavetti F, Bellomo R, Vitale C, Ponte M, Moretta L, Mingari MC: Transforming growth factor-β-induced expression of CD94/NKG2A inhibitory receptors in human T lymphocytes. Eur J Immunol 1999;29:23.

47 Gunturi A, Berg RE, Crossley E, Murray S, Forman J: The role of TCR stimulation and TGF-β in controlling the expression of CD94/NKG2A receptors on CD8 T cells. Eur J Immunol 2005;35:766–775.

48 Cone RE, Sharafieh R, O'Rourke J, Vella AT: Intracameral antigen induces Qa-1-restricted splenic regulatory (suppressor) T cells that required interferon-γ to induce suppression. Association of Research in Vision and Ophthalmology, Annual Meeting, Fort Lauderdale, 2006, abstr 5152.

49 Chattopadhyay S, O'Rourke J, Cone RE: Implication for the CD94/NKG2A-Qa-1 system in the generation and function of ocular-induced splenic CD8+ regulatory T cells. Int Immunol 2008;20:509–516.

50 Myers L, Croft M, Kwon BS, Mittler RS, Vella AT: Peptide-specific CD8 regulatory T cells use IFN-γ to elaborate TGF-β-based suppression. J Immunol 2005;174:7625–7632.

51 Sawitzki B, Kingsley CI, Oliveira V, Karim M, Herber M, Wood KJ: IFN-γ production by alloantigen-reactive regulatory T cells is important for their regulatory function in vivo. J Exp Med 2005;201:1925–1935.

52 Hachem PM, Lisbonne M, Michel L, Diem S, Roongapinun S, Lefort J, Marchal G, Herbelin A, Askenase PW, Dy M, Leite-de-Moraes MC: α-Galactosylceramide-induced iNKT cells suppress experimental allergic asthma in sensitized mice: role of IFN-γ. Eur J Immunol 2005;35:2793–2802.

53 Cone RE, Li X, Sharafieh R, O'Rourke J, Vella AT: The suppression of delayed-type hypersensitivity by CD8+ regulatory T cells requires interferon-γ. Immunology 2006;120: 112–119.

54 Keino H, Masli S, Sasaki S, Streilein JW, Stein-Streilein J: CD8+ T regulatory cells use a novel genetic program that includes CD103 to suppress Th1 immunity in eye-derived tolerance. Invest Ophthalmol Vis Sci 2006;47:1533–1542.

55 Wahl SM, Wen J, Moutsopoulos N: TGF-β: a mobile purveyor of immune privilege. Immunol Rev 2006;213: 213–227.

56 Bickerstaff AA, Xia D, Pelletier RP, Orosz CG: Mechanisms of graft acceptance: evidence that plasminogen activator controls donor-reactive delayed-type hypersensitivity responses in cardiac allograft acceptor mice. J Immunol 2000;164:5132–5139.

57 Kezuka T, Streilein JW: In vitro generation of regulatory CD8+ T cells similar to those found in mice with anterior chamber-associated immune deviation. Invest Ophthalmol Vis Sci 2000; 41:1803–1811

58 Menoret A, Myers LM, Lee S-J, Mittler RS, Rossi RJ, Vella AT: TGF-β protein processing and activity through TCR triggering of primary CD8+ T regulatory cells. J Immunol 2006;177: 6091–6097.

59 Fahlen L, Read S, Gorelik L, Hurst SD, Coffman RL, Flavell RA, Powrie F: T cells that cannot respond to TGF-β escape control by CD4+CD25+ regulatory T cells. J Exp Med 2005;201: 737–746.

60 Wohlfert EA, Gorelik L, Mittler R, Flavell RA, Clark RB: Cutting edge: deficiency in the E3 ubiquitin ligase Cbl-b results in a multifunctional defect in T cell TGF-β sensitivity in vitro and in vivo. J Immunol 2006; 176:1316–1320.

61 Kapp JA, Honjo K, Kapp LM, Xu X, Cozier A, Bucy RP: TCR transgenic CD8+ T cells activated in the presence of TGF-ß express FoxP3 and mediate linked suppression of primary immune responses and cardiac allograft rejection. Int Immunol 2006;18:1549–1562.

Robert E. Cone, PhD
Department of Immunology and the Connecticut Lions Vascular Vision Center
University of Connecticut Health Center
Farmington, CT 06030-3105 (USA)
Tel. +1 860 675 6095, Fax +1 860 675 2936, E-Mail Cone@UCHC.EDU

Blaser K (ed): T Cell Regulation in Allergy, Asthma and Atopic Skin Diseases.
Chem Immunol Allergy. Basel, Karger, 2008, vol 94, pp 150–157

Novel Therapeutic Strategies by Regulatory T Cells in Allergy

Eyad Elkord

Immunology Group, Paterson Institute for Cancer Research, University of Manchester,
Manchester, UK

Abstract

Natural CD4+CD25+FoxP3+ regulatory T cells (Treg) actively suppress physiological and pathological responses, therefore playing a critical role in controlling peripheral tolerance to self antigens and maintaining immune homeostasis. In normal individuals, natural Treg and interleukin-10-secreting Treg are able to suppress Th2 responses to allergens, whereas lower levels of Treg or defect in their functionality have been described as potential mechanisms for inducing allergic diseases. In animal models, adoptive transfer of CD4+CD25+ Treg has been shown as a promising strategy for preventing or treating allergic disorders. Recent studies show that induction of Treg activity is associated with suppression of allergic responses in allergic patients treated with specific immunotherapy. Herein, I review the potential of Treg as exciting targets for developing new immunotherapeutic strategies for treating allergic diseases.   Copyright © 2008 S. Karger AG, Basel

Immune and autoimmune responses are controlled by a fine balance between T-effector cells (Teff) and T-regulatory cells (Treg), thus generating and maintaining immune homeostasis [1]. The balance between regulatory and inflammatory immune responses to allergens is the key element for generating either immune tolerance or allergic response, and the induction of peripheral T-cell tolerance is crucial for treating allergic diseases.

In the recent few years, different populations of Treg have been described and characterized. Natural CD4+CD25+FoxP3+ Treg are generated in the thymus and require cell-cell contact for suppression. They maintain Teff responses in the periphery and their depletion results in increased Teff proliferation and consequently developing various autoimmune diseases. Signalling through the α-chain of the high-affinity interleukin (IL)-2 receptor (CD25) is essential for the differentiation and survival of Treg in vivo [2]. Indeed, CD25 is expressed on Treg as well as activated T cells, thereby limiting its utility as a specific marker for Treg. Mutations in the transcription factor FoxP3/Foxp3 are associated with severe autoimmune diseases in human and mouse. Although FoxP3 is accepted as a relatively specific marker, a definitive marker for natural Treg has not yet been identified. Clearly FoxP3 is intracellularly expressed and this limits its value for isolating viable Treg for further characterization and manipulation. In the last few years, several groups performed extensive research for identifying unique surface markers for Treg. Recently, the α chain of the IL-7 receptor (CD127) [3] and CD39 in association with CD73 [4] have been described as more specific markers expressed on FoxP3+ Treg. The identification of these recent Treg surface markers might facilitate further the investigation of Treg role in different clinical aspects, including allergic diseases.

Inducible CD4+CD25+FoxP3+ Treg can be generated in the periphery from naive CD4+ CD25– T cells under the influence of tumour growth factor (TGF)-β [5]. Inducible Treg include Tr1 and Th3, which secrete high levels of IL-10 and TGF-β, respectively. They arise from naive T cells in the periphery and exert their suppressive activity through their immunosuppressive cytokines.

Recent evidence suggests that natural and inducible Treg may directly or indirectly influence different cells involved in allergic reactions, including mast cells, basophils and eosinophils.

Role of T-Regulatory Cells in Inhibiting Allergic Diseases

Implications from Mouse Models

Although the role of natural and inducible Treg in controlling allergic diseases remains poorly understood, there is some compelling evidence from mouse models supporting their essential role in suppressing allergic diseases through cell-cell contact or increased production of IL-10 and/or TGF-β. Tr1 cells, one type of inducible Treg, are known to secrete high levels of IL-10 (therefore called IL-10-secreting Treg) with or without TGF-β production. The role of Tr1 cells in inhibiting antigen-specific Th2 responses (both proliferation and cytokine production) in vivo was confirmed by the adoptive transfer of Tr1 cell clones into an immediate hypersensitivity OVA-sensitized mice model [6]. Treating mice with a killed *Mycobacterium vaccae* suspension induces allergen-specific Treg which protect against airway inflammation in IL-10 and TGF-β-mediated mechanisms [7]. Additionally, infecting mice with helminth downregulates allergic reactions through elevated numbers of CD4+

CD25+FoxP3+ Treg and higher TGF-β and IL-10 expression in mesenteric lymph node cells [8]. Transfer of OVA peptide-specific CD4+CD25+ Treg induces IL-10-dependent inhibition of multiple pathophysiological characteristics of allergic airway disease in an OVA-sensitized mouse model [9]. Interestingly, depletion of CD4+ CD25+ T cells in vivo using anti-CD25 antibody in airway hyperresponsiveness (AHR)-resistant mice before contact with house dust mite increases several allergic-related symptoms, whereas no allergen-induced AHR are reported in AHR-susceptible mice [10]. The role of natural and inducible Treg in inhibiting allergic diseases in mouse models is illustrated in figure 1.

Evidence for Targeting Treg Cells

Some recent studies have shown that both natural and inducible Treg are key players in suppressing allergen-specific Th2 responses, and consequently inhibiting the development of allergic disorders. In healthy donors, natural CD4+CD25+ Treg suppress proliferation to self, dietary and foreign antigens [11], and their depletion from peripheral blood increases proliferation and Th2 cytokine production in response to nickel (a cause of allergic-contact dermatitis) [12]. The dominant subpopulation of allergen-specific T cells are of the IL-10-secreting Tr1 cells in non-atopic healthy individuals, while these cells are of the IL-4-secreting Th2 cells in atopic patients [1]. This confirms the important role played by IL-10-secreting Tr1 cells in controlling allergic responses. Importantly, Umetsu and co-workers [13, 14] have shown in two studies that CD4+ T cells engineered to secrete TGF-β or IL-10 are able to effectively reverse allergen-induced AHR and inflammation.

The essential role of Treg cells in suppressing allergic responses is inferred from the downregulation of Treg activity systemically and in situ in allergic patients. There has been a defect in corticosteroid-induced IL-10 production in T cells isolated from corticosteroid-resistant asthmatic

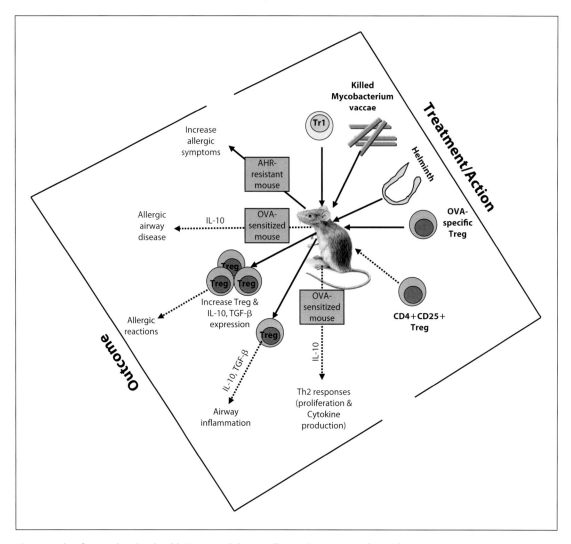

Fig. 1. Role of natural and inducible Treg in inhibiting allergic diseases as inferred from mouse models. Treg suppress allergic reactions through cell-cell contact or increased secretion of IL-10 and/or TGF-β. Depletion of CD25+ cells induces allergic symptoms in AHR-resistant mice but not in AHR-susceptible mice. Continuous arrows indicate induction; dashed arrows indicate inhibition, downregulation or depletion; mechanism of action is shown in blue.

patients compared with corticosteroid-sensitive patients [15]. Proliferation and IL-5 secretion in allergen-stimulated CD4+CD25– Teff cells from non-atopic individuals is effectively suppressed by autologous CD4+CD25+ Treg, while this suppression is significantly diminished in hay fever patients, especially during the pollen season [16]. Depleting CD4+CD25+ Treg from peripheral blood of non-atopic individuals induces a similar pattern of proliferation and Th2-cytokine production to atopic patients in response to allergen stimulation [16]. CD4+CD25high Treg frequency and suppressive activity (both proliferation and cytokine/chemokine production) are reduced in bronchoalveolar lavage fluid of asthmatic children compared to children with chronic cough or healthy controls [17]. Interestingly, inhaled corticosteroid treatment is associated with increased frequency and suppressive activity of Treg in peripheral blood and bronchoalveolar lavage fluid [17]. This study implies that pulmonary Treg might be a potential target for treating asthmatic children. Furthermore, CD4+CD25+FoxP3+ Treg infiltration was reported to be absent in atopic dermatitis lesions, despite the significant expression of Tr1 cells in the dermis [18]. Surprisingly, it has recently been reported that atopic patients with active disease have lower levels of circulating CD4+FoxP3+ T cells compared with asymptomatic control subjects with similar levels of serum IFN-γ, total IgE, and eosinophils, implying that Treg regulate unknown factors unrelated to Th1/Th2 responses [19].

Therapeutic Strategies for Modulating Treg Activity in Allergy

Manipulation of Treg for therapeutic purposes has been hindered by the inability of Treg to proliferate in vitro in different systems. Recently, large-scale in vitro expansion of human CD4+CD25^{high} Treg has been achieved following stimulation with anti-CD3/CD28 antibody-coated beads and high doses of IL-2 [20]. Hopefully, this approach will facilitate the evaluation of the expanded Treg as suppressive immunotherapeutic agents in allergic diseases. The human natural Treg display a polyclonal TCR repertoire and are therefore able to recognize a wide spectrum of antigens. However, the success of Treg-based immunotherapy was found to be vitally-dependent on antigen specificity of the Treg. Clearly, the ability to use antigen-specific Treg rather than polyclonally expanded Treg will reduce the total number of Treg required for immunotherapeutic purposes.

I have recently reviewed the potential for inducing Treg-suppressive activity and/or IL-10 secretion by different mechanisms, including FoxP3 transduction, corticosteroids (with or without β$_2$-agonists or vitamin D$_3$), rapamycin or estrogen [21]. In this review I focus on inducing Treg activity using specific immunotherapy or by targeting Toll-like receptors expressed on Treg. The potential therapeutic strategies for modulation of Treg activity in allergic diseases are summarized in table 1.

Induction of Treg Activity by Peptide-Based Immunotherapy

Allergen-specific immunotherapy (SIT), the only causative approach to treat allergy, may induce allergic reactions and anaphylaxis. However, peptide-based immunotherapy (PIT) has the potential to inhibit T-cell reaction without inducing anaphylaxis. The safety and efficiency of PIT has been demonstrated in recent clinical trials. In this approach, short synthetic peptides, which represent major T-cell epitopes derived from the allergen, are used as therapeutic vaccines against allergy. Unlike the whole protein immunotherapy, peptides induce minimum adverse symptoms related to systemic IgE release. The exact mechanism of inducing tolerance in PIT is not completely identified but the recent interest in Treg has driven re-examining the possibility of inducing/expanding populations of Treg using specific immunotherapy approaches.

Available data provide evidence that modulating immune responses to allergens by PIT is mediated by reducing Th2 responses, increasing IL-10/TGF-β production or inducing Treg activity. In normal immunity and during mucosal allergen-SIT, IL-10 and/or TGF-β secretion by allergen-specific T cells was increased, in addition to inducing allergen-specific suppressive activity in CD4+CD25+ T cells of allergic subjects by SIT [22]. Treating patients with grass pollen immunotherapy induced significantly higher IL-10 levels from the CD4+CD25+ population than untreated atopic control subjects [23]. The mechanism of action of Fel d 1 PIT in

Table 1. Summary of potential strategies for inducing Treg activity for treating allergic diseases

Method	Outcome of immune regulation
Specific immunotherapy	
Grass pollen	Increase IL-10 production in CD4+CD25+ Treg
Fel d 1 cat allergen	Induce suppressive activity in CD4+ T cells
Bee venom	Increase IL-10 production
	Increase Treg activity?
TLR ligands	
LPS (TLR4 ligand)	Induce Treg activity in CD4+ T cells
Pam3Cys (TLR2 ligand)	Increase expansion and activity of Treg
HSP60 (TLR2 ligand)	Increase IL-10/TGF-β production
	Increase Treg-suppressive activity
Flagellin (TLR5 ligand)	Increase Treg-suppressive activity
	Increase FoxP3 expression in Treg
Others	
FoxP3 transduction	Induce Treg activity in CD4+ T cells
Anti-CD3/CD28 & IL-2	Expand Treg
Glucocorticoids	Increase IL-10 production
	Increase FoxP3 expression in Treg
Glucocorticoids and β$_2$-agonist or vitamin D$_3$	Increase IL-10 production
Rapamycin or estrogen	Expand Treg
	Increase FoxP3 expression in Treg

cat-allergic asthmatic patients was investigated. One study reported that PIT alters T-cell responses to allergens through mechanisms other than changes in the suppressive activity of peripheral blood CD4+CD25+ Treg [24]. However, another study revealed that PIT induces a population of allergen-specific CD4+ T cells able to actively suppress allergen-specific proliferative responses of pretreatment CD4– T cells [25]. This study provides clear evidence that PIT induces a population of allergen-specific CD4+ T cells with functional suppressive/regulatory activity. In addition, the mechanism of action of bee venom immunotherapy may involve increased Treg activity and/or IL-10 secretion [26]. Clearly, our recent understanding of SIT mechanisms, especially the role of Treg in inducing peripheral tolerance, may drive the development of new, novel therapeutic strategies.

Induction of Treg Activity by Targeting Toll-Like Receptors

The hygiene hypothesis proposes that reduced exposure to infections in early life over the past few decades owing to declining family size, improved living standards and higher personal hygiene have reduced cross-infection, and consequently may have resulted in a more widespread of allergic diseases [27]. Therefore, exposure to microbes in early life might be an important strategy for reducing allergic disorders. Several microbial components initiate signal transduction pathways through toll-like receptors (TLR) expressed on immune cells, and the recent research on the molecular mechanisms of the hygiene hypothesis highlights the impact of TLR ligands on early priming of the immune system towards antiallergic responses. Bacterial and viral infections during early life direct the immune system toward Th1 responses, which counteract the proallergic Th2 responses and lead to the development of a balanced immune system [28]. In children, an increased concentration of house-dust endotoxin has been shown to correlate with increased Th1 responses and inverse allergen sensitization [29] and development of asthma [30]. The typical mechanistic explanations for the hygiene hypothesis have invoked the Th1/Th2 model (prevention of Th2-driven allergy by promoting Th1 responses) [31]. However, this model is contradicted by the evidence that parasitism with helminth, which induce strong Th2 responses, is also protective from allergy [31]. Furthermore, there is evidence that hygiene hypothesis applies to Th1-mediated autoimmune diseases because of the increasing incidence of autoimmune diseases in westernized countries. Therefore, strong immunological counterregulation inhibiting the development of both Th2-mediated allergic diseases and Th1-mediated autoimmune diseases was proposed as a broader mechanistic model explaining the hygiene hypothesis [31]. Some data suggest that infectious agents enhance Treg activity and/or IL-10 and TGF-β production whose effects extend beyond the responses to the invading microbe, and leading to bystander suppression of both Th1 and Th2 responses [32].

TLR might be promising targets for developing immunotherapeutic strategies for allergic diseases and asthma because of their essential role in innate and adaptive immunities by inducing the production of pro- or anti-inflammatory cytokines, and activation and/or inhibition of Teff and Treg. Stimulating T cells via their TLR enhances the suppressive activity and/or FoxP3 expression. Bacterial lipopolysaccharide (LPS), the prototypical TLR4 ligand, is suggested to have dual effect on allergic diseases by enhancing or suppressing allergic lung inflammation in mouse models. Dose and time of LPS administration might be the key factors for determining the final outcome of TLR4 ligation in the course of allergic responses [33]. Recently, it has been shown that mucosal antigen exposure in the neonatal period results in inhibition of allergic responses to environmental allergens, and newborn mice exposed to LPS develop T cells with Treg phenotype (CD25 and IL-10 expression) on sensitization and challenge [34]. LPS may act directly on TLR4 expressed on Treg [35] or indirectly by activating dendritic cells to generate different types of CD4+ T-cell responses, including Treg activity. Clearly, LPS is toxic and cannot be used in patients; therefore, some natural and synthetic non-toxic TLR4 ligands derived from LPS have been developed for clinical usage [33]. TLR2 ligands have been shown to be able to induce Treg activity by different mechanisms. Pam3Cys, a TLR2 ligand, directly act on Treg by enhancing their expansion and activity [36]. HSP60, another TLR2 ligand, increases IL-10, TGF-β and contact-dependent Treg-suppressive activity, which inhibit proliferation and proinflammatory cytokine secretion from CD4+CD25– Teff [37]. Flagellin, a TLR5 ligand, enhances the suppressive activity and FoxP3 expression in CD4+ CD25+ Treg [38]. In summary, targeting TLR by their counterpart ligands for activating Treg activity might be a promising and safe strategy for the control of allergic diseases and asthma. However, further investigation and careful follow-up of patients involved in clinical trials is still required to establish TLR ligands as effective and safe immunotherapeutic drugs.

Conclusion

Induction of peripheral T-cell tolerance to allergens is vital for generating a healthier immune response in allergic individuals. Allergen-specific Th2 immune responses are actively suppressed by Treg in non-atopic individuals, while this suppression is either missed or can be conquered by allergen exposure in atopic patients. There is increasing evidence suggesting that naturally occurring and inducible Treg cells play a significant role in controlling the development of allergic diseases in response to allergens as well as in the mechanism involved in SIT. Additionally, the common treatments for allergic diseases might exert their effect, at least in part, by promoting the generation of IL-10-producing Treg and/or inducing Treg activity. Visibly, understanding immune mechanisms controlling diseases in non-allergic individuals and evidence for reduced Treg activity in allergic patients are the key justifications for stimulating allergen-specific Treg for treating allergic diseases.

Summarizing, inducing Treg activity is an exciting approach for treating patients with allergic diseases. PIT appears to be associated with inducing functional allergen-specific Treg. Targeting Treg through their TLR might be another attractive approach for controlling allergic diseases. However, more intensive work is still required for exploring novel immunotherapies that have the potential to upregulate the activity of Treg in patients with allergic diseases. Applicable, safe and effective strategies to selectively activate and expand antigen-specific Treg in vivo and in vitro is the focus of current research in genuine attempts to develop novel pharmaceuticals for controlling or treating allergic diseases and asthma.

References

1 Akdis M, Verhagen J, Taylor A, et al: Immune responses in healthy and allergic individuals are characterized by a fine balance between allergen-specific T regulatory 1 and T-helper-2 cells. J Exp Med 2004;199:1567–1575.
2 Antony PA, Restifo NP: CD4+CD25+ T regulatory cells, immunotherapy of cancer, and interleukin-2. J Immunother 2005;28:120–128.
3 Seddiki N, Santner-Nanan B, Martinson J, et al: Expression of interleukin (IL)-2 and IL-7 receptors discriminates between human regulatory and activated T cells. J Exp Med 2006;203:1693–1700.
4 Deaglio S, Dwyer KM, Gao W, et al: Adenosine generation catalyzed by CD39 and CD73 expressed on regulatory T cells mediates immune suppression. J Exp Med 2007;204:1257–1265.
5 Chen W, Jin W, Hardegen N, et al: Conversion of peripheral CD4+CD25− naive T cells to CD4+CD25+ regulatory T cells by TGF-β induction of transcription factor FoxP3. J Exp Med 2003;198:1875–1886.
6 Cottrez F, Hurst SD, Coffman RL, Groux H: T regulatory cells 1 inhibit a Th2-specific response in vivo. J Immunol 2000;165:4848–4853.
7 Zuany-Amorim C, Sawicka E, Manlius C, et al: Suppression of airway eosinophilia by killed *Mycobacterium vaccae*-induced allergen-specific regulatory T cells. Nat Med 2002;8:625–629.

8 Wilson MS, Taylor MD, Balic A, Finney CA, Lamb JR, Maizels RM: Suppression of allergic airway inflammation by helminth-induced regulatory T cells. J Exp Med 2005;202:1199–1212.
9 Kearley J, Barker JE, Robinson DS, Lloyd CM: Resolution of airway inflammation and hyperreactivity after in vivo transfer of CD4+CD25+ regulatory T cells is interleukin-10 dependent. J Exp Med 2005;202:1539–1547.
10 Lewkowich IP, Herman NS, Schleifer KW, et al: CD4+CD25+ T cells protect against experimentally induced asthma and alter pulmonary dendritic cell phenotype and function. J Exp Med 2005;202:1549–1561.
11 Taams LS, Vukmanovic-Stejic M, Smith J, et al: Antigen-specific T cell suppression by human CD4+CD25+ regulatory T cells. Eur J Immunol 2002;32:1621–1630.
12 Cavani A, Nasorri F, Ottaviani C, Sebastiani S, De Pita O, Girolomoni G: Human CD25+ regulatory T cells maintain immune tolerance to nickel in healthy, nonallergic individuals. J Immunol 2003;171:5760–5768.
13 Hansen G, McIntire JJ, Yeung VP, et al: CD4+ T-helper cells engineered to produce latent TGF-β₁ reverse allergen-induced airway hyperreactivity and inflammation. J Clin Invest 2000;105:61–70.

14 Oh JW, Seroogy CM, Meyer EH, et al: CD4 T-helper cells engineered to produce IL-10 prevent allergen-induced airway hyperreactivity and inflammation. J Allergy Clin Immunol 2002;110:460–468.
15 Hawrylowicz C, Richards D, Loke TK, Corrigan C, Lee T: A defect in corticosteroid-induced IL-10 production in T lymphocytes from corticosteroid-resistant asthmatic patients. J Allergy Clin Immunol 2002;109:369–370.
16 Ling EM, Smith T, Nguyen XD, et al: Relation of CD4+CD25+ regulatory T-cell suppression of allergen-driven T-cell activation to atopic status and expression of allergic disease. Lancet 2004;363:608–615.
17 Hartl D, Koller B, Mehlhorn AT, et al: Quantitative and functional impairment of pulmonary CD4+CD25^hi regulatory T cells in pediatric asthma. J Allergy Clin Immunol 2007;119:1258–1266.
18 Verhagen J, Akdis M, Traidl-Hoffmann C, et al: Absence of T-regulatory cell expression and function in atopic dermatitis skin. J Allergy Clin Immunol 2006;117:176–183.
19 Orihara K, Narita M, Tobe T, et al: Circulating FoxP3+CD4+ cell numbers in atopic patients and healthy control subjects. J Allergy Clin Immunol 2007;120:960–962.

20 Godfrey WR, Ge YG, Spoden DJ, et al: In vitro-expanded human CD4+ CD25+ T-regulatory cells can markedly inhibit allogeneic dendritic cell-stimulated MLR cultures. Blood 2004;104: 453–461.

21 Elkord E: Role of regulatory T cells in allergy: implications for therapeutic strategy. Inflamm Allergy Drug Targets 2006;5:211–217.

22 Jutel M, Akdis M, Budak F, et al: IL-10 and TGF-β cooperate in the regulatory T cell response to mucosal allergens in normal immunity and specific immunotherapy. Eur J Immunol 2003;33: 1205–1214.

23 Francis JN, Till SJ, Durham SR: Induction of IL-10+CD4+CD25+ T cells by grass pollen immunotherapy. J Allergy Clin Immunol 2003;111: 1255–1261.

24 Smith TR, Alexander C, Kay AB, Larche M, Robinson DS: Cat allergen peptide immunotherapy reduces CD4+ T-cell responses to cat allergen but does not alter suppression by CD4+ CD25+ T cells: a double-blind placebo-controlled study. Allergy 2004; 59:1097–1101.

25 Verhoef A, Alexander C, Kay AB, Larche M: T cell epitope immunotherapy induces a CD4+ T cell population with regulatory activity. PLoS Med 2005;2:e78.

26 Jutel M, Akdis M, Blaser K, Akdis CA: Are regulatory T cells the target of venom immunotherapy? Curr Opin Allergy Clin Immunol 2005;5:365–369.

27 Strachan DP: Hay fever, hygiene, and household size. BMJ 1989;299: 1259–1260.

28 Yazdanbakhsh M, Kremsner PG, van Ree R: Allergy, parasites, and the hygiene hypothesis. Science 2002;296:490–494.

29 Gereda JE, Leung DY, Thatayatikom A, et al: Relation between house-dust endotoxin exposure, type 1 T-cell development, and allergen sensitisation in infants at high risk of asthma. Lancet 2000;355:1680–1683.

30 Braun-Fahrlander C, Riedler J, Herz U, et al: Environmental exposure to endotoxin and its relation to asthma in school-age children. N Engl J Med 2002;347:869–877.

31 Wills-Karp M, Santeliz J, Karp CL: The germless theory of allergic disease: revisiting the hygiene hypothesis. Nat Rev Immunol 2001;1:69–75.

32 Bach JF: The effect of infections on susceptibility to autoimmune and allergic diseases. N Engl J Med 2002;347:911–920.

33 Goldman M: Translational mini-review series on toll-like receptors: toll-like receptor ligands as novel pharmaceuticals for allergic disorders. Clin Exp Immunol 2007;147:208–216.

34 Wang Y, McCusker C: Neonatal exposure with LPS and/or allergen prevents experimental allergic airways disease: development of tolerance using environmental antigens. J Allergy Clin Immunol 2006;118:143–151.

35 Caramalho I, Lopes-Carvalho T, Ostler D, Zelenay S, Haury M, Demengeot J: Regulatory T cells selectively express toll-like receptors and are activated by lipopolysaccharide. J Exp Med 2003;197:403–411.

36 Sutmuller RP, den Brok MH, Kramer M, et al: Toll-like receptor 2 controls expansion and function of regulatory T cells. J Clin Invest 2006;116:485–494.

37 Zanin-Zhorov A, Cahalon L, Tal G, Margalit R, Lider O, Cohen IR: Heat shock protein 60 enhances CD4+ CD25+ regulatory T cell function via innate TLR2 signaling. J Clin Invest 2006;116:2022–2032.

38 Crellin NK, Garcia RV, Hadisfar O, Allan SE, Steiner TS, Levings MK: Human CD4+ T cells express TLR5 and its ligand flagellin enhances the suppressive capacity and expression of FoxP3 in CD4+CD25+ T regulatory cells. J Immunol 2005;175:8051–8059.

Dr. Eyad Elkord
Immunology Group, Paterson Institute for Cancer Research
University of Manchester, Manchester M20 4BX (UK)
Tel. +44 161 446 3192, Fax +44 161 446 3109
E-Mail eelkord@picr.man.ac.uk

Blaser K (ed): T Cell Regulation in Allergy, Asthma and Atopic Skin Diseases.
Chem Immunol Allergy. Basel, Karger, 2008, vol 94, pp 158–177

T-Cell Regulatory Mechanisms in Specific Immunotherapy

Marek Jutel[a] · Cezmi A. Akdis[b]

[a]Department of Internal Medicine and Allergology, Wroclaw Medical University, Wroclaw, Poland, and [b]Swiss Institute of Allergy and Asthma Research (SIAF), Davos, Switzerland

Abstract

Allergen-specific immunotherapy (SIT) is the only treatment which leads to a lifelong tolerance against previously disease-causing allergens due to restoration of normal immunity against allergens. The description of T-regulatory (Treg) cells being involved in prevention of sensitization to allergens has led to great interest whether they represent a major target for allergen-SIT and whether it would be possible to manipulate Treg cells to increase its efficacy. Activation-induced cell death, anergy and/or immune response modulation by Treg cells are essential mechanisms of peripheral T-cell tolerance. There is growing evidence that anergy, tolerance and active suppression are not entirely distinct, but rather represent linked mechanisms possibly involving the same cells and multiple suppressor mechanisms. Skewing of allergen-specific effector T cells to Treg cells appears as a crucial event in the control of healthy immune response to allergens and successful allergen-SIT. The Treg cell response is characterized by abolished allergen-induced specific T-cell proliferation and suppressed T-helper (Th)1- and Th2-type cytokine secretion. In addition, mediators of allergic inflammation that trigger cAMP-associated G-protein-coupled receptors, such as histamine receptor-2, may contribute to peripheral tolerance mechanisms. The increased levels of interleukin-10 and transforming growth factor-β that are produced by Treg cells potently suppress IgE production, while simultaneously increasing production of non-inflammatory isotypes IgG4 and IgA, respectively. In addition, Treg cells directly or indirectly suppress effector cells of allergic inflammation such as mast cells, basophils and eosinophils. In conclusion, peripheral tolerance to allergens is controlled by multiple active suppression mechanisms. It is associated with regulation of antibody isotypes and effector cells to the direction of a healthy immune response. By the application of the recent knowledge in Treg-dependent mechanisms of peripheral tolerance, more rational and safer approaches are awaited for the future prevention and cure of allergen hypersensitivity.

Copyright © 2008 S. Karger AG, Basel

Although it is well documented that allergen-specific immunotherapy (SIT) represents the only approach to achieve tolerance to causative allergens, its mechanism was unclear for a long time. SIT has been demonstrated to influence the deviated immune response in allergic individuals in a specific manner and eventually redirect the immune system towards normal immunity. A rise in allergen-blocking IgG antibodies, particularly of the IgG4 class [1], the generation of IgE-modulating CD8+ T cells and a decrease in release of mediators [2–5], was shown to be associated with successful SIT. Later on, SIT was found to be associated with a decrease in interleukin (IL)-4 and IL-5 production by CD4+ Th2 cells, and a shift towards increased IFN-γ production by Th1 cells [6–14]. Distinct Th1 and Th2 subpopulations of T cells counterregulate each other and play a role in distinct diseases [6, 7]. The mechanism of repolarization of specific T-cell activity from dominating Th2-type towards Th1-type as observed during VIT was a matter of controversy. A new light was shed when a further subtype of T cells, with immuno-suppressive function and cytokine profiles distinct from either Th1 and Th2 cells, termed regulatory/suppressor T cells (Treg), was described [8–10]. T-cell tolerance is characterized by functionally inactivation of the cell to antigen encounter, which remains alive for an extended period of time in an unresponsive state. In recognition of the importance of the phenomenon of immunological tolerance, the Nobel Prize in Physiology and Medicine was awarded in 1960 to Medawar [11] for discovering that skin allografts in mice and chicken can be accepted if they had been preinoculated during embryonic development with allogeneic lymphoid cells, and to Burnet [12, 13] for first proposing that exposure to antigens before the development of immune response, specifically abrogates the capacity to respond to that antigen in later life. During the last decade, this area of immunology research had become so popular and promiscuous. The overall evaluation of the studies on T-cell unresponsiveness suggests that anergy, tolerance and active suppression are not entirely distinct, but rather represent linked mechanisms possibly involving the same molecular events. The term anergy was first coined by Von Pirquet [14] in 1908 to describe the loss of delayed-type hypersensitivity to tuberculin in individuals infected with measles virus. The term was clinically accepted since then to describe negative tuberculin skin test results in conditions where it is expected to be positive. In 1980, the term 'anergy' was used to describe the specific inactivation of B cells in mice by high doses of antigen [15]. It was subsequently used for T cells to describe a phenomenon in which antigen presentation to T-cell clones in the absence of professional antigen-presenting cells induced a hyporesponsive state affecting subsequent IL-2 production and proliferation upon restimulation [16]. A variety of reversible functional limitations characterize the anergic state, including cell division, cell differentiation, and cytokine production [17, 18]. It is important to note here that in earlier studies, which are referred to as a basis for the definition of anergy/tolerance, functional unresponsiveness was analyzed by non-sophisticated assays such as antigen-induced [^{3}H]thymidine incorporation, IL-2 and total IgG production. In addition, antigens used in mouse models until the last few years contained high amounts of impurities, such as lipopolysaccharide and other innate immune response-stimulating substances, which may influence the outcome of the experiments. Although some of the biochemical steps overlap with anergy, activation-induced cell death induced by trigger of the death receptors and caspase activation represents a distinct physiological response [19, 20].

It is still not understood why exposure to allergens causes atopic disorders in some individuals, but not others, however, it is clear that strong interaction of environmental and genetic factors is involved. Four cardinal events during allergic inflammation can be classified as activation of memory/effector T cells and other effector cells such as mast cells, eosinophils and basophils, their organ-selective homing, prolonged survival and reactivation inside the allergic organs and effector functions [21]. T cells are activated by aeroallergens, food antigens, autoantigens and bacterial superantigens in allergic inflammation [22, 23]. They are under the influence of skin, lung or nose-related chemokine network and they show organ-selective homing [24–26]. A prolonged survival of the inflammatory cells and strong interaction with resident cells of the allergic organ and consequent reactivation is observed in the subepithclial tissues [27, 28]. T cells play important effector roles in atopic dermatitis and asthma with induction of hyper-IgE, eosinophil survival and mucus hyperproduction [22, 28, 29] (fig. 1). In addition, activated T cells induce bronchial epithelial cell and keratinocyte apoptosis as major tissue injury events [30–33]. Peripheral T-cell tolerance to allergens can overcome all of the above

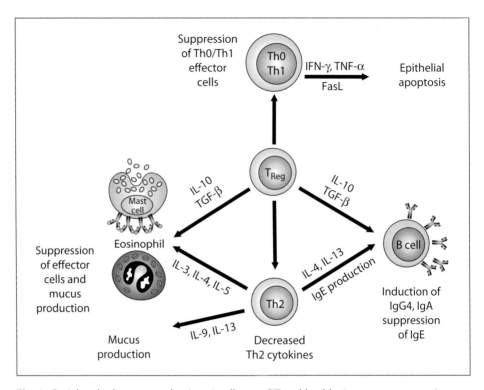

Fig. 1. Peripheral tolerance mechanisms in allergen-SIT and healthy immune response. Immune deviation towards Treg cell response is an essential step in allergen-SIT and natural allergen exposure of non-allergic individuals. Treg cells utilize multiple suppressor factors, which influence the final outcome of allergen-SIT. In addition, IL-10 and TGF-β induce IgG4 and IgA respectively from B cells as non-inflammatory Ig isotypes and suppress IgE production. These two cytokines directly or indirectly suppress effector cells of allergic inflammation such as mast cells, basophils and eosinophils. In addition, Th2 cells, which are dominated by Treg cells, can no longer induce IgE by IL-4 and IL-13, and cannot provide cytokines such as IL-3, IL-4, IL-5 and IL-9, which are required for the differentiation, survival and activity of mast cells, basophils and eosinophils, and mucus-producing cells. Furthermore, the suppressed Th0/Th1 compartment of allergic inflammation cannot mediate essential tissue injury mechanisms via IFN-γ, TNF-α and Fas-ligand (L) such as apoptosis of skin keratinocytes and bronchial epithelial cells (red line: suppression; black line: stimulation).

pathological events in allergic inflammation, because they all require T-cell activation.

The initial event responsible for the development of allergic diseases is the generation of allergen-specific CD4+ T-helper (Th) cells. The current view is that under the influence of IL-4, naive T cells activated by antigen-presenting cells differentiate into Th2 cells [34–36]. Once generated, effector Th2 cells produce IL-4, IL-5 and IL-13, and mediate several regulatory and effector functions. These cytokines induce the production of allergen-specific IgE by B cells, development and recruitment of eosinophils, production of mucus and contraction of smooth muscles [34, 35, 37]. Furthermore, the degranulation of basophils and mast cells by IgE-mediated cross-linking of receptors is the key event in type 1 hypersensitivity, which may lead to chronic allergic inflammation.

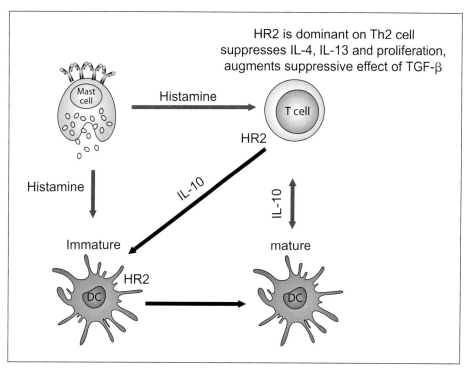

Fig. 2. Regulatory/suppressor functions of histamine by HR2. In maturing DCs, histamine enhances intracellular cAMP levels and stimulates IL-10 secretion, but suppresses IL-12 by HR2. IL-10 affects the maturation of DCs to IL-10-producing DCs and induces of IL-10-producing T cells. Th2 cells show increased expression of HR2 and T-cell proliferation and IL-4 and IL-13 production are negatively regulated by HR2. IL-10 suppresses the antigen-presentation capacity and proinflammatory cytokine synthesis of DCs. In addition, Th2 cells are more efficiently suppressed by TGF-β in the presence of histamine via HR2 (red line: suppression; black line: differentiation).

Importantly, although Th2 cells are responsible for the development of allergic diseases, Th1 cells may contribute to chronicity and effector phase in allergic diseases [30–33, 38, 39]. Distinct Th1 and Th2 2 subpopulations of T cells counterregulate each other and play a role in distinct diseases [34, 35]. In addition, recent studies have demonstrated that peripheral T-cell tolerance is crucial for a healthy immune response and successful treatment of allergic disorders [40–42]. A further subtype of T cells, with immunosuppressive function and cytokine profiles distinct from either Th1 and Th2 cells, termed regulatory/suppressor T cells (Treg), has been existence in humans has been demonstrated [41,

45, 46]. In addition to Th1 cells, Treg cells are able to inhibit the development of allergic Th2 responses [47] and play a major role in allergen-SIT [41, 42]. This review will examine allergen-specific peripheral tolerance mechanisms in humans and discuss novel ways of T-cell suppression.

Peripheral T-Cell Tolerance in Allergen-Specific Immunotherapy

The symptoms of IgE-mediated allergic reactions – such as rhinitis, conjunctivitis and asthma – can be ameliorated by temporary suppression of mediators and immune cells (by antihistamines, antileukotrienes, β₂-adrenergic receptor antagonists and corticosteroids) [48–51]. However, a more long-term solution is allergen-SIT that specifically restores a normal immunity against allergens. Allergen-SIT is most efficiently used in allergy to insect venoms and allergic rhinitis [52–56]. Despite its usage in clinical practice for nearly a century, the underlying immunological mechanisms of allergen-SIT are slowly being elucidated [40, 42, 57–61]. A rise in allergen-blocking IgG antibodies, particularly of the IgG4 class, which supposedly block allergen and IgE facilitated antigen presentation [62–64], the generation of IgE-modulating CD8+ T cells [65] and a reduction in the numbers of mast cells and eosinophils, including the release of mediators [66–68], were shown to be associated with successful allergen-SIT. Furthermore, allergen-SIT was found to be associated with a decrease in IL-4 and IL-5 production by CD4+ T cells [56, 69, 70]. Also a shift from Th2 cytokine pattern towards increased IFN-γ production in allergen-SIT of allergy to bee venom, wasp venom, grass pollen and house dust mite was observed [69, 71]. It appears however that the induction of a tolerant state in peripheral T cells represents an essential step in allergen-SIT (fig. 1) [40–42, 57]. Peripheral T-cell tolerance is characterized mainly by suppressed proliferative and cytokine responses against the major allergens and its T-cell recognition sites [57]. T-cell tolerance is initiated by autocrine action of IL-10, which is increasingly produced by the antigen-specific T cells [40, 41]. Tolerized T cells can be reactivated to produce either distinct Th1 or Th2 cytokine patterns depending on the cytokine present in the tissue microenvironment, and thus directing allergen-SIT towards successful or unsuccessful treatment [57].

Peptide immunotherapy (PIT) is another attractive approach for investigation of peripheral T-cell tolerance in humans. Short allergen peptides, either native sequences or altered peptide ligands, with amino acid substitutions do not contain epitopes for IgE cross-linking to induce anaphylaxis. There is considerable rationale for targeting T cells with synthetic peptides based on such T-cell epitopes. To date, clinical trials of PIT have been performed in two allergies [72–76]. Relatively long peptides of 27 and 35 amino acids of the major cat allergen Fel d 1 containing the T-cell epitopes or mixture of peptides spanning the whole protein sequence were used to treat allergy to cats and resulted in the induction of tolerance in IL-4-producing cells [73, 76]. In the other trial, PIT of bee venom allergy was performed with a mixture of short peptides that directly represent the T-cell epitopes [17, 12, 11], amino acids of the bee venom major allergen, phospholipase A₂ [72]. The study showed modulation of the immune response against the whole allergen, inducing specific T-cell tolerance and a decrease in the specific IgE:IgG4 ratio [72]. Single amino acid alteration in T-cell epitopes can modify specific T-cell activation and cytokine production [77]. Rodent studies suggest that, under highly controlled experimental conditions, allergic diseases can be inhibited by altered peptide ligand administration. Whether this is due to Th2 to Th1 immune deviation or the induction of Treg cells remains to be elucidated [77, 78]. Although PIT is theoretically attractive as a means to avoid IgE-mediated early phase reactions, it is important to note that serum IgE in allergic individuals may sometimes bind to relatively short linear epitopes of protein allergens [79]. A potential barrier to PIT of allergy is the apparent complexity of the allergen-specific T-cell response in terms of epitope usage and dominant epitopes in humans [80–82].

Peripheral T-Cell Tolerance to Allergens Is Associated with Regulation of Antibody Isotypes and Suppression of Effector Cells

The serum levels of specific IgE and IgG4 antibodies delineate allergic and normal immunity to allergen. Although peripheral tolerance was demonstrated in specific T cells, the capacity of B cells to produce specific IgE and IgG4 antibodies was not abolished during SIT [57]. In fact, specific serum levels of both isotypes increased during the early phase of treatment. However, the increase in antigen-specific IgG4 was more pronounced and the ratio of specific IgE to IgG4 decreased by 10- to 100-fold. Also the in vitro production of PLA-specific IgE and IgG4 antibodies by PBMC changed in parallel to the serum levels of specific isotypes. A similar change in specific isotype ratio was observed in SIT of various allergies. Moreover, IL-10, which is induced and increasingly secreted by SIT, appears to counterregulate antigen-specific IgE and IgG4 antibody synthesis [41]. IL-10 is a potent suppressor of both total and allergen-specific IgE, while it simultaneously increases IgG4 production [41, 83]. Thus, IL-10 not only generates tolerance in T cells, but it also regulates specific isotype formation and skews the specific response from an IgE- to an IgG4-dominated phenotype (fig. 1). The healthy immune response to Der p 1 demonstrated increased specific IgA and IgG4, small amounts of IgG1 and almost undetectable IgE antibodies in serum [42]. House dust mite-SIT did not significantly change specific IgE levels after 70 days of treatment, however a significant increase in specific IgA, IgG1 and IgG4 was observed [42]. The increase of specific IgA and IgG4 in serum coincides with increased transforming growth factor-β (TGF-β) and IL-10 respectively. This may account for the role of IgA and TGF-β as well as IgG4 and IL-10 in peripheral mucosal immune responses to allergens in healthy individuals [41, 84].

Despite the fact that a definite decrease in IgE antibody levels and IgE-mediated skin sensitivity normally requires several years of SIT, most patients are protected against bee stings already at an early stage of bee venom-SIT. The reason for this is that effector cells of allergic inflammation, such as mast cells, basophils and eosinophils,

require T-cell cytokines for priming, survival and activity, [85, 86] which are not efficiently provided by suppressed Th2 cells and Treg cells (fig. 1). SIT efficiently modulates the thresholds for mast cell and basophil activation and decreases immunoglobulin E-mediated histamine release [87, 88]. In addition, IL-10 was shown to reduce proinflammatory cytokine release from mast cells [89]. Furthermore, IL-10 downregulates eosinophil function and activity, and suppresses IL-5 production by human resting Th0 and Th2 cells [90]. Moreover, IL-10 inhibits endogenous GM-CSF production and CD40 expression by activated eosinophils and enhances eosinophil cell death [91].

T-Regulatory Cells

T cells that were able to suppress immune responses were described first in the early 1970s [92]. Suppressor T cells were thought to be a specialized subpopulation, the effects of which were mediated in an antigen-specific fashion [65, 93]. Unfortunately, the failure to clearly identify the mechanisms underlying immune suppression led to a collapse in the entire field in the 1980s [94]. The concept of T-cell-mediated immune suppression was started to be strongly explored the mid-1990s. Many types of suppressor T cells have been described in a number of systems, and their biology has been the subject of intensive investigation. Although many aspects of the mechanisms by which suppressor cells exert their effects remain to be elucidated, it is well established that Treg cells suppress immune responses via cell-to-cell interactions and/or the production of suppressor cytokines [40, 41, 44, 95].

Tr1 Cells

Type-1 T-regulatory (Tr1) cells are defined by their ability to produce high levels of IL-10 and TGF-β [44, 95]. Tr1 cells specific for a variety of antigens arise in vivo, but may also differentiate from naive CD4+ T cells. Tr1 cells have a low proliferative capacity which can be overcome by IL-15 [96]. Tr1 cells suppress naive and memory Th1 or Th2 responses via production of IL-10 and TGF-β [95]. The use of Tr1 cells to identify novel targets for the development of new therapeutic agents, and as a cellular therapy to modulate peripheral tolerance in allergy and autoimmunity, can be foreseen [40, 72, 97].

The generation in vitro of a Treg cell subset by stimulating naive CD4 T cells in the presence of IL-10, IFN-α or a combination of IL-4 and IL-10, has previously been reported [44, 95]. To overcome the problems in cytokine profiles of regulatory T cells, it has been demonstrated that a combination of vitamin D_3 and dexamethasone induced human and mouse naive CD4+ T cells to differentiate in vitro into regulatory T cells [98]. In contrast to the previously described in vitro derived CD4+ T cells, these cells produced only IL-10, but no IL-5 and IFN-γ, and furthermore retained a strong proliferative capacity and prevented central nervous system inflammation in an IL-10-dependent manner. There is now clear evidence that IL-10- and/or TGF-β-producing Tr1 cells are in vivo generated in humans during the early course of allergen-SIT, suggesting that high and increasing doses of allergens induce Tr1 cells in humans [41, 42, 99].

Th3 Cells
Regulatory/suppressor T-cell clones have been induced by oral feeding of low doses of antigen in a TCR-transgenic experimental encephalitis model [8, 100]. CD4+ T-cell clones isolated from mesenteric lymph nodes in orally tolerated animals produced high levels of TGF-β, and variable amounts of IL-4 and IL-10 upon activation with appropriate antigen or anti-CD3 antibody [8]. These cells functioned in vivo to suppress encephalitis induction with myelin basic protein and were designated as Th3 cells. TGF-β and IL-10 seemed critical, as treatment with neutralizing antibodies abrogated the disease-protective effects

of these cells. These Treg cells also exerted bystander immune suppression in vitro.

CD4+CD25+ Treg Cells
There is clear evidence from various animal models and human studies for an active mechanism of immune suppression, whereby a distinct subset of T cells inhibits the activation of conventional T cells in the periphery [101–104]. This Treg cell population has been determined as CD4+CD25+ T cells. The CD4+CD25+ T cells constitute 5–10% of peripheral CD4+ T cells and express the IL-2 receptor α-chain (CD25) [101]. They can prevent the development of autoimmunity indicating that the normal immune system contains a population of professional Treg cells. Elimination of CD4+CD25+ T cells leads to spontaneous development of various autoimmune diseases, such as gastritis or thyroiditis in genetically-susceptible hosts. In mice these cells have been shown to express CD45RB[low] [43]. The CD38–CD25+CD4+ CD45RB[low] subpopulation contains T cells which respond to recall antigens and produced high levels of cytokines in response to polyclonal stimulation. In contrast, the CD38+ cells within this subpopulation fail to proliferate or to produce detectable levels of cytokines, and furthermore inhibit anti-CD3-induced proliferation induced by CD38– population [105].

There are two major hypotheses concerning the generation of CD4+CD25+ Treg cells. One of these suggests that Treg cells emerge from the thymus as a distinct subset of mature T cells with defined functions [101, 103]. On the other hand, several studies have shown that Treg cells may differentiate from naive T cells in the periphery upon encountering antigens present at high concentrations [44, 98, 106]. It can be proposed that thymic differentiation accounts for Treg cells that are specific for self peptides and are devoted to the control of autoimmune responses, whereas peripheral differentiation may be required for environmental antigen-specific T cells for which an undesired immune response results in pathology.

Other T-Regulatory Cells

It has been proposed that, in addition to CD4+ T cells, CD8+ Treg cells may have a role in oral tolerance [107, 108]. Recent efforts to generate suppressor cell lines in vitro resulted in a population of CD8+CD28– T cells restricted by allogeneic HLA class I antigens which were able to prevent upregulation of B7 molecules induced by Th cells on antigen-presenting cells [109]. This resulted in the suppression of CD4+ T cells in an HLA-nonrestricted fashion [109]. Interestingly, the magnitude of a CD8+ T-cell-mediated immune response to an acute viral infection is also subject to control by CD4+CD25+ Treg cells. If natural Treg were depleted with specific anti-CD25 antibody before infection with virus, the resultant CD8+ T-cell response was significantly enhanced suggesting that controlling suppressor effects at the time of vaccination could result in more effective immunity [110].

Double negative (CD4–CD8–) TCR-αβ+ Treg cells that mediate tolerance in several experimental autoimmune diseases have been described [111]. These double negative T cells are specific for MHC class I molecules and the suppressive effect of these cells on the proliferation and cytotoxic activity of CD8+ T cells with the same antigen specificity was not mediated by cytokines, but instead was attributed to Fas-mediated apoptosis of alloreactive T cells [112].

γδ T cells with regulatory functions have also been described. A population of γδ Treg cells with a cytokine profile reminiscent of Tr1 cell clones has been isolated from tumor-infiltrating lymphocytes [113]. These Treg cells could play a role in the inhibition of immune responses to tumors [114]. It has also been shown that aerosol delivery of protein antigens resulted in the differentiation of γδ T cells with regulatory functions [113]. It has been observed that induction of tolerance by various doses of ovalbumin (OVA) was abrogated

in mice lacking TCR-δ [115]. In contrast, TCR-γδ-deficient mice have the same degree of IgE-specific unresponsiveness after aerosol priming and immunization with OVA [116].

B-Regulatory Cells

A regulatory role for IL-10-secreting B cells has been recently proposed [117]. These B cells prevented the development of arthritis and their suppressive effect was particularly IL-10-dependent, because the B cells isolated from IL-10-deficient mice failed to protect from arthritis.

Dendritic-Regulating Cells

It is generally thought that immature dendritic cells (DCs) do not appropriately activate T cells, which may lead to tolerance [118]. In normal immunity, DCs should not have any restriction in antigen presentation and they should appropriately receive maturation signals given by the surroundings of the antigen, T cells and other tissue cells, such as costimulatory ligands, cytokines, innate immune response-stimulating (i.e. toll-like receptor triggering) substances. However, there are some indications that DCs can induce peripheral T-cell tolerance and a regulatory DC subset may exist. Pulmonary DCs from mice exposed to respiratory antigen transiently produce IL-10 [119]. These phenotypically mature pulmonary DCs, which were B7hi, stimulated the development of CD4+ Tr1-like cells that also produced high amounts of IL-10. Adoptive transfer of pulmonary DCs from IL-10+/+, but not IL-10–/–, mice exposed to respiratory antigen induced antigen-specific unresponsiveness in recipient mice. In accordance with these findings, IL-10 inhibited the development of fully mature DCs, which induced a state of alloantigen-specific anergy in CD4+ T cells [120]. These studies show that IL-10 production by DCs is critical for the induction of tolerance, and that phenotypically mature regulatory DCs may exist under certain circumstances.

Table 1. Regulatory/suppressor cells and their subsets

Regulatory/suppressor cells		Suppressor mechanism[1]	References
T cells	Tr1	IL-10, TGF-β	30–35, 102–106
	Th3	TGF-β	33, 107
	CD4+CD25+ Treg	IL-10, TGF-β, CTLA-4, PD-1, GITR	108–113
	CD8+CD25+CD28–Treg	same as CD4+CD25+	114–117
	CD4–CD8– Treg	induction of apoptosis	118–119
	TCR-γδ Treg	IL-10, TGF-β	120–123
B-cell subset	B-regulatory	IL-10	124
DCs	DC-regulatory	IL-10	125–127
NK cell subset[2]	NK-regulatory	IL-10	131, 132
Macrophages		IL-10, TGF-β	131
Resident tissue cells[2]		IL-10, TGF-β	128–133

[1]Suppressor mechanisms are not conclusive. It is possible that multiple other suppressive mechanisms exist.
[2]NK cells and resident tissue cells are included in the table because of expression of suppressive cytokines by these cells.

Other Cells with a Possible Regulatory Function

It has been clearly demonstrated that natural killer cells, epithelial cells, macrophages, glial cells, etc., express suppressor cytokines such as IL-10 and TGF-β. Although their role has not been coined as professional regulatory cells, these cells may efficiently contribute to the generation and maintenance of a regulatory/suppressor type immune response [121–126]. The expression of suppressor cytokines in resident tissue cells may additionally contribute to this process (table 1).

Suppression Mechanisms of T-Regulatory Cells

A great deal of uncertainty remains about mechanisms of action of Treg cells. Initial studies have shown that Treg cells act as suppressor T cells, which downregulate effector cells and inflammation models in chronic infection, organ transplantation and autoimmunity [8, 44, 127]. Most studies have failed to find a soluble factor as a suppressive mechanism of CD4+CD25+ Treg cells. Antigen-induced proliferation of CD4+ T cells was dramatically reduced following coculture with activated Treg clones, which had been separated from the responding T cells by a Transwell insert [128]. However, in Transwell membrane cultures that separate suppressor cells and target cells, the distance between two populations is approximately 2 mm and this may influence the concentration of suppressor cytokines. Accordingly, it cannot be possible to rule out an effect of a cytokine that acts in short distances or a membrane-bound cytokine. Indeed, membrane-bound TGF-β might be one of the mechanisms of suppression of CD4+CD25+ Treg cells [129]. In contrast to CD4+CD25+ Treg cells, suppressive effects of Tr1 cells were reversed by addition of neutralizing monoclonal antibody, directed against TGF-β and IL-10, implicating the role of suppressive cytokines in the mechanism of immune suppression both in vitro and in vivo in different settings and different autoimmune as well as allergy models [42, 44, 129–131]. This suppression was a hallmark of Tr1 clones, as OVA-specific Th1 or Th2 clones, derived from the same mice, had no suppressive effects, but rather enhanced OVA-induced proliferation of naive CD4+ T cells [47].

One group of CD4+CD25+ Treg cells originate from the thymus as a distinctive subset [101, 103, 132]. Thymectomy at a very early stage of animal development induces various autoimmune diseases in genetically-susceptible animals [133, 134]. Furthermore, induction of autoimmune diseases in an immunodeficient animal model was prevented by adoptively transferred CD4+ T cells or CD4+CD8– thymocytes isolated from normal syngeneic animals. In a rat model, CD4+ Treg cells were found to be of the CD45RC^{low} phenotype and to produce IL-2 and IL-4, but not IFN-γ, upon in vitro stimulation [133]. IL-4 and TGF-β are critical in preventing autoimmunity, as neutralization of either of these two cytokines abrogates the protective response. In another study, CD4+CD25+ Treg cells from thymus were shown to exert their suppressive function via the inhibition of IL-2R α-chain in target T cells, induced by the combined activity of CTLA-4 and membrane TGF-β$_1$ [135].

Studies of this activated CD4+ T-cell subpopulation have shown that they do not proliferate upon normal TCR-mediated stimulation and suppress proliferation of other T cells. TCR stimulation was required for these cells to exert suppression of other T cells; such suppression, however, was not confined to T cells specific for the same antigen. CD4+CD25+ T cells are the only lymphocyte subpopulation in both mice and humans that express CTLA4 constitutively. The expression apparently correlates with the suppressor function of CTLA4. The addition of anti-CTLA4 antibody or its Fab (fragment of antigen binding) reverses suppression in cocultures of CD4+CD25+ and CD4+CD25– T cells [136]. Similarly, the treatment of mice, which are recipients of CD4+CD45RB^{low} T cells with these agents, abrogated the suppression of inflammatory bowel disease [137]. These studies indicate that signals that result from the engagement of CTLA4 by its ligands, CD80 or CD86, are required for the induction of suppressor activity. Under some circumstances, the engagement of CTLA4 on the CD4+CD25+ T cells by antibody or by CD80/CD86 might lead to inhibition of the TCR-derived signals that are required for the induction of suppressor activity.

Programmed death-1 (PD-1) is an immunoreceptor tyrosine-based inhibitory motif (ITIM)-containing receptor expressed upon T-cell activation. PD-1-deleted mice develop autoimmune diseases, suggesting an inhibitory role for PD-1 in immune responses [138]. Members of the B7 family, PD-L1 and PD-L2, are ligands for PD-1. PD-1:PD-L engagement on murine CD4 and CD8 T cells results in inhibition of proliferation and cytokine production. T cells stimulated with anti-CD3/PD-L1 display dramatically decreased proliferation and IL-2 production [139]. PD-1:PD-L interactions inhibit IL-2 production even in the presence of costimulation and, thus, after prolonged activation, the PD-1:PD-L inhibitory pathway dominates. Exogenous IL-2 is able to overcome PD-L1-mediated inhibition at all times, indicating that cells maintain IL-2 responsiveness.

Glucocorticoid-induced tumor-necrosis factor receptor family-related gene (TNFRSF18, GITR) is expressed by CD4+CD25+ alloantigen-specific and naturally occurring circulating Treg cells [140, 141]. Stimulation of CD25+CD4+

regulatory T cells through GITR breaks immuno-logical self-tolerance [141]. GITR is upregulated in CD4+CD25– T cells after T-cell receptor stimulation and it also functions as a survival signal for activated cells [142]. In addition, CD103 (αEβ7 integrin) and CD122 (β chain of IL-2 receptor) are highly expressed on CD4+CD25+ Treg cells, which correlates with their suppressive activity [143, 144].

An X-linked forkhead/winged helix transcription factor, FoxP3 (Scurfin) is essential for the suppressive function of CD4+CD25+ Treg cells [145, 146]. It is highly expressed in CD4+CD25+, but not CD4+CD25– Treg cells [145, 146]. It acts as a silencer of cytokine gene promoters and programs the development and function of CD4+CD25+ Treg cells [145–148]. Mutations in the FoxP3 gene in humans leads to a severe immune dysregulation with polyendocrinopathy, enteropathy and hyper-IgE known as IPEX syndrome [149].

The failure of Treg cells to proliferate after TCR stimulation in vitro has suggested they are naturally anergic. However, Treg cells expressing a transgenic TCR were shown to proliferate and accumulate locally in response to transgenically expressed tissue antigen, whereas their CD25– counterparts are depleted at such sites [150]. CD4+CD25+ Treg cells population is composed of two Treg subsets that have distinct phenotypes. Some Treg remain quiescent and have a long lifespan, in the order of months, whereas the other Treg cells (mainly the autoantigen-specific ones) divide extensively and express multiple activation markers [151].

Clinical Relevance of T-Regulatory Cells

Since the concept of professional suppressor cells is recovering interest among the immunological community, it is now time to consider how the manipulation of regulatory/suppressor T cells might be used clinically. As tumor antigens are an important group of autoantigens, the depletion of Treg cells should result in an enhanced immune response to tumor vaccines. Several studies have shown that the antibody-mediated depletion of CD25+ T cells facilitates the induction of tumor immunity [152, 153].

Currently, the relationship between the different Treg cell populations is unclear with respect to their development, and activation. However, numerous animal experiments have clearly shown that Treg cells can suppress both Th1 and Th2 responses in vivo and thereby actively suppress the development of autoimmune and allergic responses. Recent studies reported that the application of in vitro engineered allergen-specific Treg cells lines protected mice from developing allergen-induced Th2 responses [154].

In humans, there is circumstantial evidence to suggest that Treg cells play a major role in the inhibition of allergic disorders. It has been reported that IL-10 levels in the bronchoalveolar lavage fluid of asthmatic patients are lower than in healthy controls, and that T cells from children suffering from asthma also produce less IL-10 mRNA than T cells from control children [155, 156]. These findings indicate that increased IL-10 production is associated with decreased allergic reactions. As Treg cells are a major source of IL-10, it has been speculated that Treg cells secreting IL-10 are involved in the suppression of allergic Th2 responses in humans. Several human aller-gen-SIT studies supported this hypothesis [41, 72, 157]. In contrast, some studies demonstrated that increased IL-10 levels are not associated with less allergic disease [158]. IL-10 may also promote airway hyperresponsiveness [159] and even eosinophilia [160] in allergy models. In contrast to its known T-cell-suppressive activity, some reports imply a role for TGF-β in the pathogenesis of asthma, particularly in remodeling of injured lung tissue in humans [161]. A recent report indicated that the increased allergic inflammation observed after blocking of CTLA-4 is clearly associated with decreased TGF-β levels in the bronchoalveolar lavage fluid of these animals [162]. Furthermore, inhibition of experimental tracheal eosinophilia was also due to the induction of CD4+ T cells secreting TGF-β [163].

An alloantigen-independent, systemic expansion of the maternal CD4+CD25+ T cells with dominant regulatory T-cell activity has been demonstrated [164]. In addition to their function in suppressing autoimmune responses, maternal Treg cells suppressed an aggressive allogeneic response directed against the fetus. Their absence led to a failure of gestation due to immunological rejection of the fetus.

To analyze human in vivo existence of Treg cells, lymphocyte populations in human lymph nodes with a special emphasis on the CD4+ CD25+ Treg cells have been investigated [165]. CD4+CD25+ T cells constitutively coexpressed high levels of CD152. Similar to Treg cells from peripheral blood, Treg cells from lymph node were in vitro anergic and efficiently inhibited other CD4+ and CD8+ lymphocyte proliferation [165]. Treg cells may play destructive roles in cancer and chronic infectious diseases [166–171]. Further studies are needed to demonstrate in the clinic, whether in vivo generation or adoptive transfer of Treg cells and/or their related suppressive cytokines may change the course of allergy and asthma. Small molecular weight compounds that may generate Treg cells or increase their suppressive properties is an important target not only for the use in allergy and asthma, but also for transplantation and autoimmunity.

cAMP-Stimulating G-Protein-Coupled Receptors in Peripheral Tolerance

The superfamily of seven-transmembrane G-protein-coupled receptors is the largest and most diverse group of membrane-spanning proteins [172]. Within all identified human genes, approximately 1,000 encode G-protein-coupled receptors. Many established G-protein-coupled receptor systems have been successfully exploited by the pharmaceutical industry to become the target for approximately 40% of the currently available drugs [172]. As a small molecular weight monoamine that binds to four different G-protein-coupled receptors, histamine was recently demonstrated to regulate several essential events in the immune response [173, 174]. The expression of these receptors on different cells and cell subsets is regulated and, apparently, diverse effects of histamine on immune regulation are due to differential expression of these receptors and their distinct intracellular signals. Histamine receptor (HR)2 is coupled to adenylate cyclase and studies in different species and several human cells demonstrated that inhibition of characteristic features of the cells by primarily cAMP formation dominates in HR2-dependent effects of histamine [175]. Recent studies indicated that HR3 and HR4 may antagonize with HR2-mediated suppression of the cells [176–178].

Histamine actively participates in functions and activity of DC precursors as well as their immature and mature forms. Immature and mature DCs express all four HRs [179–182]. In the differentiation process of type 1 DC from monocytes, HR1 and HR3 act as positive stimulants that increase antigen-presentation capacity and proinflammatory cytokine production and Th1-priming activity. In contrast, HR2 acts as a suppressive molecule for antigen-presentation capacity, enhances IL-10 production and induces of IL-10-producing T cells [183–185].

In monocytes stimulated with toll-like receptor-triggering bacterial products, histamine inhibits the production of proinflammatory IL-1-like activity, TNF-α and IL-12, but enhances IL-10 secretion, through HR2 stimulation [185–187]. Histamine induces intracellular Ca^{2+} flux, actin polymerization, and chemotaxis in immature DCs due to stimulation of HR1 and HR3 subtypes. Maturation of DCs results in loss of these responses. In maturing DCs, however, histamine dose-dependently enhances intracellular cAMP levels and stimulates IL-10 secretion, while inhibiting production of IL-12 via HR2 [184].

It has been demonstrated that differential patterns of HR expression on Th1 and Th2 cells determine reciprocal T-cell responses following histamine stimulation [49]. Th1 cells show predominant, but not exclusive expression of HR1, while Th2 cells show increased expression of HR2. Histamine enhances Th1-type responses by triggering the HR1, whereas both Th1- and Th2-type responses are negatively regulated by HR2, due to activation of different biochemical intracellular signals [49]. In mice, deletion of HR1 results in suppression of IFN-γ and dominant secretion of Th2 cytokines (IL-4 and IL-13). HR2-deleted mice show upregulation of both Th1 and Th2 cytokines. In addition, histamine stimulation induced IL-10 secretion through HR2 [188]. Increased IL-10 production in both DCs and T cells may account for an important regulatory mechanism in the control of inflammatory functions through histamine. In accordance with this phenomenon, it has recently been demonstrated that histamine supports the suppressive effect of TGF-β on T cells via HR2 [189]. Th2 cells are more affected by histamine-enhanced TGF-β suppression, which is particularly important for the regulation of allergen-specific T cells in allergic immune responses.

Clinical Evidence for T-Regulatory Function of Histamine Receptors

Considerable evidence has emerged to suggest that histamine participates in the immune regulation of the inflammatory response in several diseases. Histamine interferes with the peripheral tolerance induced during SIT in several pathways. Histamine induces the production of IL-10 by DCs [184]. In addition, histamine induces IL-10 production by Th2 cells [188]. Furthermore, histamine enhances the suppressive activity of TGF-β on T cells [189]. All three of these effects are mediated via HR2, which is relatively highly expressed on Th2 cells and suppresses IL-4 and IL-13 production and T-cell proliferation [49]. Apparently, these recent findings suggest that HR2 may represent an essential receptor that participates in peripheral tolerance or active suppression of inflammatory/immune responses.

The long-term protection from honeybee stings by terfenadine premedication during rush immunotherapy with honeybee venom in a double-blind, placebo-controlled trial was analyzed [190]. After an average of 3 years, 41 patients were re-exposed to honeybee stings. Surprisingly, none of 20 patients who had been given HR1 antihistamine premedication, but 6 of 21 given placebo, had a systemic allergic reaction to the re-exposure by either a field sting or a sting challenge. This highly significant difference suggests that antihistamine premedication during the initial dose-increase phase may have enhanced the long-term efficacy of immunotherapy. Expression of HR1 on T lymphocytes is strongly reduced during ultrarush immunotherapy, which may lead to a dominant expression and function of tolerance-inducing HR2. This indicates a positive role of histamine in immune regulation during SIT [191].

Selective HR2 antagonists have attracted interest because of their potential immune response-modifying activity [192]. Most data suggest that cimetidine has a stimulatory effect on the immune system, possibly by blocking the receptors on subsets of T lymphocytes and inhibiting HR2-induced immune suppression. Cimetidine has also been used to restore immune functions in patients with malignant disorders, HIV/AIDS and other viral infections [193–195]. Although their systemic usage may cause side effects such as ulcer development, together these findings are tempting to investigate local usage of selective agonists of HR2 and antagonists of HR3 and HR4 in the treatment of allergic diseases. Apparently, due to same signal transduction patterns,

β_2-adrenergic receptors may function similar to HR2 in humans [196, 197]. The role of histamine and other redundant G-protein-coupled receptors in the regulation of immune/inflammatory pathways in allergic inflammation remain to be intensely focused in future studies.

Conclusion

There is growing evidence supporting the role for Treg cells and/or immunosuppressive cytokine-IL-10 as a mechanism, by which venom-SIT and healthy immune response to venoms is mediated leading to both suppression of Th2 responses, ensuring a well-balanced immune response and a switch from IgE to IgG4 antibody production (fig. 1). Peripheral T-cell tolerance is the key immunological mechanism in healthy immune response to self and non-infectious, non-self antigens. This phenomenon is clinically well documented in allergy, autoimmunity, transplantation, tumor and infection. There is growing evidence supporting the role for Treg cells and/or immunosuppressive cytokines as a mechanism, by which allergen-SIT and healthy immune response to allergens is mediated (fig. 1). In addition to the treatment of established allergy, it is essential to consider prophylactic approaches before initial sensitization has taken place. Preventive vaccines that induce Treg responses can be developed. Allergen-specific Treg cells may in turn dampen both the Th1 and Th2 cells and cytokines, ensuring a well-balanced immune response. Enhancement of the number and activity of Treg cells could be an obvious goal for the suppression of allograft rejection, graft-versus-host disease and autoimmunity. Treg cells may not be always responsible for healthy immune response, because several studies have shown that they may be responsible for the chronicity of infections and tumor tolerance. Treg cell populations have proven possible, but difficult to grow, expand and clone in vitro. A crucial area for future studies is the identification of drugs, cytokines or costimulatory molecules that induce the growth while preserving the suppressor function of the Treg cells. These mechanisms can be better used by improvement of current treatment using recombinant allergens or peptide therapy. The elaboration of more efficacious desensitization methods including rapid protocols and antihistamine pretreatment also hold a promise for further development.

References

1 Hussain R, Poindexter RW, Ottesen EA: Control of allergic reactivity in human filariasis. Predominant localization of blocking antibody to the IgG4 subclass. J Immunol 1992;148:2731–2739.
2 Creticos PS: Immunological changes associated with immunotherapy; in Greenberger PA (ed): Immunotherapy of IgE-Mediated Disorders. Philadelphia, Saunders, 1992, pp 13–37.
3 Jutel M, Müller UM, Fricker M, Rihs S, Pichler W, Dahinden C: Influence of bee venom immunotherapy on degranulation and leukotriene generation in human blood basophils. Clin Exp Allergy 1996;26:112–118.
4 Rak S, Rowhagen O, Venge P: The effect of immunotherapy on bronchial hyperresponsiveness and eosinophil cationic protein in pollen allergic patients. J Allergy Clin Immunol 1988; 82:470–480.
5 Wetterwald A, Skvaril F, Müller U, Blaser K: Isotypic and idiotypic characterization of anti-bee venom phospholipase A$_2$ antibodies. Arch Allergy Appl Immunol 1985;77:195–197.
6 Akdis CA, Akdis M, Blesken T, Wymann D, Alkan SS, Müller U, et al: Epitope specific T-cell tolerance to phospholipase A$_2$ in bee venom immunotherapy and recovery by IL-2 and IL-15 in vitro. J Clin Invest 1996;98:1676–1683.
7 Akdis CA, Blesken T, Akdis M, Wuthrich B, Blaser K: Role of interleukin-10 in specific immunotherapy. J Clin Invest 1998;102:98–106.
8 Chen Y, Kuchroo VK, Inobe J, Hafler DA, Weiner HL: Regulatory T cell clones induced by oral tolerance: suppression of autoimmune encephalomyelitis. Science 1994;265:1237–1240.

9   Powrie F, Correa-Oliveira R, Mauze S, Coffman RL: Regulatory interactions between CD45RB^{high} and CD45RB^{low} CD4+ T cells are important for the balance between protective and pathogenic cell-mediated immunity. J Exp Med 1994;179:589–600.

10 Groux H, O'Garra A, Bigler M, Rouleau M, Antonenko S, De Vries JE, et al: A CD4+ T-cell subset inhibits antigen-specific T-cell responses and prevents colitis. Nature 1997;389:737–742.

11 Billingham RE, Brent L, Medawar PB: Actively acquired tolerance of foreign cells. Nature 1953;172:603–606.

12 Burnet F: The Nobel Lectures in Immunology. The Nobel Prize for Physiology or Medicine, 1960. Immunologic recognition of self. Scand J Immunol 1991;33:3–13.

13 Burnet FM: The Production of Antibodies. Melbourne, Macmillan, 1949.

14 Pirquet V: Das Verhalten der kutanen Tuberkulin-Reaktion während der Masern. Münch Med Wochenschr 1908; 34:1297–1300.

15 Nossal GJ, Pike BL: Clonal anergy: persistence in tolerant mice of antigen-binding B lymphocytes incapable of responding to antigen or mitogen. Proc Natl Acad Sci USA 1980;77:1602–1606.

16 Lamb JR, Skidmore BJ, Green N, Chiller JM, Feldman M: Induction of tolerance in influenza virus-immune T lymphocyte clones with synthetic peptides of influenza hemagglutinin. J Exp Med 1983;157:1434–1447.

17 Faith A, Akdis CA, Akdis M, Simon H-U, Blaser K: Defective TCR stimulation in anergized type 2 T helper cells correlates with abrogated p56(lck) and ZAP-70 tyrosine kinase activities. J Immunol 1997;159:53–60.

18 Schwartz RH: T cell anergy. Annu Rev Immunol 2003;21:305–334.

19 Dhein J, Walczak H, Bäumler C, Debatin KM, Krammer PH: Autocrine T-cell suicide mediated by APO-1(Fas/CD95). Nature 1995;373:438–441.

20 Brunner T, Mogil RJ, LaFace D, Jin Yoo N, Mahboubi A, Echeverri F, et al: Cell-autonomous Fas (CD95)/Fas-ligand interaction mediates activation-induced apoptosis in T-cell hybridomas. Nature 1995;373:441–444.

21 Akdis CA, Akdis M, Trautmann A, Blaser K: Immune regulation in atopic dermatitis. Curr Opin Immunol 2000; 12:641–646.

22 Akdis M, Simon H-U, Weigl L, Kreyden O, Blaser K, Akdis CA: Skin homing (cutaneous lymphocyte-associated antigen-positive) CD8+ T cells respond to superantigen and contribute to eosinophilia and IgE production in atopic dermatitis. J Immunol 1999;163: 466–475.

23 Abernathy-Carver KJ, Sampson HA, Picker LJ, Leung DYM: Milk-induced eczema is associated with the expansion of T cells expressing cutaneous lymphocyte antigen. J Clin Invest 1995; 95:913–918.

24 Klunker S, Trautmann A, Akdis M, Verhagen J, Schmid-Grendelmeier P, Blaser K, et al: A second step of chemotaxis after transendothelial migration: keratinocytes undergoing apoptosis release IP-10, Mig and iTac for T cell chemotaxis towards epidermis in atopic dermatitis. J Immunol 2003;171:1078–1084.

25 Luster AD: The role of chemokines in linking innate and adaptive immunity. Curr Opin Immunol 2002;14:129–135.

26 Gutierrez-Ramos JC, Lloyd C, Kapsenberg ML, Gonzalo JA, Coyle AJ: Non-redundant functional groups of chemokines operate in a coordinate manner during the inflammatory response in the lung. Immunol Rev 2000;177:31–42.

27 Akdis M, Trautmann A, Klunker S, Daigle I, Kücüksezer UC, Deglmann W, et al: T helper (Th)2 predominance in atopic diseases is due to preferential apoptosis of circulating memory/effector Th1 cells. FASEB J 2003;17:1026–1035.

28 Simon H-U, Blaser K: Inhibition of programmed eosinophil death: a key pathogenic event for eosinophilia. Immunol Today 1995;16:53–55.

29 Whittaker L, Niu N, Temann UA, Stoddard A, Flavell RA, Ray A, et al: Interleukin-13 mediates a fundamental pathway for airway epithelial mucus induced by CD4 T cells and interleukin-9. Am J Respir Cell Mol Biol 2002;27:593–602.

30 Trautmann A, Akdis M, Kleemann D, Altznauer F, Simon HU, Graeve T, et al: T-cell-mediated Fas-induced keratinocyte apoptosis plays a key pathogenetic role in eczematous dermatitis. J Clin Invest 2000;106:25–35.

31 Trautmann A, Schmid-Grendelmeier P, Krüger K, Crameri R, Akdis M, Akkaya A, et al: T cells and eosinophils cooperate in the induction of bronchial epithelial apoptosis in asthma. J Allergy Clin Immunol 2002;109:329–337.

32 Trautmann A, Akdis M, Brocker EB, Blaser K, Akdis CA: New insights into the role of T cells in atopic dermatitis and allergic contact dermatitis. Trends Immunol 2001;22:530–532.

33 Trautmann A, Akdis M, Schmid-Grendelmeier P, Disch R, Brocker EB, Blaser K, et al: Targeting keratinocyte apoptosis in the treatment of atopic dermatitis and allergic contact dermatitis. J Allergy Clin Immunol 2001; 108:839–846.

34 Romagnani S: Lymphokine production by human T cells in disease states. Annu Rev Immunol 1994;12:227–257.

35 Mosmann TR, Sad S: The expanding universe of T-cell subsets: Th1, Th2 and more. Immunol Today 1996;17:142–146.

36 Rincon M, Anguita J, Nakamura T, Fikrig E, Flavell RA: Interleukin (IL)-6 directs the differentiation of IL-4-producing CD4+ T cells. J Exp Med 1997; 185:461–469.

37 Corry DB: IL-13 in allergy: home at last. Curr Opin Immunol 1999;11:610–614.

38 Yssel H, Groux H: Characterization of T cell subpopulations involved in the pathogenesis of asthma and allergic diseases. Int Arch Allergy Immunol 2000;121:10–18.

39 El Biaze M, Boniface S, Koscher V, Mamessier E, Dupuy P, Milhe F, et al: T cell activation, from atopy to asthma: more a paradox than a paradigm. Allergy 2003;58:844–853.

40 Akdis CA, Blaser K: IL-10-induced anergy in peripheral T cell and reactivation by microenvironmental cytokines: two key steps in specific immunotherapy. FASEB J 1999;13: 603–609.

41 Akdis CA, Blesken T, Akdis M, Wüthrich B, Blaser K: Role of IL-10 in specific immunotherapy. J Clin Invest 1998;102:98–106.

42 Jutel M, Akdis M, Budak F, Aebischer-Casaulta C, Wrzyszcz M, Blaser K, et al: IL-10 and TGF-β cooperate in the regulatory T cell response to mucosal allergens in normal immunity and specific immunotherapy. Eur J Immunol 2003;33:1205–1214.

43 Powrie F, Correa-Oliveira R, Mauze S, Coffman RL: Regulatory interactions between CD45RB^high and CD45RB^low CD4+ T cells are important for the balance between protective and pathogenic cell-mediated immunity. J Exp Med 1994;179:589–600.

44 Groux H, O'Garra A, Bigler M, Rouleau M, Antonenko S, de Vries JE, et al: A CD4+ T-cell subset inhibits antigen-specific T-cell responses and prevents colitis. Nature 1997;389:737–742.

45 Taams LS, Smith J, Rustin MH, Salmon M, Poulter LW, Akbar AN: Human anergic/suppressive CD4+CD25+ T cells: a highly differentiated and apoptosis-prone population. Eur J Immunol 2001;31:1122–1131.

46 Jonuleit H, Schmitt E, Schuler G, Knop J, Enk AH: Induction of interleukin-10-producing, nonproliferating CD4+ T cells with regulatory properties by repetitive stimulation with allogeneic immature human dendritic cells. J Exp Med 2000;192:1213–1222.

47 Cottrez F, Hurst SD, Coffman RL, Groux H: T regulatory cells 1 inhibit a Th2-specific response in vivo. J Immunol 2000;165:4848–4853.

48 Bousquet J: Global initiative for asthma (GINA) and its objectives. Clin Exp Allergy 2000;30(suppl 1):2–5.

49 Jutel M, Watanabe T, Klunker S, Akdis M, Thomet OAR, Malolepszy J, et al: Histamine regulates T-cell and antibody responses by differential expression of H1 and H2 receptors. Nature 2001;413:420–425.

50 Holgate ST: Asthma: more than an inflammatory disease. Curr Opin Allergy Clin Immunol 2002;2:27–29.

51 Kussebi F, Karamloo F, Akdis M, Blaser K, Akdis CA: Advances in immunological treatment of allergy. Curr Med Chem 2003;2:297–308.

52 Müller UR, Mosbech H: Position paper: Immunotherapy with hymenoptera venoms. Allergy 1993;48:36–46.

53 Bousquet J, Lockey R, Malling HJ, Alvarez-Cuesta E, Canonica GW, Chapman MD, et al: Allergen immunotherapy: therapeutic vaccines for allergic diseases. World Health Organization. American Academy of Allergy, Asthma and Immunology. Ann Allergy Asthma Immunol 1998; 81:401–405.

54 Walker SM, Varney VA, Gaga M, Jacobson MR, Durham SR: Grass pollen immunotherapy: efficacy and safety during a 4-year follow-up study. Allergy 1995;50:405–413.

55 Varney VA, Gaga M, Frew AJ, Aber VR, Kay AB, Durham SR: Usefulness of immunotherapy in patients with severe summer hay fever uncontrolled by antiallergic drugs. BMJ 1991;302: 265–269.

56 Durham SR, Walker SM, Varga EM, Jacobson MR, O'Brien F, Noble W, et al: Long-term clinical efficacy of grass-pollen immunotherapy. N Engl J Med 1999;341:468–475.

57 Akdis CA, Akdis M, Blesken T, Wymann D, Alkan SS, Muller U, et al: Epitope-specific T cell tolerance to phospholipase A_2 in bee venom immunotherapy and recovery by IL-2 and IL-15 in vitro. J Clin Invest 1996;98:1676–1683.

58 Durham SR, Till SJ: Immunological changes associated with allergen immunotherapy. J Allergy Clin Immunol 1998;102:157–164.

59 Rolland JM, Douglass J, O'Hehir RE: Allergen immunotherapy: current and new therapeutic strategies. Expert Opin Investig Drugs 2000;9:515–527.

60 Ebner C: Immunological mechanisms operative in allergen-specific immunotherapy. Int Arch Allergy Immunol 1999;119:1–5.

61 Akdis CA, Blaser K: Mechanisms of allergen-specific immunotherapy. Allergy 2000;55:522–530.

62 Flicker S, Steinberger P, Norderhaug L, Sperr WR, Majlesi Y, Valent P, et al: Conversion of grass pollen allergen-specific human IgE into a protective IgG1 antibody. Eur J Immunol 2002; 32:2156–2162.

63 Wetterwald A, Skvaril F, Muller U, Blaser K: Isotypic and idiotypic characterization of anti-bee venom phospholipase A_2 antibodies. Int Arch Allergy Appl Immunol 1985;77:195–197.

64 Van Neerven RJ, Wikborg T, Lund G, Jacobsen B, Brinch-Nielsen A, Arnved J, et al: Blocking antibodies induced by specific allergy vaccination prevent the activation of CD4+ T cells by inhibiting serum-IgE-facilitated allergen presentation. J Immunol 1999;163:2944–2952.

65 Rocklin RE, Sheffer A, Greineder DK, Melmon KL: Generation of antigen-specific suppressor cells during allergy desensitization. N Engl J Med 1980; 302:1213–1219.

66 Creticos PS, Adkinson NF Jr, Kagey-Sobotka A, Proud D, Meier HL, Naclerio RM, et al: Nasal challenge with ragweed pollen in hay fever patients. Effect of immunotherapy. J Clin Invest 1985;76:2247–2253.

67 Rak S, Lowhagen O, Venge P: The effect of immunotherapy on bronchial hyper-responsiveness and eosinophil cationic protein in pollen-allergic patients. J Allergy Clin Immunol 1988; 82:470–480.

68 Otsuka H, Mezawa A, Ohnishi M, Okubo K, Seki H, Okuda M: Changes in nasal metachromatic cells during allergen immunotherapy. Clin Exp Allergy 1991;21:115–119.

69 Jutel M, Pichler WJ, Skrbic D, Urwyler A, Dahinden C, Muller UR: Bee venom immunotherapy results in decrease of IL-4 and IL-5 and increase of IFN-γ secretion in specific allergen-stimulated T-cell cultures. J Immunol 1995;154:4187–4194.

70 Secrist H, Chelen CJ, Wen Y, Marshall JD, Umetsu DT: Allergen immunotherapy decreases interleukin-4 production in CD4+ T cells from allergic individuals. J Exp Med 1993;178:2123–2130.

71 Bellinghausen I, Metz G, Enk AH, Christmann S, Knop J, Saloga J: Insect venom immunotherapy induces interleukin-10 production and a Th2- to-Th1 shift, and changes surface marker expression in venom-allergic subjects. Eur J Immunol 1997;27:1131–1139.

72 Müller U, Akdis CA, Fricker M, Akdis M, Blesken T, Bettens F, Blaser K: Successful immunotherapy with T-cell epitope peptides of bee venom phospholipase A2 induces specific T-cell anergy in patients allergic to bee venom. J Allergy Clin Immunol 1998;101:747–754.

73 Marcotte GV, Braun CM, Norman PS, Nicodemus CF, Kagey-Sobotka A, Lichtenstein LM, et al: Effects of peptide therapy on ex vivo T-cell responses. J Allergy Clin Immunol 1998;101:506–513.

74 Von Garnier C, Astori M, Kettner A, Dufour N, Heusser C, Corradin G, et al: Allergen derived long peptide immunotherapy down-regulates specific IgE response and protects from anaphylaxis. Eur J Immunol 2000;30:1638–1645.

75 Haselden BM, Kay AB, Larche M: Immunoglobulin E-independent major histocompatibility complex-restricted T cell peptide epitope-induced late asthmatic reactions. J Exp Med 1999;189:1885–1894.

76 Oldfield WL, Larche M, Kay AB: Effect of T-cell peptides derived from Fel d 1 on allergic reactions and cytokine production in patients sensitive to cats: a randomised controlled trial. Lancet 2002;360:47–53.

77 Faith A, Akdis CA, Akdis M, Joss A, Wymann D, Blaser K: An altered peptide ligand specifically inhibits Th2 cytokine synthesis by abrogating TCR signaling. J Immunol 1999;162:1836–1842.

78 Janssen EM, van Oosterhout AJ, van Rensen AJ, van Eden W, Nijkamp FP, Wauben MH: Modulation of Th2 responses by peptide analogues in a murine model of allergic asthma: amelioration or deterioration of the disease process depends on the Th1 or Th2 skewing characteristics of the therapeutic peptide. J Immunol 2000;164: 580–588.

79 Banerjee B, Kanitpong K, Fink JN, Zussman M, Sussman GL, Kelly KJ, et al: Unique and shared IgE epitopes of Hev b 1 and Hev b 3 in latex allergy. Mol Immunol 2000;37:789–798.

80 Woodfolk JA, Sung SS, Benjamin DC, Lee JK, Platts-Mills TA: Distinct human T cell repertoires mediate immediate and delayed-type hypersensitivity to the Trichophyton antigen, Tri r 2. J Immunol 2000;165:4379–4387.

81 Grabie N, Karin N: Expansion of neonatal tolerance to self in adult life. II. Tolerance preferentially spreads in an intramolecular manner. Int Immunol 1999;11:907–913.

82 Rolland JM, O'Hehir RE: Immunotherapy of allergy: anergy, deletion, and immune deviation. Curr Opin Immunol 1998;10:640–645.

83 Punnonen J, De Waal Malefyt R, Van Vlasselaer P, Gauchat J-F, De Vries JE: IL-10 and viral IL-10 prevent IL-4-induced IgE synthesis by inhibiting the accessory cell function of monocytes. J Immunol 1993;151:1280–1289.

84 Sonoda E, Matsumoto R, Hitoshi Y, Ishii T, Sugimoto M, Araki S, et al: Transforming growth factor-β induces IgA production and acts additively with interleukin-5 for IgA production. J Exp Med 1989;170:1415–1420.

85 Walker C, Virchow J-C, Bruijnzeel PLB, Blaser K: T cell subsets and their soluble products regulate eosinophilia in allergic and nonallergic asthma. J Immunol 1991;146:1829–1835.

86 Schleimer RP, Derse CP, Friedman B, Gillis S, Plaut M, Lichtenstein LM, et al: Regulation of human basophil mediator release by cytokines. I. Interaction with anti-inflammatory steroids. J Immunol 1989;143:1310–1327.

87 Treter S, Luqman M: Antigen-specific T cell tolerance down-regulates mast cell responses in vivo. Cell Immunol 2000;206:116–124.

88 Shim YK, Kim BS, Cho SH, Min KU, Hong SJ: Allergen-specific conventional immunotherapy decreases immunoglobulin E-mediated basophil histamine releasability. Clin Exp Allergy 2003;33:52–57.

89 Marshall JS, Leal-Berumen I, Nielsen L, Glibetic M, Jordana M: Interleukin (IL)-10 Inhibits long-term IL-6 production but not preformed mediator release from rat peritoneal mast cells. J Clin Invest 1996;97:1122–1128.

90 Schandane L, Alonso-Vega C, Willems F, Gerard C, Delvaux A, Velu T, et al: B7/CD28-dependent IL-5 production by human resting T cells is inhibited by IL-10. J Immunol 1994;152:4368–4374.

91 Ohkawara Y, Lim KG, Glibetic M, Nakano K, Dolovich J, Croitoru K, et al: CD40 expression by human peripheral blood eosinophils. J Clin Invest 1996; 97:1761–1766.

92 Gershon RK, Kondo K: Cell interactions in the induction of tolerance: the role of thymic lymphocytes. Immunology 1970;18:723–737.

93 Lee WY, Sehon AH: Abrogation of reaginic antibodies with modified proteins. Nature 1977;267:618–620.

94 Green DR, Webb DR: Saying the 'S' word in public. Immunol. Today 1993; 14:523–525.

95 Levings MK, Sangregorio R, Galbiati F, Squadrone S, de Waal Malefyt R, Roncarolo MG: IFN-α and IL-10 induce the differentiation of human type 1 T regulatory cells. J Immunol 2001;166:5530–5539.

96 Bacchetta R, Sartirana C, Levings MK, Bordignon C, Narula S, Roncarolo MG: Growth and expansion of human T regulatory type 1 cells are independent from TCR activation but require exogenous cytokines. Eur J Immunol 2002; 32:2237–2245.

97 Roncarolo MG, Bacchetta R, Bordignon C, Narula S, Levings MK: Type 1 T regulatory cells. Immunol Rev 2001;182:68–79.

98 Barrat FJ, Cua DJ, Boonstra A, Richards DF, Crain C, Savelkoul HF, et al: In vitro generation of interleukin-10-producing regulatory CD4+ T cells is induced by immunosuppressive drugs and inhibited by T-helper (Th) type 1 and Th2-inducing cytokines. J Exp Med 2002;195:603–616.

99 Nasser SM, Ying S, Meng O, Kay AB, Ewan PW: Interleukin-10 levels increase in cutaneous biopsies of patients undergoing wasp venom immunotherapy. Eur J Immunol 2001; 31:3704–3713.

100 Chen Y, Inobe J, Kuchroo VK, Baron JL, Janeway CA Jr, Weiner HL: Oral tolerance in myelin basic protein T-cell receptor transgenic mice: suppression of autoimmune encephalomyelitis and dose-dependent induction of regulatory cells. Proc Natl Acad Sci USA 1996;93:388–391.

101 Sakaguchi S, Sakaguchi N, Asano M, Itoh M, Toda M: Immunologic self-tolerance maintained by activated T cells expressing IL-2 receptor α-chains (CD25). Breakdown of a single mechanism of self-tolerance causes various autoimmune diseases. J Immunol 1995;155:1151–1164.

102 Shevach EM: CD4+ CD25+ suppressor T cells: more questions than answers. Nat Rev Immunol 2002;2:389–400.

103 Wood KJ, Sakaguchi S: Regulatory T cells in transplantation tolerance. Nat Rev Immunol 2003;3:199–210.

104 Read S, Powrie F: CD4+ regulatory T cells. Curr Opin Immunol 2001;13: 644–649.

105 Read S, Mauze S, Asseman C, Bean A, Coffman R, Powrie F: CD38+ CD45RB^{low} CD4+ T cells: a population of T cells with immune regulatory activities in vitro. Eur J Immunol 1998;28:3435–3447.

106 Weiner HL: Induction and mechanism of action of transforming growth factor-β-secreting Th3 regulatory cells. Immunol Rev 2001;182:207–214.

107 Ke Y, Kapp JA: Oral antigen inhibits priming of CD8+ CTL, CD4+ T cells, and antibody responses while activating CD8+ suppressor T cells. J Immunol 1996;156:916–921.

108 Weiner HL: Oral tolerance for the treatment of autoimmune diseases. Annu Rev Med 1997;48:341–351.

109 Ciubotariu R, Colovai AI, Pennesi G, Liu Z, Smith D, Berlocco P, et al: Specific suppression of human CD4+ Th cell responses to pig MHC antigens by CD8+CD28– regulatory T cells. J Immunol 1998;161:5193–5202.

110 Suvas S, Kumaraguru U, Pack CD, Lee S, Rouse BT: CD4+CD25+ T cells regulate virus-specific primary and memory CD8+ T cell responses. J Exp Med 2003;198:889–901.

111 Strober S, Cheng L, Zeng D, Palathumpat R, Dejbakhsh-Jones S, Huie P, et al: Double negative (CD4–CD8– αβ+) T cells which promote tolerance induction and regulate autoimmunity. Immunol Rev 1996;149:217–230.

112 Zhang ZX, Yang L, Young KJ, DuTemple B, Zhang L: Identification of a previously unknown antigen-specific regulatory T cell and its mechanism of suppression. Nat Med 2000;6:782–789.

113 Hanninen A, Harrison LC: γδ T cells as mediators of mucosal tolerance: the autoimmune diabetes model. Immunol Rev 2000;173:109–119.

114 Seo N, Tokura Y, Takigawa M, Egawa K: Depletion of IL-10- and TGF-β-producing regulatory γδ T cells by administering a daunomycin-conjugated specific monoclonal antibody in early tumor lesions augments the activity of CTLs and NK cells. J Immunol 1999; 163:242–249.

115 Ke Y, Pearce K, Lake JP, Ziegler HK, Kapp JA: γδ T lymphocytes regulate the induction and maintenance of oral tolerance. J Immunol 1997;158:3610–3618.

116 Seymour BW, Gershwin LJ, Coffman RL: Aerosol-induced immunoglobulin-E unresponsiveness to ovalbumin does not require CD8+ or T-cell receptor-γ/δ+ T cells or interferon-γ in a murine model of allergen sensitization. J Exp Med 1998;187:721–731.

117 Mauri C, Gray D, Mushtaq N, Londei M: Prevention of arthritis by interleukin-10-producing B cells. J Exp Med 2003; 197:489–501.

118 Reid CD: The biology and clinical applications of dendritic cells. Transfus Med 1998;8:77–86.

119 Akbari O, DeKruyff RH, Umetsu DT: Pulmonary dendritic cells producing IL-10 mediate tolerance induced by respiratory exposure to antigen. Nat Immunol 2001;2:725–731.

120 Steinbrink K, Wolfl M, Jonuleit H, Knop J, Enk A: Induction of tolerance by IL-10-treated dendritic cells. J Immunol 1997;159:4772–4780.

121 Morganti-Kossmann MC, Kossmann T, Brandes ME, Mergenhagen SE, Wahl SM: Autocrine and paracrine regulation of astrocyte function by transforming growth factor-β. J Neuroimmunol 1992;39:163–173.

122 Kao JY, Gong Y, Chen CM, Zheng QD, Chen JJ: Tumor-derived TGF-β reduces the efficacy of dendritic cell/tumor fusion vaccine. J Immunol 2003;170:3806–3811.

123 Rivas JM, Ullrich SE: Systemic suppression of delayed-type hypersensitivity by supernatants from UV-irradiated keratinocytes. An essential role for keratinocyte-derived IL-10. J Immunol 1992;149:3865–3871.

124 Lidstrom C, Matthiesen L, Berg G, Sharma S, Ernerudh J, Ekerfelt C: Cytokine secretion patterns of NK cells and macrophages in early human pregnancy decidua and blood: implications for suppressor macrophages in decidua. Am J Reprod Immunol 2003; 50:444–452.

125 Dowdell KC, Cua DJ, Kirtkman E, Stohlman SA: NK cells regulate CD4 responses prior to antigen encounter. J Immunol 2003;171:234–239.

126 Kitamura M, Suto T, Yokoo T, Shimizu F, Fine LG: Transforming growth factor-β₁ is the predominant paracrine inhibitor of macrophage cytokine synthesis produced by glomerular mesangial cells. J Immunol 1996;156:2964–2971.

127 Qin S, Cobbold SP, Pope H, Elliott J, Kioussis D, Davies J, et al: 'Infectious' transplantation tolerance. Science 1993; 259:974–977.

128 Thornton AM, Shevach EM: CD4+ CD25+ immunoregulatory T cells suppress polyclonal T cell activation in vitro by inhibiting interleukin-2 production. J Exp Med 1998;188:287–296.

129 Nakamura K, Kitani A, Strober W: Cell contact-dependent immunosuppression by CD4+CD25+ regulatory T cells is mediated by cell surface-bound transforming growth factor-β. J Exp Med 2001;194:629–644.

130 Levings MK, Bachetta R, Schulz U, Roncarolo MG: The role of IL-10 and TGF-β in the differentiation and effector function of T regulatory cells. Int Arch Allergy Appl Immunol 2002;129: 263–276.

131 Akdis CA, Joss A, Akdis M, Faith A, Blaser K: A molecular basis for T cell suppression by IL-10:CD28-associated IL-10 receptor inhibits CD28 tyrosine phosphorylation and phosphatidylinositol 3-kinase binding. FASEB J 2000; 14:1666–1669.

132 Itoh M, Takahashi T, Sakaguchi N, Kuniyasu Y, Shimizu J, Otsuka F, et al: Thymus and autoimmunity: production of CD25+CD4+ naturally anergic and suppressive T cells as a key function of the thymus in maintaining immunologic self-tolerance. J Immunol 1999;162:5317–5326.

133 Fowell D, Mason D: Evidence that the T cell repertoire of normal rats contains cells with the potential to cause diabetes. Characterization of the CD4+ T cell subset that inhibits this autoimmune potential. J Exp Med 1993; 177:627–636.

134 Asano M, Toda M, Sakaguchi N, Sakaguchi S: Autoimmune disease as a consequence of developmental abnormality of a T cell subpopulation. J Exp Med 1996;184:387–396.

135 Annunziato F, Cosmi L, Liotta F, Lazzeri E, Manetti R, Vanini V, et al: Phenotype, localization, and mechanism of suppression of CD4+CD25+ human thymocytes. J Exp Med 2002; 196:379–387.

136 Takahashi T, Tagami T, Yamazaki S, Uede T, Shimizu J, Sakaguchi N, et al: Immunologic self-tolerance maintained by CD25+CD4+ regulatory T cells constitutively expressing cytotoxic T lymphocyte-associated antigen 4. J Exp Med 2000;192:303–310.

137 Read S, Malmstrom V, Powrie F: Cytotoxic T lymphocyte-associated antigen 4 plays an essential role in the function of CD25+CD4+ regulatory cells that control intestinal inflammation. J Exp Med 2000;192:295–302.

138 Nishimura H, Nose M, Hiai H, Minato N, Honjo T: Development of lupus-like autoimmune diseases by disruption of the PD-1 gene encoding an ITIM motif-carrying immunoreceptor. Immunity 1999;11:141–151.

139 Carter L, Fouser LA, Jussif J, Fitz L, Deng B, Wood CR, et al: PD-1:PD-L inhibitory pathway affects both CD4+ and CD8+ T cells and is overcome by IL-2. Eur J Immunol 2002;32:634–643.

140 McHugh RS, Whitters MJ, Piccirillo CA, Young DA, Shevach EM, Collins M, et al: CD4+CD25+ immunoregulatory T cells: gene expression analysis reveals a functional role for the glucocorticoid-induced TNF receptor. Immunity 2002;16:311–323.

141 Shimizu J, Yamazaki S, Takahashi T, Ishida Y, Sakaguchi S: Stimulation of CD25+CD4+ regulatory T cells through GITR breaks immunological self-tolerance. Nat Immunol 2002;3: 135–142.

142 Nocentini G, Giunchi L, Ronchetti S, Krausz LT, Bartoli A, Moraca R, et al: A new member of the tumor necrosis factor/nerve growth factor receptor family inhibits T cell receptor-induced apoptosis. Proc Natl Acad Sci USA 1997;94:6216–6221.

143 Lehmann J, Huehn J, de la Rosa M, Masyzna F, Kretschmer U, Krenn V, et al: Expression of the integrin αEβ7 identifies unique subsets of CD25+ as well as CD25– regulatory T cells. Proc Natl Acad Sci USA 2002;99:13031–13036.

144 Levings MK, Sangregorio R, Roncarolo MG: Human CD25+CD4+ T regulatory cells suppress naive and memory T cell proliferation and can be expanded in vitro without loss of function. J Exp Med 2001;193:1295–1302.

145 Khattri R, Cox T, Yasayko SA, Ramsdell F: An essential role for Scurfin in CD4+CD25+ T regulatory cells. Nat Immunol 2003;4:337–342.

146 Fontenot JD, Gavin MA, Rudensky AY: Foxp3 programs the development and function of CD4+CD25+ regulatory T cells. Nat Immunol 2003;4:330–336.

147 Kanangat S, Blair P, Reddy R, Daheshia M, Godfrey V, Rouse BT, et al: Disease in the Scurfy mouse is associated with overexpression of cytokine genes. Eur J Immunol 1996;26:161–165.

148 Schubert LA, Jeffrey E, Zhang Y, Ramsdell F, Ziegler SF: Scurfin (FoxP3) acts as a repressor of transcription and regulates T cell activation. J Biol Chem 2001;276:37672–37679.

149 Wildin RS, Ramsdell F, Peake J, Faravelli F, Casanova JL, Buis TN, et al: X-linked neonatal diabetes mellitus, enteropathy and endocrinopathy syndrome is the human equivalent of mouse scurfy. Nat Genet 2001;27:18–20.

150 Walker LS, Chodos A, Eggena M, Dooms H, Abbas AK: Antigen-dependent proliferation of CD4+ CD25+ regulatory T cells in vivo. J Exp Med 2003;198: 249–258.

151 Fisson S, Darrasse-Jeze G, Litvinova E, Septier F, Klatzmann D, Liblau R, et al: Continuous activation of autoreactive CD4+ CD25+ regulatory T cells in the steady state. J Exp Med 2003;198: 737–746.

152 Sutmuller RP, van Duivenvoorde LM, van Elsas A, Schumacher TN, Wildenberg ME, Allison JP, et al: Synergism of cytotoxic T lymphocyte-associated antigen-4 blockade and depletion of CD25+ regulatory T cells in antitumor therapy reveals alternative pathways for suppression of autoreactive cytotoxic T lymphocyte responses. J Exp Med 2001;194:823–832.

153 Shimizu J, Yamazaki S, Sakaguchi S: Induction of tumor immunity by removing CD25+CD4+ T cells: a common basis between tumor immunity and autoimmunity. J Immunol 1999;163:5211–5218.

154 Hansen G, McIntire JJ, Yeung VP, Berry G, Thorbecke GJ, Chen L, et al: CD4+ T helper cells engineered to produce latent TGF-β₁ reverse allergen-induced airway hyperreactivity and inflammation. J Clin Invest 2000;105:61–70.

155 Borish L, Aarons A, Rumbyrt J, Cvietusa P, Negri J, Wenzel S: Interleukin-10 regulation in normal subjects and patients with asthma. J Allergy Clin Immunol 1996;97:1288–1296.

156 Koning H, Neijens HJ, Baert MR, Oranje AP, Savelkoul HF: T cells subsets and cytokines in allergic and non-allergic children. II. Analysis and IL-5 and IL-10 mRNA expression and protein production. Cytokine 1997;9:427–436.

157 Pierkes M, Bellinghausen I, Hultsch T, Metz G, Knop J, Saloga J: Decreased release of histamine and sulfidoleukotrienes by human peripheral blood leukocytes after wasp venom immunotherapy is partially due to induction of IL-10 and IFN-γ production of T cells. J Allergy Clin Immunol 1999;103:326–332.

158 Tillie-Leblond I, Pugin J, Marquette CH, Lamblin C, Saulnier F, Brichet A, et al: Balance between proinflammatory cytokines and their inhibitors in bronchial lavage from patients with status asthmaticus. Am J Respir Crit Care Med 1999;159:487–494.

159 Makela MJ, Kanehiro A, Borish L, Dakhama A, Loader J, Joetham A, et al: IL-10 is necessary for the expression of airway hyperresponsiveness but not pulmonary inflammation after allergic sensitization. Proc Natl Acad Sci USA 2000;97:6007–6012.

160 Yang X, Wang S, Fan Y, Han X: IL-10 deficiency prevents IL-5 overproduction and eosinophilic inflammation in a murine model of asthma-like reaction. Eur J Immunol 2000;30:382–391.

161 Vignola AM, Chanez P, Chiappara G, Merendino A, Pace E, Rizzo A, et al: Transforming growth factor-β expression in mucosal biopsies in asthma and chronic bronchitis. Am J Respir Crit Care Med 1997;156:591–599.

162 Hellings PW, Vandenberghe P, Kasran A, Coorevits L, Overbergh L, Mathieu C, et al: Blockade of CTLA-4 enhances allergic sensitization and eosinophilic airway inflammation in genetically predisposed mice. Eur J Immunol 2002;32:585–594.

163 Haneda K, Sano K, Tamura G, Shirota H, Ohkawara Y, Sato T, et al: Transforming growth factor-β secreted from CD4+ T cells ameliorates antigen-induced eosinophilic inflammation. A novel high-dose tolerance in the trachea. Am J Respir Cell Mol Biol 1999;21:268–274.

164 Aluvihare VR, Kallikourdis M, Betz AG: Regulatory T cells mediate maternal tolerance to the fetus. Nat Immunol 2004;5:266–271.

165 Battaglia A, Ferrandina G, Buzzonetti A, Malinconico P, Legge F, Salutari V, et al: Lymphocyte populations in human lymph nodes. Alterations in CD4+ CD25+ T regulatory cell phenotype and T-cell receptor Vβ repertoire. Immunology 2003;110:304–312.

166 Wolf AM, Wolf D, Steurer M, Gastl G, Gunsilius E, Grubeck-Loebenstein B: Increase of regulatory T cells in the peripheral blood of cancer patients. Clin Cancer Res 2003;9:606–612.

167 Antony PA, Restifo NP: Do CD4+ CD25+ immunoregulatory T cells hinder tumor immunotherapy. J Immunother 2002;25:202–206.

168 Turner J, Gonzalez-Juarro M, Ellis DL, Basaraba RJ, Kipnis A, Orme IM, et al: In vivo IL-10 production reactivates chronic pulmonary tuberculosis in C57BL/6 mice. J Immunol 2002;169:6343–6351.

169 Casaulta C, Schoni MH, Weichel M, Crameri R, Jutel M, Daigle I, et al: IL-10 controls *Aspergillus fumigatus*- and *Pseudomonas aeruginosa*-specific T-cell response in cystic fibrosis. Pediatr Res 2003;53:313–319.

170 Belkaid Y, Hoffmann KF, Mendez S, Kamhawi S, Udey MC, Wynn TA, et al: The role of interleukin (IL)-10 in the persistence of *Leishmania major* in the skin after healing and the therapeutic potential of anti-IL-10 receptor antibody for sterile cure. J Exp Med 2001; 194:1497–1506.

171 Redpath S, Ghazal P, Gascoigne NR: Hijacking and exploitation of IL-10 by intracellular pathogens. Trends Microbiol 2001;9:86–92.

172 Wilson S, Bergsma DJ: Orphan G-protein-coupled receptors: novel drug targets for the pharmaceutical industry. Drug Des Discov 2000;17:105–114.

173 Jutel M, Watanabe T, Akdis M, Blaser K, Akdis CA: Immune regulation by histamine. Curr Opin Immunol 2002; 14:735–740.

174 Akdis CA, Blaser K: Histamine in the immune regulation of allergic inflammation. J Allergy Clin Immunol 2003; 112:15–22.

175 Del Valle J, Gantz I: Novel insights into histamine H_2 receptor biology. Am J Physiol 1997;273:G987–G996.

176 Lovenberg TW, Roland BL, Wilson SJ, Jiang X, Pyati J, Huvar A, et al: Cloning and functional expression of the human histamine H_3 receptor. Mol Pharmacol 1999;55:1101–1107.

177 Dimitriadou V, Rouleau A, Dam Trung Tuong M, Newlands GJ, Miller HR, Luffau G, et al: Functional relationship between mast cells and C-sensitive nerve fibres evidenced by histamine H_3-receptor modulation in rat lung and spleen. Clin Sci (Lond) 1994;87: 151–163.

178 Nakamura T, Itadani H, Hidaka Y, Ohta M, Tanaka K: Molecular cloning and characterization of a new human histamine receptor, HH4R. Biochem Biophys Res Commun 2000;279:615–620.

179 Idzko M, la Sala A, Ferrari D, Panther E, Herouy Y, Dichmann S, et al: Expression and function of histamine receptors in human monocyte-derived dendritic cells. J Allergy Clin Immunol 2002;109:839–846.

180 Gutzmer R, Langer K, Lisewski M, Mommert S, Rieckborn D, Kapp A, et al: Expression and function of histamine receptors 1 and 2 on human monocyte-derived dendritic cells. J Allergy Clin Immunol 2002;109:524–531.

181 Caron G, Delneste Y, Roelandts E, Duez C, Herbault N, Magistrelli G, et al: Histamine induces CD86 expression and chemokine production by human immature dendritic cells. J Immunol 2001;166:6000–6006.

182 Gantner F, Sakai K, Tusche MW, Cruikshank WW, Center DM, Bacon KB: Histamine h4 and h2 receptors control histamine-induced interleukin-16 release from human CD8+ T cells. J Pharmacol Exp Ther 2002;303:3000–3007.

183 Caron G, Delneste Y, Roelandts E, Duez C, Bonnefoy JY, Pestel J, et al: Histamine polarizes human dendritic cells into Th2 cell-promoting effector dendritic cells. J Immunol 2001;167:3682–3686.

184 Mazzoni A, Young HA, Spitzer JH, Visintin A, Segal DM: Histamine regulates cytokine production in maturing dendritic cells, resulting in altered T cell polarization. J Clin Invest 2001; 108:1865–1873.

185 Van der Pouw Kraan TC, Snijders A, Boeije LC, de Groot ER, Alewijnse AE, Leurs R, et al: Histamine inhibits the production of interleukin-12 through interaction with H_2 receptors. J Clin Invest 1998;102:1866–1873.

186 Vannier E, Dinarello CA: Histamine enhances interleukin (IL)-1-induced IL-1 gene expression and protein synthesis via H_2 receptors in peripheral blood mononuclear cells. Comparison with IL-1 receptor antagonist. J Clin Invest 1993;92:281–287.

187 Elenkov IJ, Webster E, Papanicolaou DA, Fleisher TA, Chrousos GP, Wilder RL: Histamine potently suppresses human IL-12 and stimulates IL-10 production via H_2 receptors. J Immunol 1998;161:2586–2593.

188 Osna N, Elliott K, Khan MM: Regulation of interleukin-10 secretion by histamine in Th2 cells and splenocytes. Int Immunopharmacol 2001;1:85–96.

189 Kunzmann S, Mantel P-Y, Wohlfahrt JG, Akdis M, Blaser K, Schmidt-Weber CB: Histamine enhances TGF-β_1-mediated suppression of Th2 responses. FASEB J 2003;17:1089–1095.

190 Müller U, Hari Y, Berchtold E: Premedication with antihistamines may enhance efficacy of specific allergen immunotherapy. J Allergy Clin Immunol 2001;107:81–86.

191 Jutel M, Zak-Nejmark T, Wrzyyszcz M, Malolepszy J: Histamine receptor expression on peripheral blood CD4+ lymphocytes is influenced by ultrarush bee venom immunotherapy. Allergy 1997;52(suppl 37):88.

192 Gifford R, Schmidke J: Cimetidine-induced augmentation of human lymphocyte blastogenesis: comparison with levamisole in mitogen stimulation. Surg Forum 1979;30:113–115.

193 Tomita K, Izumi K, Okabe S: Roxatidine- and cimetidine-induced angiogenesis inhibition suppresses growth of colon cancer implants in syngeneic mice. J Pharmacol Sci 2003;93:321–330.

194 Bourinbaiar AS, Jirathitikal V: Low-cost anti-HIV compounds: potential application for AIDS therapy in developing countries. Curr Pharm Des 2003; 9:1419–1431.

195 Mitsuishi T, Iida K, Kawana S: Cimetidine treatment for viral warts enhances IL-2 and IFN-γ expression but not IL-18 expression in lesional skin. Eur J Immunol 2003;13:153–169.

196 Benovic J: β_2-Adrenergic receptor signaling pathways. J Allergy Clin Immunol 2002;110:S229-S235.

197 Roth M, Johnson PR, Rudiger JJ, King GG, Ge Q, Burgess JK, et al: Interaction between glucocorticoids and β_2-agonists on bronchial airway smooth muscle cells through synchronised cellular signalling. Lancet 2002;360:1293–1299.

Dr. Marek Jutel
Department of Internal Medicine and Allergology
Wroclaw Medical University, Traugutta 57
PL–50-417 Wroclaw (Poland)
Tel. +48 71 341 7123, Fax +48 71 341 7830, E-Mail mjutel@ak.am.wroc.pl

Blaser K (ed): T Cell Regulation in Allergy, Asthma and Atopic Skin Diseases.
Chem Immunol Allergy. Basel, Karger, 2008, vol 94, pp 178–188

Control and Regulation of Peripheral Tolerance in Allergic Inflammatory Disease: Therapeutic Consequences

Lequn Li · Vassiliki A. Boussiotis

Division of Hematology/Oncology, Department of Medicine, Beth Israel Deaconess
Medical Center, Harvard Medical School, Boston, Mass., USA

Abstract

During the past few years there has been significant progress in understanding the mechanisms by which abnormal T-cell responses are generated in allergic diseases. Peripheral T-cell tolerance to environmental antigens is crucial for a healthy immune response and avoidance of allergy. The balance between T-helper (Th)2 cells and T-regulatory (Treg) cells has a critical role in the generation of immune responses to environmental antigens. Allergic individuals display an aberrant activation and expansion of Th2 cells. It appears that aberrant activation of Th2 cells in allergy is secondary to impaired mechanisms of peripheral T-cell tolerance that is normally mediated by antigen-specific T-cell anergy, Treg cells and suppressive cytokines, IL-10 and TGF-β. Therefore, a most appealing therapy for allergic diseases would be an allergen-specific immunotherapy that reduces Th2 cytokine production and promotes induction of anergy, Treg and suppressor cytokines. Such novel therapeutic approaches include the use of recombinant allergen-derived peptides, recombinant DNA technology and adjuvants. These approaches are employed individually or in combination in order to induce T-cell anergy and to utilize innate immunity in order to alter the balance of Th1- and Th2-type cytokines and generate or expand Treg in vivo.

Copyright © 2008 S. Karger AG, Basel

Pathobiology of the Allergic Inflammatory Response

The term allergy implies an often familial tendency to manifest conditions such as asthma, rhinitis, urticaria and eczematous dermatitis, alone or in combination. The induction of allergic diseases requires sensitization of a predisposed individual to specific antigen. This sensitization can occur anytime in life, although the greatest propensity for development of allergic diseases appears to occur in childhood and early adolescence. Exposure of a susceptible individual to an allergen results in processing of the allergen by antigen presenting cells (APC), including macrophages and dendritic cells (DCs) located throughout the body at surfaces that contact the outside environment, such as nose, lungs, eyes, skin and intestine. These APC process the allergen protein and present the epitope-bearing peptides via their MHC to particular T-cell subsets. T-cell responses depend both on cognate recognition through various ligand/receptor interactions and on the cytokine microenvironment, with IL-4 directing a Th2 response and interferon (IFN)-γ a Th1 profile. T cells can potentially induce several responses to an allergen, including those typical for contact dermatitis, known as Th1-type response, and those mediated by IgE, known as the Th2-allergic response. The Th2 response is associated with activation of specific B cells that transform into plasma cells. Synthesis and release into the serum of allergen-specific IgE by plasma cells result in sensitization of IgE Fc receptor-bearing cells, including mast cells and basophils, which subsequently are capable of becoming activated upon exposure to the specific allergen (fig. 1) [1, 2].

The mast cell is the key effector cell of the biological response in allergic diseases. Interaction of specific antigen with receptor-bound IgE results in clustering of the receptors to initiate signal transduction through the src family tyrosine kinase, Lyn. Lyn phosphorylates the canonical immunoreceptor tyrosine-based activation motifs (ITAMs) of the β- and γ-receptor chain, resulting in recruitment of more active Lyn and of the Syk/Zap-70 family kinases. The two phosphorylated tyrosines in the ITAMs function as binding sites for the tandem SH2 domains within these kinases. It appears that Syk activates not only phospholipase Cγ, but also phosphatidylinositol-3-kinase to provide phosphatidyl-3,4,5-triphosphate, which allows membrane targeting of the Tec family kinase (Btk and Itk) and their activation by Lyn. The resulting Tec kinase-dependent phosphorylation of phospholipase Cγ with cleavage of its phospholipid membrane substrate provides inositol 1,4,5-triphosphate (IP$_3$) and 1,2-diacylglycerols (1,2-DAGs) so as to mobilize intracellular calcium and activate protein kinase C. The subsequent opening of calcium-regulate activated channels provides the sustained elevations of intracellular calcium required to recruit the mitogen-activated protein (MAP) kinases, JNK and p38, which provide cascades to augment arachidonic acid release and to mediate nuclear translocation of transcription factors for various cytokines. The calcium ion-dependent activation of phospholipases cleaves membrane phospholipids to generate lysophospholipids, which like 1,2-DAG, are fusigenic and may facilitate the fusion of the secretory granule perigranular membrane with the cell membrane, a step that releases the membrane-free granule containing the preformed or primary mediators of mast cell effects.

The cellular component of the inflammatory response is elicited by preformed secretory granule-associated and membrane-derived lipid mediators of the mast cells [2]. The later mediators specifically arachidonic acid that is subsequently converted to sequential intermediates prostaglandin (PG)G$_2$ and PGH$_2$, which is then converted to PGD$_2$, the predominant mast cell prostanoid, and important mediator of allergic responses. In addition to prostaglandins, inflammatory responses are augmented and sustained by the release of cytokines that originated from mast cells or T cells in the local microenvironment. Activation of human skin mast cells in situ elicits TNF-α production and release, which in turn induces endothelial cell responses favoring leukocyte adhesion. Activation of mast cells also results in production of IL-4 and even more prominently IL-5, although the major sources of these cytokines along with GM-CSF are Th2 cells.

Regulation of Peripheral T-Cell Tolerance and Aberrations in Allergic Diseases

Although central tolerance is the major mechanism to establish the T-cell repertoire by positive and negative selection mechanisms, thymic deletion of harmful T-cell populations is incomplete. Therefore, the immune system has developed mechanisms that deal with tolerance in the peripheral lymphoid organs providing the necessary

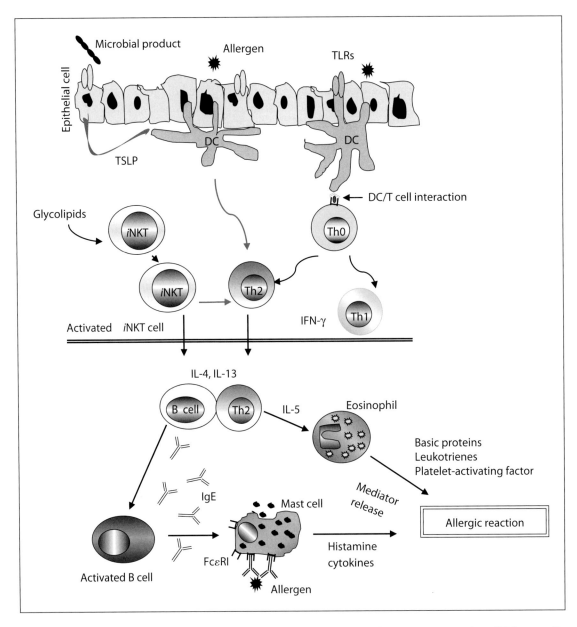

Fig. 1. Mechanisms promoting allergic reaction. After allergen encounter, DCs promote generation of Th2-type cells. This function of DCs is further enhanced by TSLP produced by epithelial cells. Th2-type cytokines, IL-4 and IL-13, provide signals to B cells to switch activated B cells to produce allergen-specific IgE isotype. IgE binding to high-affinity IgE receptors (FcεRI) on mast cells results in the release of preformed and newly generated mediators from these cells, which, consequently, generate symptoms of the allergic response. In asthma, pulmonary iNKT cells are activated by glycolipid antigens resulting in secretion of IL-4 and IL-13, but not IFN-γ. iNKT cells might amplify the function of allergen-specific Th2 cells or may be the direct source of Th2-type cytokines.

safety net to prevent aberrant immune responses. Peripheral tolerance is regulated by T-cell intrinsic and extrinsic mechanisms. Intrinsic mechanisms involve T-cell anergy, phenotype skewing and apoptosis, whereas extrinsic mechanisms involve T-cell regulation by T-regulatory cells (Treg), suppressive cytokines, mainly IL-10 and TGF-β, and by APC. During the past 5 years there has been significant progress in our understanding of the mechanisms by which abnormal T-cell responses are generated in allergic diseases [1, 2]. Early studies had focused on the imbalanced Th2- to Th1-type cytokine responses as the cause of allergy. However, recent work has demonstrated that T-cell tolerance to environmental antigens is crucial for a healthy immune response and avoidance of allergy [3].

T-Cell Anergy

Tolerance to environmental allergens can be influenced by many events, including induction of anergy, deletion and altered presentation by APC. Allergy may be secondary to impaired peripheral tolerance due to impaired anergization of allergen-specific T cells. In support of this hypothesis, using DRB1*0401 tetramers loaded with the major epitope of rye grass allergen Lol p 1, Macaubas et al. [4] detected allergen-specific CD4+ T cells in the peripheral blood of DRB1*0401 rye grass-allergic individuals following ex vivo expansion with allergen. These tetramer-positive cells produced IL-4 but little IFN-γ. By contrast, no rye grass tetramer-positive cells were expanded in cultures from HLA-DR*0401 non-allergic individuals, even after incubation with IL-2. These results indicate that in normal individuals allergen-specific T cells are present at low levels and differ significantly in their requirement for ex vivo expansion from those present in allergic individuals, suggesting that they may be anergic and incapable of responding not only to the specific antigen, but also to critical T-cell growth

factors like IL-2. This event is impaired in allergic individuals.

Consistent with these studies supporting that allergy may result from impaired induction of T-cell anergy, recent work has provided evidence that development of allergic asthma might be associated with activation of a potent costimulatory pathway mediated by TIM-1 (T cell, immunoglobulin and mucin) [5]. It is well established that one of the anergy-inducing mechanisms involves the lack of appropriate costimulation at a certain time in the life of a T cell. TIM-1, a cell surface molecule expressed preferentially by Th2 cells, is encoded by an important asthma susceptibility gene. TIM-1 is a potent costimulatory molecule that mediates enhanced cytokine production and loss of tolerance. In humans, the hepatitis A virus (HAV) binds to TIM-1. Importantly, infection by HAV may protect individuals from atopy if they carry a particular variant of the gene encoding TIM-1 [6]. Exposure to HAV is associated with poor hygiene, large family size and attendance at daycare centers, all factors that are inversely associated with atopy [7]. This observation not only supports the notion that costimulation may be directly involved in the allergic response, but also suggests that TIM-mediated pathway may represent a novel therapeutic target in allergic asthma.

Suppressive Cytokines (IL-10, TGF-β)
IL-10 is a major suppressive cytokine involved in the physiologic regulation of immunosuppression and T-cell tolerance. Several lines of evidence indicate that the tolerant state of allergen-specific T cells is related to the presence of IL-10 [reviewed in 1]. The cellular origin of IL-10 was demonstrated as being the antigen-specific T-cell population and activated CD4+CD25+ T cells as well as monocytes and B cells. It was proposed that IFN-γ, IL-4- and IL-10-secreting allergen-specific CD4+ T cells resemble Th1, Th2 and Tr1-like cells, respectively [8]. Healthy and allergic individuals exhibit all three subsets, but in different proportions. In healthy individuals, Tr1

cells represent the dominant subset for common environmental allergens, whereas a high frequency of allergen-specific IL-4-secreting T cells (Th2-like) is found in allergic individuals. IL-10 not only induces tolerance in T cells, but also is a potent suppressor of total and allergen-specific IgE, while it simultaneously increases production of IgG4. It has been determined that T cells from children suffering from asthma produce less IL-10 mRNA than T cells from control children. Conversely, schistosoma infection in Gabonese children is associated with increased serum levels of IL-10 and a decreased incidence of immediate hypersensitivity to house dust mite antigens [7]. These observations suggested that a change in the dominant T-cell subsets might lead to the development of allergy or to recovery from the allergic inflammatory response.

TGF-β is produced during antigenic stimulation of T lymphocytes and suppresses T-cell responses providing a strong evidence for the autocrine TGF-β regulatory function in T cells. Genetic approaches have indicated that endogenous TGF-β has a significant role in inhibiting proliferation of antigen-experienced cells and in regulating tolerance induction and maintenance of T-cell quiescence. TGF-$β_1$-deficient mice develop a hyperactivated CD4+ T-cell phenotype and die at 3–4 weeks of age of a rapidly wasting syndrome [9]. The role of TGF-β in the development and the immunosuppressive function of Treg and the precise mechanism via which it mediates its suppressive effects on T-cell activation remain controversial. However, TGF-β appears to induce IgA production, thereby regulating mucosal immune tolerance [10]. Recent studies indicate that Treg cells, induced by exposure of the respiratory mucosa to antigen, expressed membrane-bound TGF-β and mediated immunosuppression by activating the Notch1-hairy and enhancer of split 1 (Notch 1-HES1) axis in target cells, suggesting that TGF-β-Notch1 pathway is crucial in regulating tolerance in the lungs [11].

Natural and Adaptive Treg Cells
Natural CD25+ Treg cells develop in the thymus, although they might expand in the periphery upon antigen exposure. Adaptive Treg cells are induced by immunization with antigen or by exposure to the environment. Treg cells can inhibit allergen-induced airway hypersensitivity by IL-10-dependent mechanisms or by inhibiting antigen presentation by DCs. The number of CD25+ Treg cells that inhibit allergen-induced tissue pathology in an antigen non-specific manner increases greatly during gastrointestinal nematode infection, suggesting a mechanism by which infection might inhibit the development of allergy [12]. The well-documented, longstanding observation that the incidence of infections inversely correlates to the incidence of atopic allergy and asthma [7] may be mediated via the generation and/or expansion of adoptive Treg during the infectious process.

Mechanisms Promoting the Inflammatory Response in Allergic Diseases

Although experimental and clinical evidence provide strong support that impaired immunosuppressive and tolerance mechanisms are involved in the pathobiology of allergic diseases, the role of factors that actively promote the allergic response should not be underestimated. Abnormal production of soluble factors like TNF-α, TSLP, and IL-25, or activation of natural killer T-cell compartment (iNKT) cells, may result in development of allergic disease by overcoming the capacity of suppressive mechanisms of peripheral tolerance to prevent the enhanced immune response.

Tumor Necrosis Factor-α
TNF-α is a cytokine produced by T cells and mast cells. TNF-α is involved in the gut inflammatory process in Crohn disease, where treatment with soluble TNF-α receptor and anti-TNF-α antibodies and soluble TNF-α receptor has the highest

success rate. TNF-α may also be involved in asthma as supported by the promising results of a recent clinical study, in which patients with refractory asthma were treated with soluble TNF-α receptor [13].

Thymic Stromal Lymphopoietin

Thymic stromal lymphopoietin (TSLP) was first described in 1994 as a novel IL-7-like cytokine involved in T- and B-cell differentiation [14]. Produced in Hassall's corpuscles, TSLP has a critical role in the positive selection of natural Treg cells in the thymus. However, TSLP appears to also be important in the periphery, where it promotes development of Th2 cells by DCs. Interestingly, TSLP is expressed at high levels in the lungs of patients who have asthma and over-expression of TSLP in the lungs of mice results in severe allergic airway inflammation. Expression of TSLP by skin keratinocytes in mice results in the development of a condition that resembles atopic dermatitis. Interestingly, TSLP is also produced by gut epithelial cells leading to the development of tolerogenic DC, which release IL-10 and IL-6 but not IL-12 and promote polarization of T cells toward a non-inflammatory Th2 response. Strikingly, this mechanism is impaired in patients with Crohn disease, in which expression of TSLP in epithelial cells is undetectable [15].

Interleukin-25

IL-25(IL-17E), a proinflammatory factor produced by mast cells and Th2 cells, is known to mediate production of large quantities of Th2 cytokines. IL-25 might also enhance Th2 responses by actively inhibiting IFN γ and IL-17 production thereby limiting pathologic (Th1-biased) inflammation at mucosal sites. Because IL-25 enhances Th2 cytokine production, it might also enhance the development of allergic inflammatory responses at mucosal sites inducing eosinophilia, airway hyperreactivity and increased mucus production [16].

Natural Killer T Cells

A cellular population that is part of the innate immune system has received much attention during the past year: the invariant T-cell receptor iNKT. Several years ago, iNKT cells were shown to be required for the development of allergen-induced airway hyperreactivity in mouse models of asthma. More recently, the activation of iNKT cells was shown to induce allergen-induced airway hyperreactivity when activated with glycolipid antigens, specifically α-galacosyl-ceramide (α-Gal-Cer) or glycolipids from the membranes of lipopolysaccharide-negative *Sphingomonas paucimobilis* bacteria [17]. When the frequency and distribution of iNKT cells was assessed in the lungs and in the circulating blood of patients with moderate-to-severe persistent asthma, it was determined that 60% of the pulmonary CD4+ CD3+ cells in the lungs of these patients were not class II MHC-restricted CD4+ T cells, but rather iNKT cells [18]. These iNKT cells produced IL-4 and IL-13, but not IFN-γ, suggesting that these cells might have been mistakenly identified in the past as conventional CD4+ Th2 cells. The mechanisms by which the Th2-like subset of iNKT cells enters or expands in the lungs are under investigation. Clarification of these mechanisms will provide an exciting novel therapeutic target in the treatment of asthma.

Immunotherapeutic Approaches for Regulation of T-Cell Tolerance in Allergic Diseases

It is a longstanding observation that activation of innate immunity appears to protect against allergic diseases. The reciprocal downregulation of Th1 cells by Th2 cytokines and the Th2 cells by Th1 cytokines raised the possibility that these cytokines are involved in infection-mediated protection against allergy [7]. A second potential protective mechanism is antigenic competition, in which the immune response to an antigen is decreased by a concomitant immune response against an unrelated antigen. However, the precise mechanism of antigenic competition has never been identified. Recently, it was determined that bacteria and viruses could protect against immune disorders by signaling through toll-like receptors (TLRs). TLR2 serves as a receptor for peptidoglycan and bacterial lipoproteins, TLR4 as a receptor for Gram-negative lipopolysaccharide, TLR5 as a receptor for flagellin, and TLR9 as a receptor for the CpG motif of bacterial DNA. When they bind these bacterial ligands, TLRs stimulate mononuclear cells to produce cytokines, some of which could downregulate allergic and autoimmune responses [19]. These recent developments may change our view on allergy-specific immunotherapy.

Allergen-specific immunotherapy, also called hyposensitization or desensitization, has been used for the treatment of allergic disease for nearly 100 years. This approach consists of administration of increasing concentrations of extracts of allergen over a long period. The mode of action of specific immunotherapy is complex. It is thought that IgG 'blocking' antibodies compete with IgE for allergen. They may also prevent the aggregation of complexes of IgE and the α-chain of the high-affinity IgE receptor (FcεRI-α) on mast cells by altering the steric conformation. In addition, they may interfere with antigen trapping by IgE bound to antigen-presenting cells [20]. Specific immunotherapy induces a shift from the production of Th2-type cytokines IL-4 and IL-5 to the production of Th1-type cytokines IFN-γ and IL-12. In addition, immunotherapy can induce activation of cells secreting IL-10, which leads to long-term hyporesponsiveness of allergen-specific CD4+ T cells, decreases the level of IgE, decreases the number of mast cells, and inhibits the production of eosinophils [20].

Based on the improvement of our understanding on the regulation of productive T-cell responses versus T-cell tolerance and the recent advances of biotechnology, newer immunotherapeutic approaches have been designed (fig. 2). Induction of anergy of allergen-specific T cells by the use of allergen-specific peptides or altered peptide ligands may provide a successful approach to control aberrant T-cell responses in allergic diseases. Short, allergen-derived peptides can induce T-cell anergy but, because of their short length, are unable to cross-link IgE and induce anaphylaxis. Recombinant DNA technology has enabled the cloning of many allergens and the generation of synthetic peptides. The use of mixtures of allergen-derived peptides elected on the basis of their ability to bind to common MHC class II molecules has great efficacy, since they are recognized by T cells of most individuals in the population. Mixtures of recombinant allergen-specific peptides have been successfully used in clinical trials for bee venom-, grass pollen- and cat-allergic individuals [21–23]. Treated patients developed strong allergen-specific IgG1 and IgG4 antibody responses and exhibited a significant reduction in the frequency and intensity of their symptoms. Development of peripheral T-cell tolerance to whole allergens was detected in patients from these trials. Peptide immunotherapy induced generation of Tr1 cells and simultaneous increase in IL-10, while IL-4, IL-5, IL-13 and IFN-γ levels were reduced [24].

With new technology, genetical engineering of several recombinant allergens into one chimeric protein became available. In two recent in vivo mouse studies, two different chimeric proteins of the major honey bee venom allergens, which preserved the entire T-cell epitopes, were used for vaccination. With both vaccines, IgE cross-linking leading to mast cell and basophil mediator release was profoundly reduced [25, 26]. Using a genetically modified derivative of the major birch pollen allergen Bet v 1, a clinical trial demonstrated that Bet v 1-specific IgG1, IgG2, and IgG4 were significantly increased whereas Bet v 1-reactive IL-5- and IL-13-producing cells were diminished [27]. These studies provide challenging support for future clinical trials.

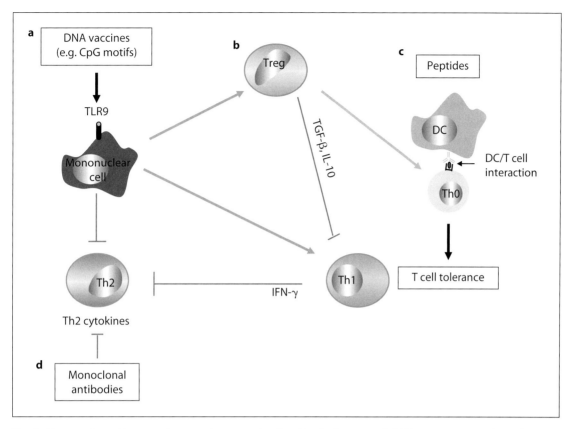

Fig. 2. Targets of novel immunotherapeutic approaches for allergic diseases. **a, b** DNA vaccines using plasmid vectors containing genes that encode allergens or CpG motifs can enhance Th1-mediated responses, decrease Th2-mediated responses, and induce antigen-specific adaptive Treg cells that produce IL-10. **c** Treatment with allergen-specific peptides or altered peptide ligands can induce antigen-specific T-cell anergy. **d** The products of aberrant Th2 cell activation can be targeted by strategies to block IgE synthesis and use of IL-4- and IL-5-specific monoclonal antibodies.

DNA vaccines have also been employed for treatment of allergic diseases. Plasmid vectors containing genes that encode allergens injected into animals either before or after allergen challenge can enhance Th1-mediated responses, markedly decrease Th2-mediated responses and suppress the allergic inflammatory response. Virus-like particles such as the yeast-derived Ty can also induce IFN-γ producing CD8+ T cells and suppress Th2-mediated response [reviewed in 1]. Other approaches include administration of CpG motifs such as GACGTC, which induce strong Th1-mediated responses, either alone or in combination with allergen proteins [28]. As mentioned above, CpG motifs may work by activating TLR9. When administered into the lungs, CpG oligonucleotides can inhibit Th2 cytokine production. This occurs first by inhibition of DC antigen presentation to Th2 cells and second by inhibiting production of cytokines by mast cells and basophils [29]. Further supporting the role of TLR-mediating signaling in protecting against allergic diseases, it was observed that intestinal microflora might provide anti-inflammatory effect and enhance tolerance by signaling through TLR4 [30]. In contrast, elimination of commensal bacteria with broad-spectrum antibiotics prevents development of oral tolerance and enhances allergic sensitization and susceptibility to intestinal inflammation [30, 31].

Other immunological therapeutic approaches are targeting the products of aberrant Th2 cell activation in allergic diseases. These approaches include strategies to block IgE synthesis or function and to interrupt the Th2-dependent allergic cascade. Treatment with a recombinant humanized monoclonal antibody against IgE (rhuMAB-E25, or omalizumab) virtually eliminated IgE and markedly decreased the expression of FcεRI on basophils [32]. To interrupt the Th2-dependent allergic cascade, inhibition of IL-4 and IL-5 is under investigation. Treatment with soluble recombinant IL-4 receptor moderately improved severe atopic asthma [33]. In monkeys a monoclonal antibody against IL-5 almost completely eliminated eosinophilia and airway hyperresponsiveness. However, a study in patients with mild asthma showed that a humanized monoclonal antibody against IL-5 abolished eosinophils in blood and reduced the number of eosinophils in sputum but had no apparent effect on the allergen-induced late-phase asthmatic reaction or non-specific airway hyperresponsiveness [34].

Recently, it became clear that lack of peripheral tolerance in allergy is caused not only due impaired anergy induction and overactivation of allergen-specific Th2 cells, but also due to Treg cell deficiency. Therefore, a most appealing therapy would be an allergen-specific immunotherapy that reduces Th2 cytokine production and enhances development of Treg. Based on this notion, several approaches have been developed to induce protective immunity, including subcutaneous or sublingual administration of antigen, immunization with allergen peptides and use of adjuvant such as *Listeria monocytogenes* [12]. Allergen-specific immunotherapy with antigen peptides or with adjuvant can induce antigen-specific adaptive Treg cells that produce IL-10 [35, 36]. Importantly, loss of Treg cells might be caused by the use of corticosteroids. Specifically, corticosteroids, an established drug for the treatment of exacerbations of asthma and allergy, appear to block the development of T-cell tolerance and the function of DCs that induce antigen-specific adaptive Treg cells [37]. These results suggest that treatment with corticosteroids in patients with allergy and asthma could potentially enhance Th2 responses and could adversely affect the long-term course of allergic diseases and asthma. These observations may have significant implications in our treatment choices for allergic diseases in the future.

Conclusions and Future Directions

During the past 5 years, much progress has been made in our understanding of the specific mechanisms that control the allergic inflammatory response both in a positive and negative manner. We now know that impaired mechanisms of allergen-specific response include lack of T-cell anergy and suppression mediated via Treg and suppressive cytokines. These newly identified mechanisms can be targeted for therapeutic purposes. Utilization of innate immunity and toll-like receptors for in vivo expansion of Treg and generation of Th1 cytokines, will be exciting a promising novel therapeutic approach for the treatment of allergic diseases. In contrast, the novel mechanisms positively regulating the allergic response including TSLP, IL-25, TNF-α, TIM proteins and iNKT cells can be therapeutic targets for inhibition, in order to eliminate or suppress the inflammatory process and prevent or reverse the exacerbation of allergic diseases.

References

1 Umetsu DT, Dekruyff RH: Immune dysregulation in asthma. Curr Opin Immunol 2006;18:727–732.

2 Kay AB: Allergy and allergic diseases. First of two parts. N Engl J Med 2001; 344:30–37.

3 Jutel M, Akdis M, Blaser K, Akdis CA: Mechanisms of allergen-specific immunotherapy – T-cell tolerance and more. Allergy 2006;61:796–807.

4 Macaubas C, Wahlstrom J, Galvao da Silva AP, Forsthuber TG, Sonderstrup G, Kwok WW, DeKruyff RH, Umetsu DT: Allergen-specific MHC class II tetramer+ cells are detectable in allergic, but not in nonallergic, individuals. J Immunol 2006;176:5069–5077.

5 Umetsu SE, Lee WL, McIntire JJ, Downey L, Sanjanwala B, Akbari O, Berry GJ, Nagumo H, Freeman GJ, Umetsu DT, DeKruyff RH: TIM-1 induces T cell activation and inhibits the development of peripheral tolerance. Nat Immunol 2005;6:447–454.

6 McIntire JJ, Umetsu SE, Macaubas C, Hoyte EG, Cinnioglu C, Cavalli-Sforza LL, Barsh GS, Hallmayer JF, Underhill PA, Risch NJ, Freeman GJ, DeKruyff RH, Umetsu DT: Immunology: hepatitis A virus link to atopic disease. Nature 2003;425:576.

7 Bach JF: The effect of infections on susceptibility to autoimmune and allergic diseases. N Engl J Med 2002; 347:911–920.

8 Akdis M, Verhagen J, Taylor A, Karamloo F, Karagiannidis C, Crameri R, Thunberg S, Deniz G, Valenta R, Fiebig H, Kegel C, Disch R, Schmidt-Weber CB, Blaser K, Akdis CA: Immune responses in healthy and allergic individuals are characterized by a fine balance between allergen-specific T regulatory 1 and T-helper 2 cells. J Exp Med 2004;199:1567–1575.

9 Shull MM, Ormsby I, Kier AB, Pawlowski S, Diebold RJ, Yin M, Allen R, Sidman C, Proetzel G, Calvin D, et al: Targeted disruption of the mouse transforming growth factor-β_1 gene results in multifocal inflammatory disease. Nature 1992;359:693–699.

10 Sonoda E, Matsumoto R, Hitoshi Y, Ishii T, Sugimoto M, Araki S, Tominaga A, Yamaguchi N, Takatsu K: Transforming growth factor-β induces IgA production and acts additively with interleukin-5 for IgA production. J Exp Med 1989;170:1415–1420.

11 Ostroukhova M, Qi Z, Oriss TB, Dixon-McCarthy B, Ray P, Ray A: Treg-mediated immunosuppression involves activation of the Notch-HES1 axis by membrane-bound TGF-β. J Clin Invest 2006;116:996–1004.

12 Wilson MS, Taylor MD, Balic A, Finney CA, Lamb JR, Maizels RM: Suppression of allergic airway inflammation by helminth-induced regulatory T cells. J Exp Med 2005;202:1199–1212.

13 Berry MA, Hargadon B, Shelley M, Parker D, Shaw DE, Green RH, Bradding P, Brightling CE, Wardlaw AJ, Pavord ID: Evidence of a role of tumor necrosis factor-α in refractory asthma. N Engl J Med 2006;354:697–708.

14 Liu YJ: Thymic stromal lymphopoietin: master switch for allergic inflammation. J Exp Med 2006;203:269–273.

15 Rimoldi M, Chieppa M, Salucci V, Avogadri F, Sonzogni A, Sampietro GM, Nespoli A, Viale G, Allavena P, Rescigno M: Intestinal immune homeostasis is regulated by the crosstalk between epithelial cells and dendritic cells. Nat Immunol 2005;6:507–514.

16 Hurst SD, Muchamuel T, Gorman DM, Gilbert JM, Clifford T, Kwan S, Menon S, Seymour B, Jackson C, Kung TT, Brieland JK, Zurawski SM, Chapman RW, Zurawski G, Coffman RL: New IL-17 family members promote Th1 or Th2 responses in the lung: in vivo function of the novel cytokine IL-25. J Immunol 2002;169:443–453.

17 Meyer EH, Goya S, Akbari O, Berry GJ, Savage PB, Kronenberg M, Nakayama T, DeKruyff RH, Umetsu DT: Glycolipid activation of invariant T cell receptor + NK T cells is sufficient to induce airway hyperreactivity independent of conventional CD4+ T cells. Proc Natl Acad Sci USA 2006;103:2782–2787.

18 Akbari O, Faul JL, Hoyte EG, Berry GJ, Wahlstrom J, Kronenberg M, DeKruyff RH, Umetsu DT: CD4+ invariant T-cell-receptor+ natural killer T cells in bronchial asthma. N Engl J Med 2006;354:1117–1129.

19 Akira S, Takeda K, Kaisho T: Toll-like receptors: critical proteins linking innate and acquired immunity. Nat Immunol 2001;2:675–680.

20 Durham SR, Till SJ: Immunologic changes associated with allergen immunotherapy. J Allergy Clin Immunol 1998;102:157–164.

21 Muller U, Akdis CA, Fricker M, Akdis M, Blesken T, Bettens F, Blaser K: Successful immunotherapy with T-cell epitope peptides of bee venom phospholipase A$_2$ induces specific T-cell anergy in patients allergic to bee venom. J Allergy Clin Immunol 1998; 101:747–754.

22 Jutel M, Jaeger L, Suck R, Meyer H, Fiebig H, Cromwell O: Allergen-specific immunotherapy with recombinant grass pollen allergens. J Allergy Clin Immunol 2005;116:608–613.

23 Oldfield WL, Larche M, Kay AB: Effect of T-cell peptides derived from Fel d 1 on allergic reactions and cytokine production in patients sensitive to cats: a randomised controlled trial. Lancet 2002;360:47–53.

24 Larche M, Wraith DC: Peptide-based therapeutic vaccines for allergic and autoimmune diseases. Nat Med 2005; 11:S69–S76.

25 Karamloo F, Schmid-Grendelmeier P, Kussebi F, Akdis M, Salagianni M, von Beust BR, Reimers A, Zumkehr J, Soldatova L, Housley-Markovic Z, Muller U, Kundig T, Kemeny DM, Spangfort MD, Blaser K, Akdis CA: Prevention of allergy by a recombinant multi-allergen vaccine with reduced IgE binding and preserved T cell epitopes. Eur J Immunol 2005;35:3268–3276.

26 Kussebi F, Karamloo F, Rhyner C, Schmid-Grendelmeier P, Salagianni M, Mannhart C, Akdis M, Soldatova L, Markovic-Housley Z, Von Beust BR, Kundig T, Kemeny DM, Blaser K, Crameri R, Akdis CA: A major allergen gene-fusion protein for potential usage in allergen-specific immunotherapy. J Allergy Clin Immunol 2005;115: 323–329.

27 Gafvelin G, Thunberg S, Kronqvist M, Gronlund H, Gronneberg R, Troye-Blomberg M, Akdis M, Fiebig H, Purohit A, Horak F, Reisinger J, Niederberger V, Akdis CA, Cromwell O, Pauli G, Valenta R, van Hage M: Cytokine and antibody responses in birch-pollen-allergic patients treated with genetically modified derivatives of the major birch pollen allergen Bet v 1. Int Arch Allergy Immunol 2005;138: 59–66.

28 Tighe H, Corr M, Roman M, Raz E: Gene vaccination: plasmid DNA is more than just a blueprint. Immunol Today 1998;19:89–97.

29 Hessel EM, Chu M, Lizcano JO, Chang B, Herman N, Kell SA, Wills-Karp M, Coffman RL: Immunostimulatory oligonucleotides block allergic airway inflammation by inhibiting Th2 cell activation and IgE-mediated cytokine induction. J Exp Med 2005;202: 1563–1573.

30 Bashir ME, Louie S, Shi HN, Nagler-Anderson C: Toll-like receptor-4 signaling by intestinal microbes influences susceptibility to food allergy. J Immunol 2004;172:6978–6987.

31 Rakoff-Nahoum S, Paglino J, Eslami-Varzaneh F, Edberg S, Medzhitov R: Recognition of commensal microflora by toll-like receptors is required for intestinal homeostasis. Cell 2004;118: 229–241.

32 MacGlashan DW Jr, Bochner BS, Adelman DC, Jardieu PM, Togias A, McKenzie-White J, Sterbinsky SA, Hamilton RG, Lichtenstein LM: Down-regulation of FcεRI expression on human basophils during in vivo treatment of atopic patients with anti-IgE antibody. J Immunol 1997;158: 1438–1445.

33 Borish LC, Nelson HS, Lanz MJ, Claussen L, Whitmore JB, Agosti JM, Garrison L: Interleukin-4 receptor in moderate atopic asthma. A phase I/II randomized, placebo-controlled trial. Am J Respir Crit Care Med 1999;160:1816–1823.

34 Leckie MJ, ten Brinke A, Khan J, Diamant Z, O'Connor BJ, Walls CM, Mathur AK, Cowley HC, Chung KF, Djukanovic R, Hansel TT, Holgate ST, Sterk PJ, Barnes PJ: Effects of an interleukin-5 blocking monoclonal antibody on eosinophils, airway hyperresponsiveness, and the late asthmatic response. Lancet 2000;356:2144–2148.

35 Verhoef A, Alexander C, Kay AB, Larche M: T cell epitope immunotherapy induces a CD4+ T-cell population with regulatory activity. PLoS Med 2005;2:e78.

36 Frick OL, Teuber SS, Buchanan BB, Morigasaki S, Umetsu DT: Allergen immunotherapy with heat-killed *Listeria monocytogenes* alleviates peanut and food-induced anaphylaxis in dogs. Allergy 2005;60:243–250.

37 Stock P, Akbari O, DeKruyff RH, Umetsu DT: Respiratory tolerance is inhibited by the administration of corticosteroids. J Immunol 2005;175: 7380–7387.

Vassiliki A. Boussiotis, MD, PhD
Harvard Institutes of Medicine, HIM 924
77 Louis Pasteur Avenue, Boston, MA 02115 (USA)
Tel. +1 617 667 8563, Fax +1 617 667 3299
E-Mail vboussio@bidmc.harvard.edu

Blaser K (ed): T Cell Regulation in Allergy, Asthma and Atopic Skin Diseases.
Chem Immunol Allergy. Basel, Karger, 2008, vol 94, pp 189–200

Lung Dendritic Cells: Targets for Therapy in Allergic Disease

Bart N. Lambrecht[a,b] · Hamida Hammad[a]

[a]Department of Respiratory Diseases, University Hospital Ghent, Ghent, Belgium, and
[b]Department of Pulmonary Medicine, Erasmus MC, Rotterdam, The Netherlands

Abstract

Dendritic cells (DCs) are crucial in determining the functional outcome of allergen encounter in the lung. Antigen presentation by myeloid DCs leads to Th2 sensitization typical of allergic disease, whereas antigen presentation by plasmacytoid DCs serves to dampen inflammation. It is increasingly clear that DCs have an antigen presenting function beyond sensitization. DCs therefore constitute a novel target for the development of antiallergic therapy aimed at the origin of the inflammatory cascade. A careful study of DC biology and of the receptors expressed by lung DCs has provided a framework for the discovery of novel antiallergic compounds.   Copyright © 2008 S. Karger AG, Basel

General Function of Dendritic Cells in the Immune System: Induction of Immunity

Dendritic cells (DCs) were originally described by their capacity to efficiently process and present antigens and to prime naive T cells [1]. Over the last three decades, multiple DC subtypes have been defined, differing in phenotype, localization and immune function [2]. In the most general view, immature DCs are situated in the periphery at sites of antigen exposure. Here,

DCs are specialized in antigen recognition and uptake. A degree of discrimination between harmless antigen and dangerous pathogens can be inferred form their expression of pathogen-associated molecular pattern receptors (such as the toll-like receptors (TLRs)). Under homeostatic conditions and particularly upon recognition of pathogens, DCs subsequently migrate to the T-cell area of draining nodes, where they screen the repertoire of naive T cells for antigen-specific T cells directed against the pathogen. Upon cognate TCR-MHC- peptide interaction, DCs subsequently form more stable interactions, and optimally induce T-cell effector function by providing costimulatory molecules and T-cell stimulatory and T-cell survival cytokines. In homeostatic conditions, only harmless antigens or self antigens are being presented to T cells. Because these antigens fail to induce the complete maturation of DCs, they induce the abortive T-cell proliferation and/or lead to a T-cell response in which regulatory T cells (Tregs) are induced. This system allows for dangerous antigens to be eliminated, while avoiding overt immune-mediated damage in response to harmless environmental and self antigens.

Function of Lung Dendritic Cells: Induction of Tolerance in Steady-State and Bridging Innate and Adaptive Immunity

Immature DCs are distributed throughout the lung and are at the focal control point determining the induction of pulmonary immunity or tolerance [3–6]. Airway DCs form a dense network in the lung ideally placed to sample inhaled antigens, by forming tight junctions with airway epithelial cells and extending their dendrites into the airway lumen, analogous to the situation in the gut. Indeed, lamina propria DCs were found to depend on the chemokine receptor CX3CR1 to form transepithelial dendrites, which enable the cells to directly sample luminal antigens. Thus, CX3CR1-dependent processes, which control host interactions of specialized DCs with commensal and pathogenic bacteria, may regulate immunological tolerance and inflammation. Whether a similar CX3CR1-dependent mechanism exists in the lung remains to be shown [7].

Following antigen uptake across the airway epithelial barrier, DCs migrate to draining mediastinal LNs to stimulate naive T cells [8, 9]. As most allergens are immunologically inert proteins, the usual outcome of their inhalation is tolerance. In a true sense this means that when the antigen is subsequently given to mice in an adjuvant setting (e.g. in combination with the Th2 adjuvant alum) it no longer induces an immunological response that leads to effector cells causing inflammation [10–12]. This is best shown for the model antigen ovalbumin (OVA). When given to the airways of naive mice, it induces tolerance to a subsequent immunization with OVA in adjuvant, and effectively inhibits the development of airway inflammation, a feature of true immunological tolerance [10, 12]. This tolerance is mediated in part by deletion of Ag-reactive T cells as well as induction and/or expansion of Tregs in the mediastinal nodes [4, 11–13], is dominant and can be transferred to other mice by adoptive transfer.

It was therefore long enigmatic how sensitization to natural allergens occurred. An important discovery was the fact that most clinically important allergens, such as the major Der p 1 allergen from HDM, are proteolytic enzymes that can directly activate DCs or epithelial cells to break the process of tolerance and promote Th2 responses [14, 15]. However, other allergens, such as the experimental allergen OVA, do not have any intrinsic activating properties. For these antigens, contaminating molecules or environmental exposures (respiratory viruses, air pollution) might pull the trigger on DC activation [16]. Eisenbarth et al. [17] showed that low level TLR4 agonists admixed with harmless OVA prime DCs to induce a Th2 response, by inducing their full maturation, yet not their production of interleukin (IL)-12. This process has been recently described as being dependent on the activation of the adaptor molecule MyD88 in pulmonary DCs [18]. This is clinically important information as most natural allergens such as HDM, cockroach and animal dander contain endotoxin and undoubtedly other TLR agonists [19].

From the above it seems that the decision between tolerance or immunity (in the lungs) is controlled by the degree of maturity of myeloid DCs (mDCs) interacting with naive T cells, a process driven by signals from the innate immune system [6, 20]. It is often claimed that induction of tolerance is a function of 'immature' DCs, meaning that these cells lack the expression of high levels of MHC, adhesion and costimulatory molecules. It has indeed been shown that immature mDCs induce abortive T-cell proliferation in responding T cells and induce Tregs [3, 12, 21]. Another level of complexity arose when it was shown that (respiratory) tolerance might be a function of a subset of plasmacytoid DCs (pDCs) [10, 22]. pDCs depletion from mice using antibodies led to a break in inhalational tolerance to OVA and to development of asthmatic inflammation [10]. For more detailed discussion on this topic, see de Heer et al. [6] and Hammad and Lambrecht [23]. If pDCs promote tolerance and mDCs immunity, it is logical to assume that the balance between both subsets is tightly controlled. In support, the administration of Flt-3 ligand, a cytokine that induces the differentiation of pDCs, to sensitized mice reduced all the features of asthma [24], whereas administration of GM-CSF expanded mDCs and strongly enhanced sensitization and inflammation [25]. Xanthou et al. [26] demonstrated using osteopontin-deficient mice and using blocking antibodies that the secreted form of osteopontin promoted respiratory sensitization to inhaled antigen, an effect mediated by alteration of pDC to mDC balance. Along the same lines, the mucosal adjuvant cholera toxin has the capacity to break inhalational tolerance and promote Th2 sensitization to inhaled harmless antigens by promoting mDC over pDC balance [22].

Dendritic Cells in Established Allergic Airway Inflammation

Not only do DCs play a role in the primary immune response to inhaled allergens, they are also crucial for the outcome of the effector phase in asthma. Indeed, the number of CD11b+ mDCs is increased in the conducting airways and lung interstitium of sensitized and challenged mice during the acute phase of the response [27, 28]. Similar findings have been reported in the rat [29]. The mechanisms for this enhanced recruitment are that DC precursors, most likely at the monocyte stage of development, are attracted from the bone marrow, via the bloodstream to the lung in a CCR2-dependent and generally CCR5- and CCR6-independent way [30]. However, during the chronic phase of the pulmonary response, induced by prolonged exposure to a large number of aerosols, respiratory tolerance develops through

unclear mechanisms. During this regulatory phase, the number of mDCs in the lungs steadily decreased, and this was associated with a reduction of BHR. Inflammation however reappeared when mDCs were given [31]. The role of mDCs in the secondary immune response was further supported by the fact that their depletion at the time of allergen challenge abrogated all the features of asthma, including airway inflammation, goblet cell hyperplasia and bronchial hyperresponsiveness [9, 32]. Again the defect was restored by intratracheal injection of CD11b+ inflammatory mDCs, but not other APCs such as macrophages. The same effects were observed when DCs were depleted in the nose in an animal model for allergic rhinitis [33]. It therefore seems that inflammatory mDCs are both necessary and sufficient for secondary immune responses to allergen. The reasons for this could be manifold. Costimulatory molecules expressed by DCs could play a crucial role in established asthma. Pulmonary DCs upregulate the expression of CD40, CD80, CD86, ICOS-L, PD-L1 and PD-L2 during eosinophilic airway inflammation, particularly upon contact with Th2 cells [10, 29, 32, 34]. Costimulatory molecules might be involved in activation of effector T cells in the tissues. In allergen-challenged mice, mDCs might also be a prominent source of the chemokines CCL17 and CCL22, involved in attracting CCR4+ Th2 cells to the airways [35, 36]. The production of chemokines by lung DC subsets is furthermore differentially regulated, CD11b+ inflammatory DCs being the most prominent source of proinflammatory chemokines [37]. The proallergic cytokine thymic stromal lymphopoeitin (TSLP) induces the production of large amounts of CCL17 by mDCs, thus contributing to the recruitment of a large number of Th2 cells to the airways, explaining how it may act to enhance inflammation [38].

In humans, allergen challenge leads to an accumulation of myeloid, but not pDCs to the airways of asthmatics, concomitantly with a reduction in circulating CD11c+ cells, showing that these cells are recruited from the bloodstream in response to allergen challenge [39, 40]. A recent report suggests that pDCs are also recruited into the BAL fluid, but are poor APCs [41]. The exact role of pDCs in ongoing allergen-specific responses in asthma is currently unknown. It was shown that pDCs accumulate in the nose, but not lungs, of allergen-challenged atopics [42]. In stable asthma, the number of CD1a+ DCs is increased in the airway epithelium and lamina propria, and these numbers are reduced by treatment with inhaled corticosteroids [43]. Based on the above argumentation in mice studies of asthma, it is very likely that part of the efficacy of inhaled steroids might be due to their effects in dampening airway DC function.

Control of Lung DC Function by Regulatory T Cells

Induction of DC maturation and provision of peptide MHC to T cells is not sufficient to generate effector cells [44]. During generation of an efficient effector immune response, DCs have to overcome suppression by Tregs, and the dominant way by which they seem to do this is by producing the cytokine IL-6 that counteracts the suppression by naturally occurring CD4+ CD25+ Tregs [45]. The lung DCs of mice with allergic inflammation produce enhanced amounts of IL-6 [46]. Established airway inflammation seems to be regulated by Tregs expressing membrane transforming growth factor-β (TGF-β) [12] or secreting bioactive TGF-β, and possibly IL-10 [47]. This is a pleiotropic cytokine with significant anti-inflammatory and immunosuppressive properties in the lungs, as reduced expression of this cytokine exacerbates airway pathology in an asthma model [12]. Several papers now support the concept that Tregs alter airway DC function. Mice lacking the transcription factor RunX3, involved in downstream TGF-β

signaling, spontaneously develop asthma features [48]. In the lungs of these mice, there is a strong increase in the number of alveolar mDCs, displaying a mature phenotype with increased expression of MHC II, OX40 ligand, and CCR7 [49] and demonstrating an increased immunostimulatory capacity. Moreover, RunX3–/– DCs are able to mount inflammatory responses to otherwise harmless inhaled antigens, possibly through their lack of responsiveness to locally secreted TGF-β [48]. In mice normally resistant to HDM-induced asthma and AHR (C3H mice), Treg cell depletion similarly led to increased numbers of pulmonary mDCs with elevated expression of MHCII, CD80, and CD86, and an increased capacity to stimulate T-cell proliferation and Th2 cytokine production. In normally susceptible A/J mice, Tregs did not suppress inflammation and AHR. These data suggest therefore that resistance to allergen-driven AHR is mediated in part by CD4+CD25+ Treg cell suppression of DC activation and that the absence of this regulatory pathway contributes to susceptibility [50]. In the rat it was shown that Tregs also control the level of CD86 expression on lung DCs and are responsible for the tolerance to inhaled allergen that occurs upon repeated exposure to allergens [51]. In humans with allergy, there is a reduction in the number and possibly function of Tregs [52], but it is unclear at present whether this would also lead to altered function of DCs in these patients.

Perpetuation of Allergic Inflammation and Remodeling: A Role for Cytokine-Driven Activation of DCs?

According to current thinking, epithelial dysfunction, either intrinsic to asthma or caused by persistent inflammation, leads to epithelial release of profibrotic cytokines such as epidermal growth factor and TGF-β acting on fibroblasts and smooth muscle cells, disturbing the equilibrium between epithelial destruction and growth and repair. The exact consequences of this epithelial remodeling, myofibroblast differentiation, altered matrix distribution and neovascularization on the functioning of the airway DCs are currently unknown.

Chronically inflamed asthmatic epithelium might release growth factors such as GM-CSF, VEGF or TSLP that profoundly influence DC survival and/or function. TSLP is a 140-amino-acid IL-7-like four-helix-bundle cytokine that has potent DC-modulating capacities, by binding its receptor complex, composed of the IL-7 receptor and the TSLP receptor. [53, 54]. TSLP can directly activate DCs to prime naive CD4+ T cells to differentiate into proinflammatory Th2 cells that secrete IL-4, IL-5, IL-13 and TNF-α, but not IL-10, and express the prostaglandin D_2 receptor CRTH2 (chemoattractant receptor-homologous molecule expressed on TH2 cells) – a T-cell phenotype that is also found in asthmatic airways [55, 56]. The way by which this polarization occurs has been studied in detail (fig. 1). The polarization of Th2 cells induced by TSLP-matured DCs is further enhanced by IL-25, which is produced by epithelial cells, basophils and eosinophils [57]. A recent report showed that airway epithelial cells can produce IL-25 in response to an innate immune response to allergen [58]. In addition to its effects on DCs, TSLP can also activate human mast cells to produce Th2-associated effector cytokines in the absence of T cells or IgE crosslinking [59]. The most convincing evidence for a role for TSLP in DC-driven Th2 cell development came from studies in mice that conditionally overexpressed TSLP in the lungs. These mice mounted a vigorous DC-driven primary Th2 cell response in the airways. By contrast, *Tlspr−/−* mice fail to develop an antigen-specific Th2 cell inflammatory response in the airways unless they are supplemented with wild-type CD4+ T cells [38, 60]. Taken together, these data suggest that TSLP produced by the lung epithelium might represent a crucial factor that can initiate allergic responses at the epithelial cell

surface. Therefore it will be very important to study how the production of TSLP by epithelial cells and other inflammatory cells is regulated. TSLP production can be induced by ligands that activate TLR2, TLR3, TLR8 and TLR9, by the proinflammatory cytokines TNF, IL-1α and IL-1β, and by the proallergic cytokines IL-4 and IL-13 [61]. In the airways of patients with asthma, the levels of TSLP are increased, but it is not yet known whether exposure to enzymatically active allergens stimulates TSLP release [62].

Finally, many inflammatory cell types such as mast cells, basophils, eosinophils and even platelets are recruited to the airways in chronic asthma. These cells release many mediators such as cytokines, neuropeptides, enzymes, and lipid mediators that may also profoundly influence DC function and in this way might perpetuate ongoing inflammation [5]. As only one example, it is known that histamine and PGD_2, both released by mast cells upon IgE crosslinking, reduce the potential of DCs to produce bioactive IL-12, and in this way contribute to Th2 polarization [63, 64]. Extracellular ATP might be released by platelets upon allergen challenge. Neutralization of ATP via administration of the enzyme apyrase or the broad-spectrum P2 receptor antagonist suramin reduced all the cardinal features of asthma by interfering with DC function, although the precise receptor involved has not been elucidated [65]. How exactly ATP promotes DC-driven airway inflammation and how its blockade suppresses asthma is insufficiently known at present. Strikingly, the levels of the major eosinophil (CCL11, CCL24) and Th2 lymphocyte (CCL17, CCL22) selective chemokines were not reduced upon apyrase treatment, suggesting that ATP more likely controls responsiveness of inflammatory cells to chemokine gradients, as recently suggested by in vitro studies using apyrase to reduce neutrophil chemotaxis [66]. In vitro experiments suggested that purinergic signaling has potent chemotactic effects on immature DCs in humans [67] and

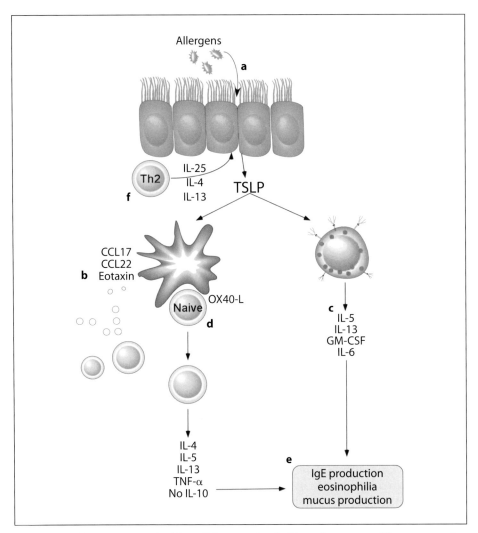

Fig. 1. TSLP takes center stage in driving DC maturation for Th2 cell responses. Allergens as well as effector T-helper 2 (Th2) cell-associated cytokines and loss of epithelium barrier function can trigger the production of thymic stromal lymphopoeitin (TSLP) by airway epithelial cells. Allergen triggering of protease-activated receptor 2 (PAR2) or by contaminating endotoxin acting on toll-like receptors (TLRs) triggers the activation of *Tslp* gene transcription (**a**). TSLP induces immediate innate immune functions in dendritic cells (DCs) leading to chemokine-driven recruitment of Th2 cells and eosinophils to the airways, possibly providing a source for polarizing Th2 cell-associated cytokines (**b**). In mast cells, there is immediate release of the Th2 effector cytokines that can attract and activate eosinophils in a T-cell-independent way (**c**). Following innate immune induction, TSLP triggers the maturation of DCs so that they migrate to the mediastinal lymph nodes and induce the polarization of inflammatory Th2 cells in an OX40L-dependent fashion. In contrast to most other triggers that induce DC maturation, TSLP-induced maturation is not accompanied by the production of IL-12, thereby explaining Th2 cell polarization (**d**). The effector cytokines produced by adaptive Th2 cells and mast cells trigger the salient features of asthma (**e**). Effector cytokines can also perpetuate TSLP-driven inflammation by further triggering the release of TSLP by airway epithelial cells. This process is enhanced by epithelial production of the proallergenic cytokine IL-25 (**f**).

Lambrecht · Hammad

mice [68]. In support, ATP administration induced a marked increase in the DC chemokine CCL20, a predominant chemokine attracting immature DCs into the mucosa. The subsequent enhanced migration of ATP exposed lung DCs to the mediastinal LN was explained by the upregulation of the CCR7 chemokine receptor, involved in directing the interest of maturing DCs to the T-cell area of the node. Alternatively, ATP might promote Th2 responses by formation of the inflammasome, a multimeric intracellular complex of signaling molecules that lead to caspase-1 activation and activation of the IL-1 family of cytokines (IL-1β, IL-18 and possibly IL-33). The formation of the inflammasome has been shown to occur following triggering by ATP of the P2X7 receptor, widely expressed on murine and human DCs, in conjunction with TLR triggering [69–71]. Clearly, blockade of ATP might also affect other inflammatory cells. Nucleotides cause the release of inflammatory mediators such as eosinophil cationic protein, radical oxygen intermediates and IL-8 from human eosinophils [71, 72].

Dendritic Cells as Drug Targets in Allergic Diseases

If DCs are so crucial in mounting immune responses during ongoing inflammation in the lung, nose and skin, then interfering with their function could constitute a novel form of treatment for allergic diseases. Additionally, pharmacological modification of DCs might fundamentally reset the balance of the allergic immune response in favor of Tregs and thus lead to a more long-lasting effect on the natural course of allergic disease. Steroids are currently the cornerstone of anti-inflammatory treatment in allergic disease. Inhaled steroids reduce the number of lung and nose DCs in patients with allergic asthma and allergic rhinitis [23]. Steroids might also interfere with a GITRL-driven induction of the enzyme

indoleamine 2,3-dioxygenase in pDCs, thus broadly suppressing inflammation [73]. Inhaled steroids reduce the number of lung and nose DCs in patients with AA and AD, whereas local application of steroids to the skin of AD patients reduces the influx of DCs [43, 74]. The immunosuppressant drug tacrolimus is currently in use for topical treatment for AD. It suppresses the expression of MHCII and costimulatory molecules and FcεRI on LC from AD patients in vitro and reduces the number of IDECs in lesional skin.

Recently, several other new molecules have surfaced that may alter DC function in allergic inflammation and thus treat disease. Many of these compounds were first discovered by their potential to interfere with DC-driven Th2 sensitization. The sphingosine-1-P analogue FTY720 is currently used in clinical trials for multiple sclerosis and transplant rejection. When given locally to the lungs of mice with established inflammation, it strongly reduced inflammation by suppressing the T-cell stimulatory capacity and migratory behavior of lung DCs, without the commonly observed lymphopenia when the drug is given orally [75]. FTY720 inhibited the potential of DCs to form stable synapses with naive Ag-specific T cells as well as Th2 effector cells, possibly explaining how these drugs might work to inhibit allergic inflammation.

Selective agonists of particular prostaglandin series receptors might suppress DC function. Prostaglandin D_2 has pleiotropic effects in the immune system, due to its activity on the DP1 and DP2 (also known as CRTH2) receptor, widely expressed on immune cells. The airways of chimeric DP1–/– deficient mice have more mature DCs, pointing to a suppressing role of endogenously released PGD_2 on DC function [68]. The DP1 agonist BW245C strongly suppressed the spontaneous migration of lung DCs to the mediastinal LN [64]. More importantly, BW245C suppressed airway inflammation and bronchial hyperreactivity when given to allergic mice by inhibiting the maturation of lung DCs. In the presence of BW245C, DCs induced the formation of FoxP3+ induced Tregs from FoxP3− antigen-specific T cells [76]. A very similar mechanism was described for inhaled iloprost, a prostacyclin analogue acting on the IP receptor expressed by lung DCs [68, 77].

As the number and activation status of lung CD11b+ DCs during secondary challenge seems critical for controlling allergic inflammation, studying the factors that control recruitment, survival or egress from the lung during allergic inflammation will be important, as this might reveal therapeutic targets. In an elegant study using mixed bone marrow chimeras in which half the hematopoietic cells were CCR2−/− and half were CCR2+/+, it was shown by Robays et al. [30] that CCR2 (and not CCR5 or CCR6) is crucial for releasing DC precursors from the bone marrow and attracting them into allergically inflamed lung. This was unexpected, as CCR6 is generally seen as the chemokine receptor attracting immature DCs into peripheral tissues. Lung mDCs use CCR7 ligands and CCR8 for emigration to the draining lymph node, but not the leukotriene C4 transporter multidrug-related protein-1 as they do in the skin [78]. Unexpectedly, disruption of CCR7-selective chemokines in paucity of lymphocyte T-cell (plt) mutant mice, deficient in CCL21 and CCL19, airway inflammation and Th2 activity were enhanced [79]. Still, increased numbers of mDCs could be found in the draining lymph node of these mice. So, other factors than CCR7 ligands are involved in the migration of DCs to the draining LN, including other chemokine receptors [78]. Eicosanoid lipid mediators, like prostaglandins and leukotrienes, can also influence the migration of lung DCs [76]. Leukotriene LTB$_4$ promoted the migration of immature and mature skin DCs, but these effects seem to be indirect [80]. It will be important to study if well-known inducers of LTB$_4$ in the lungs, such as the environmental biopolymer chitin, derived from fungi, helminths and insects, also induce DC migration [81].

Some novel drugs are emerging that effect DC function without a clear mechanism of action. A specific small molecule compound (VAF347) that blocks the function of B cells and DCs was shown to be effective in suppressing allergic airway inflammation in a mouse model of asthma [82]. Finally, specific inhibitors of *syk* kinase were shown to suppress DC function and cure established inflammation [83]. More detailed information on the interactions between DCs, other inflammatory cells and epithelial cells will undoubtedly lead to the discovery of more potentially interesting drugs. In this regard, blocking the interaction of TSLP and GMCSF with its respective receptor through small molecule inhibitor or blocking antibodies might prove very useful. Ideally, novel drugs for asthma should also try to restore epithelial barrier function, as this might reduce the threshold for allergen recognition.

Conclusion

DCs are crucial in determining the functional outcome of allergen encounter in the lung, nose and skin and antigen presentation by mDCs leads to Th2 sensitization typical of allergic disease. It is increasingly clear that DCs have an antigen presenting function beyond sensitization. DCs therefore constitute a novel target for the development of antiallergic therapy aimed at the origin of the inflammatory cascade.

Acknowledgements

The author is supported by an Odysseus grant of the FWO Vlaanderen and by a VIDI grant of the Dutch Organization for Scientific Research.

References

1 Steinman RM, Cohn ZA: Identification of a novel cell type in peripheral lymphoid organs of mice. I. Morphology, quantitation, tissue distribution. J Exp Med 1973;137:1142–1162.

2 Shortman K, Liu YJ: Mouse and human dendritic cell subtypes. Nat Rev Immunol 2002;2:151–161.

3 Akbari O, DeKruyff RH, Umetsu DT: Pulmonary dendritic cells producing IL-10 mediate tolerance induced by respiratory exposure to antigen. Nat Immunol 2001;2:725–731.

4 Akbari O, Freeman GJ, Meyer EH, Greenfield EA, Chang TT, Sharpe AH, Berry G, DeKruyff RH, Umetsu DT: Antigen-specific regulatory T cells develop via the ICOS-ICOS ligand pathway and inhibit allergen-induced airway hyperreactivity. Nat Med 2002; 8:1024–1032.

5 Lambrecht BN, Hammad H: Taking our breath away: dendritic cells in the pathogenesis of asthma. Nat Rev Immunol 2003;3:994–1003.

6 De Heer HJ, Hammad H, Kool M, Lambrecht BN: Dendritic cell subsets and immune regulation in the lung. Semin Immunol 2005;17:295–303.

7 Niess JH, Brand S, Gu X, Landsman L, Jung S, McCormick BA, Vyas JM, Boes M, Ploegh HL, Fox JG, Littman DR, Reinecker HC: CX3CR1-mediated dendritic cell access to the intestinal lumen and bacterial clearance. Science 2005;307:254–258.

8 Vermaelen KY, Carro-Muino I, Lambrecht BN, Pauwels RA: Specific migratory dendritic cells rapidly transport antigen from the airways to the thoracic lymph nodes. J Exp Med 2001; 193:51–60.

9 Lambrecht BN, Salomon B, Klatzmann D, Pauwels RA: Dendritic cells are required for the development of chronic eosinophilic airway inflammation in response to inhaled antigen in sensitized mice. J Immunol 1998;160: 4090–4097.

10 De Heer HJ, Hammad H, Soullie T, Hijdra D, Vos N, Willart MA, Hoogsteden HC, Lambrecht BN: Essential role of lung plasmacytoid dendritic cells in preventing asthmatic reactions to harmless inhaled antigen. J Exp Med 2004;200:89–98.

11 Van Hove CL, Maes T, Joos GF, Tournoy KG: Prolonged inhaled allergen exposure can induce persistent tolerance. Am J Respir Cell Mol Biol 2007; 36:573–584.

12 Ostroukhova M, Seguin-Devaux C, Oriss TB, Dixon-McCarthy B, Yang L, Ameredes BT, Corcoran TE, Ray A: Tolerance induced by inhaled antigen involves CD4+ T cells expressing membrane-bound TGF-β and FoxP3. J Clin Invest 2004;114:28–38.

13 Hintzen G, Ohl L, del Rio ML, Rodriguez-Barbosa JI, Pabst O, Kocks JR, Krege J, Hardtke S, Forster R: Induction of tolerance to innocuous inhaled antigen relies on a CCR7-dependent dendritic cell-mediated antigen transport to the bronchial lymph node. J Immunol 2006;177:7346–7354.

14 Hammad H, Charbonnier AS, Duez C, Jacquet A, Stewart GA, Tonnel AB, Pestel J: Th2 polarization by Der p 1 pulsed monocyte-derived dendritic cells is due to the allergic status of the donors. Blood 2001;98:1135–1141.

15 Kheradmand F, Kiss A, Xu J, Lee SH, Kolattukudy PE, Corry DB: A protease-activated pathway underlying Th cell type 2 activation and allergic lung disease. J Immunol 2002;169:5904–5911.

16 Dahl ME, Dabbagh K, Liggitt D, Kim S, Lewis DB: Viral-induced T helper type 1 responses enhance allergic disease by effects on lung dendritic cells. Nat Immunol 2004;5:337–343.

17 Eisenbarth SC, Zhadkevich A, Ranney P, Herrick CA, Bottomly K: IL-4-dependent Th2 collateral priming to inhaled antigens independent of toll-like receptor 4 and myeloid differentiation factor 88. J Immunol 2004;172:4527–4534.

18 Piggott DA, Eisenbarth SC, Xu L, Constant SL, Huleatt JW, Herrick CA, Bottomly K: MyD88-dependent induction of allergic Th2 responses to intranasal antigen. J Clin Invest 2005; 115:459–467.

19 Braun-Fahrlander C, Riedler J, Herz U, Eder W, Waser M, Grize L, Maisch S, Carr D, Gerlach F, Bufe A, Lauener RP, Schierl R, Renz H, Nowak D, von Mutius E: Environmental exposure to endotoxin and its relation to asthma in school-age children. N Engl J Med 2002; 347:869–877.

20 Herrick CA, Bottomly K: To respond or not to respond? T cells in allergic asthma. Nat Rev Immunol 2003;3: 405–412.

21 Brimnes MK, Bonifaz L, Steinman RM, Moran TM: Influenza virus-induced dendritic cell maturation is associated with the induction of strong T cell immunity to a coadministered, normally nonimmunogenic protein. J Exp Med 2003;198:133–144.

22 Oriss TB, Ostroukhova M, Seguin-Devaux C, Dixon-McCarthy B, Stolz DB, Watkins SC, Pillemer B, Ray P, Ray A: Dynamics of dendritic cell phenotype and interactions with CD4+ T cells in airway inflammation and tolerance. J Immunol 2005;174:854–863.

23 Hammad H, Lambrecht BN: Recent progress in the biology of airway dendritic cells and implications for understanding the regulation of asthmatic inflammation. J Allergy Clin Immunol 2006;118:331–336.

24 Edwan JH, Perry G, Talmadge JE, Agrawal DK: Flt-3 Ligand reverses late allergic response and airway hyperresponsiveness in a mouse model of allergic inflammation. J Immunol 2004; 172:5016–5023.

25 Stampfli MR, Wiley RE, Scott Neigh G, Gajewska BU, Lei XF, Snider DP, Xing Z, Jordana M: GM-CSF transgene expression in the airway allows aerosolized ovalbumin to induce allergic sensitization in mice. J Clin Invest 1998;102:1704–1714.

26 Xanthou G, Alissafi T, Semitekolou M, Simoes DC, Economidou E, Gaga M, Lambrecht BN, Lloyd CM, Panoutsakopoulou V: Osteopontin has a crucial role in allergic airway disease through regulation of dendritic cell subsets. Nat Med 2007;13:570–578.

27 Van Rijt LS, Prins JB, deVries VC, Leenen PJ, Thielemans K, Hoogsteden HC, Lambrecht BN: Allergen-induced accumulation of airway dendritic cells is supported by an increase in CD31[hi] Ly-6C[neg] hematopoietic precursors. Blood 2002;100:3663–3671.

28 Vermaelen K, Pauwels R: Accelerated airway dendritic cell maturation, trafficking, and elimination in a mouse model of asthma. Am J Respir Cell Mol Biol 2003;29:405–409.

29 Huh JC, Strickland DH, Jahnsen FL, Turner DJ, Thomas JA, Napoli S, Tobagus I, Stumbles PA, Sly PD, Holt PG: Bidirectional interactions between antigen-bearing respiratory tract dendritic cells (DCs) and T cells precede the late phase reaction in experimental asthma: DC activation occurs in the airway mucosa but not in the lung parenchyma. J Exp Med 2003;198:19–30.

30 Robays LJ, Maes T, Lebecque S, Lira SA, Kuziel WA, Brusselle GG, Joos GF, Vermaelen KV: Chemokine receptor CCR2 but not CCR5 or CCR6 mediates the increase in pulmonary dendritic cells during allergic airway inflammation. J Immunol 2007;178:5305–5311.

31 Koya T, Kodama T, Takeda K, Miyahara N, Yang ES, Taube C, Joetham A, Park JW, Dakhama A, Gelfand EW: Importance of myeloid dendritic cells in persistent airway disease after repeated allergen exposure. Am J Respir Crit Care Med 2006;173:42–55.

32 Van Rijt LS, Jung S, Kleinjan A, Vos N, Willart M, Duez C, Hoogsteden HC, Lambrecht BN: In vivo depletion of lung CD11c+ dendritic cells during allergen challenge abrogates the characteristic features of asthma. J Exp Med 2005;201:981–991.

33 KleinJan A, Willart M, van Rijt LS, Braunstahl GJ, Leman K, Jung S, Hoogsteden HC, Lambrecht BN: An essential role for dendritic cells in human and experimental allergic rhinitis. J Allergy Clin Immunol 2006;118:1117–1125.

34 Van Rijt LS, Vos N, Willart M, Kleinjan A, Coyle AJ, Hoogsteden HC, Lambrecht BN: Essential role of dendritic cell CD80/CD86 costimulation in the induction, but not reactivation, of TH2 effector responses in a mouse model of asthma. J Allergy Clin Immunol 2004;114:166–173.

35 Kohl J, Baelder R, Lewkowich IP, Pandey MK, Hawlisch H, Wang L, Best J, Herman NS, Sproles AA, Zwirner J, Whitsett JA, Gerard C, Sfyroera G, Lambris JD, Wills-Karp M: A regulatory role for the C5a anaphylatoxin in type 2 immunity in asthma. J Clin Invest 2006;116:783–796.

36 Vermaelen K, Cataldo D, Tournoy KG, Maes T, Dhulst A, Louis R, Foidart J-M, Noel A, Pauwels RA: Matrix metalloproteinse-9-mediated dendritic cell recruitment into the airways is a critical step in mouse model of asthma. J Immunol 2003;171:1016–1022.

37 Beaty SR, Rose CE Jr, Sung SS: Diverse and potent chemokine production by lung CD11b[hi] dendritic cells in homeostasis and in allergic lung inflammation. J Immunol 2007;178:1882–1895.

38 Zhou B, Comeau MR, De Smedt T, Liggitt HD, Dahl ME, Lewis DB, Gyarmati D, Aye T, Campbell DJ, Ziegler SF: Thymic stromal lymphopoietin as a key initiator of allergic airway inflammation in mice. Nat Immunol 2005;6:1047–1053.

39 Upham JW, Denburg JA, O'Byrne PM: Rapid response of circulating myeloid dendritic cells to inhaled allergen in asthmatic subjects. Clin Exp Allergy 2002;32:818–823.

40 Jahnsen FL, Moloney ED, Hogan T, Upham JW, Burke CM, Holt PG: Rapid dendritic cell recruitment to the bronchial mucosa of patients with atopic asthma in response to local allergen challenge. Thorax 2001;56:823–826.

41 Bratke K, Lommatzsch M, Julius P, Kuepper M, Kleine HD, Luttmann W, Christian Virchow J: Dendritic cell subsets in human bronchoalveolar lavage fluid after segmental allergen challenge. Thorax 2007;62:168–175.

42 Jahnsen FL, Lund-Johansen F, Dunne JF, Farkas L, Haye R, Brandtzaeg P: Experimentally induced recruitment of plasmacytoid (CD123[high]) dendritic cells in human nasal allergy. J Immunol 2000;165:4062–4068.

43 Moller GM, Overbeek SE, Van Helden-Meeuwsen CG, Van Haarst JM, Prens EP, Mulder PG, Postma DS, Hoogsteden HC: Increased numbers of dendritic cells in the bronchial mucosa of atopic asthmatic patients: downregulation by inhaled corticosteroids. Clin Exp Allergy 1996;26:517–524.

44 Sporri R, Reis e Sousa C: Inflammatory mediators are insufficient for full dendritic cell activation and promote expansion of CD4+ T cell populations lacking helper function. Nat Immunol 2005;6:163–170.

45 Doganci A, Eigenbrod T, Krug N, De Sanctis GT, Hausding M, Erpenbeck VJ, Haddad el B, Lehr HA, Schmitt E, Bopp T, Kallen KJ, Herz U, Schmitt S, Luft C, Hecht O, Hohlfeld JM, Ito H, Nishimoto N, Yoshizaki K, Kishimoto T, Rose-John S, Renz H, Neurath MF, Galle PR, Finotto S: The IL-6R α chain controls lung CD4+CD25+ Treg development and function during allergic airway inflammation in vivo. J Clin Invest 2005;115:313–325.

46 Dodge IL, Carr MW, Cernadas M, Brenner MB: IL-6 production by pulmonary dendritic cells impedes Th1 immune responses. J Immunol 2003;170:4457–4464.

47 Kearley J, Barker JE, Robinson DS, Lloyd CM: Resolution of airway inflammation and hyperreactivity after in vivo transfer of CD4+CD25+ regulatory T cells is interleukin-10 dependent. J Exp Med 2005;202:1539–1547.

48 Fainaru O, Woolf E, Lotem J, Yarmus M, Brenner O, Goldenberg D, Negreanu V, Bernstein Y, Levanon D, Jung S, Groner Y: Runx3 regulates mouse TGF-β-mediated dendritic cell function and its absence results in airway inflammation. EMBO J 2004;23:969–979.

49 Fainaru O, Shseyov D, Hantisteanu S, Groner Y: Accelerated chemokine receptor 7-mediated dendritic cell migration in Runx3 knockout mice and the spontaneous development of asthma-like disease. Proc Natl Acad Sci USA 2005;102:10598–10603.

50 Lewkowich IP, Herman NS, Schleifer KW, Dance MP, Chen BL, Dienger KM, Sproles AA, Shah JS, Kohl J, Belkaid Y, Wills-Karp M: CD4+CD25+ T cells protect against experimentally induced asthma and alter pulmonary dendritic cell phenotype and function. J Exp Med 2005;202:1549–1561.

51 Strickland DH, Stumbles PA, Zosky GR, Subrata LS, Thomas JA, Turner DJ, Sly PD, Holt PG: Reversal of airway hyperresponsiveness by induction of airway mucosal CD4+CD25+ regulatory T cells. J Exp Med 2006;203:2649–2660.

52 Kuipers H, Lambrecht BN: The interplay of dendritic cells, Th2 cells and regulatory T cells in asthma. Curr Opin Immunol 2004;16:702–708.

53 Liu YJ, Soumelis V, Watanabe N, Ito T, Wang YH, Malefyt Rde W, Omori M, Zhou B, Ziegler SF: TSLP: an epithelial cell cytokine that regulates T cell differentiation by conditioning dendritic cell maturation. Annu Rev Immunol 2007;25:193–219.

54 Leonard WJ: TSLP: finally in the limelight. Nat Immunol 2002;3:605–607.

55 Ito T, Wang YH, Duramad O, Hori T, Delespesse GJ, Watanabe N, Qin FX, Yao Z, Cao W, Liu YJ: TSLP-activated dendritic cells induce an inflammatory T helper type 2 cell response through OX40 ligand. J Exp Med 2005;202: 1213–1223.

56 Wang YH, Ito T, Wang YH, Homey B, Watanabe N, Martin R, Barnes CJ, McIntyre BW, Gilliet M, Kumar R, Yao Z, Liu YJ: Maintenance and polarization of human TH2 central memory T cells by thymic stromal lymphopoietin-activated dendritic cells. Immunity 2006;24:827–838.

57 Wang YH, Angkasekwinai P, Lu N, Voo KS, Arima K, Hanabuchi S, Hippe A, Corrigan CJ, Dong C, Homey B, Yao Z, Ying S, Huston DP, Liu YJ: IL-25 augments type 2 immune responses by enhancing the expansion and functions of TSLP-DC-activated Th2 memory cells. J Exp Med 2007;204:1837–1847.

58 Angkasekwinai P, Park H, Wang YH, Wang YH, Chang SH, Corry DB, Liu YJ, Zhu Z, Dong C: Interleukin-25 promotes the initiation of proallergic type 2 responses. J Exp Med 2007;204: 1509–1517.

59 Allakhverdi Z, Comeau MR, Jessup HK, Yoon BR, Brewer A, Chartier S, Paquette N, Ziegler SF, Sarfati M, Delespesse G: Thymic stromal lymphopoietin is released by human epithelial cells in response to microbes, trauma, or inflammation and potently activates mast cells. J Exp Med 2007; 204:253–258.

60 Al-Shami A, Spolski R, Kelly J, Keane-Myers A, Leonard WJ: A role for TSLP in the development of inflammation in an asthma model. J Exp Med 2005;202: 829–839.

61 Bogiatzi SI, Fernandez I, Bichet JC, Marloie-Provost MA, Volpe E, Sastre X, Soumelis V: Cutting edge: proinflammatory and Th2 cytokines synergize to induce thymic stromal lymphopoietin production by human skin keratinocytes. J Immunol 2007;178: 3373–3377.

62 Ying S, O'Connor B, Ratoff J, Meng Q, Mallett K, Cousins D, Robinson D, Zhang G, Zhao J, Lee TH, Corrigan C: Thymic stromal lymphopoietin expression is increased in asthmatic airways and correlates with expression of Th2-attracting chemokines and disease severity. J Immunol 2005;174: 8183–8190.

63 Idzko M, la Sala A, Ferrari D, Panther E, Herouy Y, Dichmann S, Mockenhaupt M, Di Virgilio F, Girolomoni G, Norgauer J: Expression and function of histamine receptors in human monocyte-derived dendritic cells. J Allergy Clin Immunol 2002; 109:839–846.

64 Hammad H, de Heer HJ, Souillie T, Hoogsteden HC, Trottein F, Lambrecht BN: Prostaglandin D_2 modifies airway dendritic cell migration and function in steady-state conditions by selective activation of the DP receptor. J Immunol 2003;171:3936–3940.

65 Idzko M, Hammad H, van Nimwegen M, Kool M, Willart MA, Muskens F, Hoogsteden HC, Luttmann W, Ferrari D, Di Virgilio F, Virchow JC Jr, Lambrecht BN: Extracellular ATP triggers and maintains asthmatic airway inflammation by activating dendritic cells. Nat Med 2007;13:913–919.

66 Chen Y, Corriden R, Inoue Y, Yip L, Hashiguchi N, Zinkernagel A, Nizet V, Insel PA, Junger WG: ATP release guides neutrophil chemotaxis via P2Y2 and A3 receptors. Science 2006;314: 1792–1795.

67 Idzko M, Dichmann S, Ferrari D, Di Virgilio F, la Sala A, Girolomoni G, Panther E, Norgauer J: Nucleotides induce chemotaxis and actin polymerization in immature but not mature human dendritic cells via activation of pertussis toxin-sensitive P2y receptors. Blood 2002;100:925–932.

68 Idzko M, Hammad H, van Nimwegen M, Kool M, Vos N, Hoogsteden HC, Lambrecht BN: Inhaled iloprost suppresses the cardinal features of asthma via inhibition of airway dendritic cell function. J Clin Invest 2007;117: 464–472.

69 Mariathasan S, Weiss DS, Newton K, McBride J, O'Rourke K, Roose-Girma M, Lee WP, Weinrauch Y, Monack DM, Dixit VM: Cryopyrin activates the inflammasome in response to toxins and ATP. Nature 2006;440:228–232.

70 Ogura Y, Sutterwala FS, Flavell RA: The inflammasome: first line of the immune response to cell stress. Cell 2006;126:659–662.

71 Ferrari D, Pizzirani C, Adinolfi E, Lemoli RM, Curti A, Idzko M, Panther E, Di Virgilio F: The P2X7 receptor: a key player in IL-1 processing and release. J Immunol 2006;176: 3877–3883.

72 Idzko M, Panther E, Bremer HC, Sorichter S, Luttmann W, Virchow CJ Jr, Di Virgilio F, Herouy Y, Norgauer J, Ferrari D: Stimulation of P2 purinergic receptors induces the release of eosinophil cationic protein and interleukin-8 from human eosinophils. Br J Pharmacol 2003;138:1244–1250.

73 Grohmann U, Volpi C, Fallarino F, Bozza S, Bianchi R, Vacca C, Orabona C, Belladonna ML, Ayroldi E, Nocentini G, Boon L, Bistoni F, Fioretti MC, Romani L, Riccardi C, Puccetti P: Reverse signaling through GITR ligand enables dexamethasone to activate IDO in allergy. Nat Med 2007;13: 579–586.

74 Holm AF, Fokkens WJ, Godthelp T, Mulder PG, Vroom TM, Rijntjes E: Effect of 3 months' nasal steroid therapy on nasal T cells and Langerhans' cells in patients suffering from allergic rhinitis. Allergy 1995;50:204–209.

75 Idzko M, Hammad H, van Nimwegen M, Kool M, Muller T, Soullie T, Willart MA, Hijdra D, Hoogsteden HC, Lambrecht BN: Local application of FTY720 to the lung abrogates experimental asthma by altering dendritic cell function. J Clin Invest 2006; 116:2935–2944.

76 Hammad H, Kool M, Soullie T, Narumiya S, Trottein F, Hoogsteden HC, Lambrecht BN: Activation of the D prostanoid 1 receptor suppresses asthma by modulation of lung dendritic cell function and induction of regulatory T cells. J Exp Med 2007;204: 357–367.

77 Zhou W, Hashimoto K, Goleniewska K, O'Neal JF, Ji S, Blackwell TS, Fitzgerald GA, Egan KM, Geraci MW, Peebles RS: Prostaglandin I_2 analogs inhibit proinflammatory cytokine production and T cell stimulatory function of dendritic cells. J Immunol 2007;178:702–710.

78 Jakubzick C, Tacke F, Llodra J, van Rooijen N, Randolph GJ: Modulation of dendritic cell trafficking to and from the airways. J Immunol 2006;176: 3578–3584.

79 Grinnan D, Sung SS, Dougherty JA, Knowles AR, Allen MB, Rose CE 3rd, Nakano H, Gunn MD, Fu SM, Rose CE Jr: Enhanced allergen-induced airway inflammation in paucity of lymph node T cell (plt) mutant mice. J Allergy Clin Immunol 2006;118:1234–1241.

80 Del Prete A, Shao WH, Mitola S, Santoro G, Sozzani S, Haribabu B: Regulation of dendritic cell migration and adaptive immune response by leukotriene B_4 receptors: a role for LTB_4 in up-regulation of CCR7 expression and function. Blood 2007;109: 626–631.

81 Reese TA, Liang HE, Tager AM, Luster AD, Van Rooijen N, Voehringer D, Locksley RM: Chitin induces accumulation in tissue of innate immune cells associated with allergy. Nature 2007; 447:92–96.

82 Ettmayer P, Mayer P, Kalthoff F, Neruda W, Harrer N, Hartmann G, Epstein MM, Brinkmann V, Heusser C, Woisetschlager M: A novel low molecular weight inhibitor of dendritic cells and B cells blocks allergic inflammation. Am J Respir Crit Care Med 2006; 173:599–606.

83 Matsubara S, Koya T, Takeda K, Joetham A, Miyahara N, Pine P, Masuda ES, Swasey CH, Gelfand EW: Syk activation in dendritic cells is essential for airway hyperresponsiveness and inflammation. Am J Respir Cell Mol Biol 2006;34:426–433.

Bart N. Lambrecht, MD, PhD
Department of Respiratory Diseases
Laboratory of Mucosal Immunology, MRB1, University Hospital Ghent
De Pintelaan 185, BE–9000 Ghent (Belgium)
Tel. +32 9 332 87 84, Fax +32 9 332 94 76, E-Mail bart.lambrecht@ugent.be

Blaser K (ed): T Cell Regulation in Allergy, Asthma and Atopic Skin Diseases.
Chem Immunol Allergy. Basel, Karger, 2008, vol 94, pp 201–210

Antigen-Based Therapies Targeting the Expansion of Regulatory T Cells in Autoimmune and Allergic Disease

Melanie D. Leech[a] · Stephen M. Anderton[a,b]

[a]University of Edinburgh, Institute of Immunology and Infection Research, School of Biological Sciences, and [b]Centre for Inflammation Research, Edinburgh, UK

Abstract

Between 5 and 10% of the European population suffer from autoimmune disease, whilst allergic disorders affect an even higher frequency, and both these forms of immunopathology have increased markedly in recent decades. The need for more precise and effective therapeutic strategies drives the investigation of antigen-based tolerance in rodent models and in patients. The identification of the key role T-regulatory cells (Tregs) play in avoidance of immunopathology focused on either self or environmental antigens has led to a need to determine whether established and novel tolerance-inducing strategies are in fact expanding antigen-reactive Treg populations. Here we review recent data from mouse and man. A consistent thread is that, both in T-helper (Th)1/Th17-driven autoimmune disease and in Th2-driven allergic disease, antigen-based tolerance induction often promotes an antigen-reactive IL-10 T-cell population whilst reducing the pathogenic response. Whether these IL-10-producing cells are from the 'natural' Treg population that expresses the forkhead box p3 (Foxp3) transcription factor is less clear, and often they are not. We discuss some recent studies that might provide insight into how best to expand these protective T cells and highlight some outstanding issues requiring further investigation.

Copyright © 2008 S. Karger AG, Basel

The Need for Precise Treatments for Autoimmune and Allergic Disease

Organ-specific autoimmune diseases are commonly (although not always) characterized by a proinflammatory (Th1 and Th17) assault leading to macrophage activation, release of complement-activating and Fc receptor-binding autoantibodies and subsequent tissue damage [1]. Allergic airway disease and asthma are inflammatory diseases of the respiratory mucosa in which inhaled allergen(s) trigger the release of Th2 cytokines (IL-4, IL-5, IL-9, IL-10 and IL-13) leading to airway hyperactivity, mastocytosis, eosinophilia, goblet cell hyperplasia and IgE secretion [2, 3]. There is currently no cure for any autoimmune disease and although the current generation of biologics can have an impressive efficacy in certain diseases, their long-term effects on immune protection from infection and neoplasia remain unknown. Likewise, current therapeutics for allergic disease often rely on global immunosuppression. There is therefore a powerful case for generating more precise, disease-specific therapeutic regimens and in this regard the development of reliable antigen-based approaches to establish immune tolerance remains a holy grail. To target specifically those T lymphocytes that drive autoimmune or allergic disease, the obvious choice is to develop antigen-based approaches, and this has been done in rodent models of allergic and autoimmune disease [4, 5]. The potent capacity of 'natural' regulatory T cells expressing Foxp3 to suppress the spontaneous development of immunopathology has highlighted their key role in maintaining tissue integrity [6]. They are therefore the subject of intense interest as potential targets for immunotherapy because potentiation of their function might be expected to ameliorate established autoimmune or allergic pathology. Here we discuss recent data indicating that this may be achievable using antigen-based regimens.

T-Regulatory Cells in the Natural Resolution of Autoimmune and Allergic Inflammation

Our starting point is that, if T-regulatory cells (Tregs) are to be developed as therapeutic targets to turn-off autoimmune and allergic inflammation, there should be evidence that they can do this naturally in self-limiting inflammatory models. On this point it is notable that most of the 'classical' experiments defining the indispensable function of Tregs used models from which they were serendipitously excluded, for example by neonatal thymectomy, or by transfer of T-cell populations devoid of Tregs into immunodeficient hosts [6]. These models were therefore identifying a role for Tregs in preventing spontaneous immunopathology, i.e. the Tregs were most likely acting to prevent the priming of the deleterious immune response. Reversing an ongoing inflammatory immune reaction, which is of course the requirement in established human disease, poses a greater challenge. Recent work from

our own laboratory indicates that Tregs can play a critical role in the resolution of organ-specific autoimmune and allergic inflammation.

Experimental autoimmune encephalomyelitis (EAE) is the primary laboratory model of multiple sclerosis (MS) sharing various pathological indications. EAE can be induced in C57BL/6 mice by immunization with myelin oligodendrocyte glycoprotein (MOG) and is driven by Th1 and/or Th17 CD4+ T cells. In our hands this gives a monophasic course of central nervous system (CNS) inflammation which spontaneously enters resolution ~8–10 days after first clinical signs. IL-10-deficient mice show exacerbated disease. We identified the major source of this immunosuppressive cytokine in the CNS of wild-type mice as CD4+CD25+Foxp3+ T cells. Most strikingly the frequency of these Tregs in the CNS rose sharply, correlating precisely with the recovery phase, and mice that were depleted of Tregs lost the ability to recover. Tregs therefore make an indispensable contribution to the natural recovery from CNS inflammation in this model [7]. We have recently reported a similar role of Tregs in the resolution of murine-allergic airway disease [8]. C57BL/6 mice sensitized to the Der p 1 allergen from house dust mite (HDM) develop airway inflammation characterized by eosinophilia, goblet cell hyperplasia, IgE, IgG1 and Th2 cytokine expression in the lung following intratracheal Der p 1 challenge. The inflammation is evident 2 days after challenge, peaking at days 4–6 before decline to full resolution by day 21. Similar to the situation in the inflamed CNS in EAE, peak CD4+Foxp3+ cell numbers within the inflamed lung correlate with the switch to the resolution phase. Importantly, Treg depletion after sensitization led to exacerbation of all the inflammatory parameters (except recall IL-10 responses to Der p 1) upon challenge. The conclusion from these studies is that Tregs can play a crucial role in the natural resolution of autoimmune and allergic inflammation (fig. 1). If we can expand their numbers and/or function therapeutically,

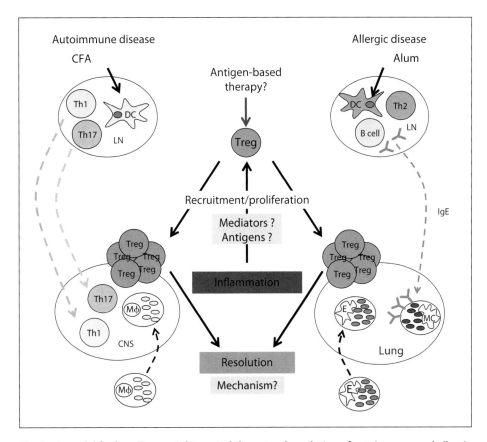

Fig. 1. A model for how Tregs might control the natural resolution of autoimmune and allergic inflammatory disease. Experimental models of autoimmune disease can be induced by immunization with autoantigen. The PAMPs contained in complete Freund's adjuvant (CFA) condition the antigen presenting dendritic cells (DC) to provoke a Th1 and/or Th17 response. These effector T cells migrate to the target organ (here depicted as the CNS as would be the case in EAE) to establish an inflammatory lesion with extensive macrophage recruitment. Allergic sensitization follows immunization with allergen in alum. This establishes a Th2 response that drives production of IgE (and perhaps IgG1). Subsequent airway challenge with allergen leads to degranulation of specific IgE-coated mast cells (MC), recruitment of other immune cells including eosinophils (E) and resulting inflammation. In either disease model, release of inflammatory mediators/chemokines attracts Tregs that proliferate rapidly in the inflamed tissue and suppress the inflammation leading to resolution. This model is based on our own data from CNS and allergic airway inflammation [7, 8, 31]. Important outstanding questions are: (**a**) How do Tregs suppress inflammation in the affected organ? (**b**) Which inflammatory mediators drive Treg recruitment and proliferation? (**c**) Which antigen(s) in the inflamed organ do the Tregs recognize? And, crucially, (**d**) can we expand these disease protective Tregs using antigen-based therapics? This model addresses how Tregs might function in the inflamed organ. It should be noted that Tregs can also regulate effector lymphocyte function in the lymphoid organs.

we may be able to have a positive influence on established inflammatory disorders that do not spontaneously resolve. From studies using the transfer of pre-formed Tregs, it is evident that Tregs that recognize a disease-relevant autoantigen are by far the most potent at suppressing autoimmune diabetes [9] and EAE [S.M.A., unpubl. observations]. To stimulate the in vivo expansion of the most effective Treg population will therefore require an antigen-based approach, rather than a generalized Treg-expanding modality. Also, the use of antigen will of course limit the risk of inadvertently prompting suppression of essential antimicrobial or antitumour immunity.

Antigen-Based Therapy for Autoimmune and Allergic Disease

A large range of rodent models of autoimmune and allergic disease are available. There are many models of induced autoimmune diseases (EAE is an example) in which defined autoantigens, or peptides thereof, are used for immunization usually in combination with complete Freund's adjuvant to drive a Th1 and/or Th17 autoaggressive response, which may or may not be accompanied by pathogenic autoantibody production. Rodent models of allergic disease are generally induced by sensitization with one or more injections of protein antigen usually in alum to provoke a Th2 response, followed by one or more challenges with the antigen in soluble form to elicit inflammation. The fact that most of these autoimmune and allergic models are induced with a defined (auto)antigen makes antigen-based treatment strategies straightforward.

There is an extensive literature documenting the use of antigen to silence pathologic T- and B-cell responses to defined autoantigens and allergens [reviewed in 5, 10, 11]. Antigen is generally administered in the absence of adjuvant. A favoured route for delivery of intact protein antigens has been via oral gavage, and there is a long history to the study of oral tolerance [12]. In many models the definition of the immunodominant T-cell epitopes has allowed the therapeutic use of short synthetic peptides. Furthermore, a range of T-cell receptor (TCR) transgenic mice provide a source of naive T cells that can be tracked during the evolution of either immunity or tolerance. The range of T-cell epitopes that have been defined in autoimmune disease is best exemplified in EAE which, depending on the strain of mouse used, can be induced with MOG, myelin basic protein (MBP), or proteolipid protein (PLP) and each of these CNS autoantigens contains multiple epitopes (although selection of these epitopes for T-cell recognition is determined by the MHC haplotype of the mouse used). There are now TCR transgenic mice available that recognize epitopes from MBP, PLP and MOG and that can be used for adoptive transfer in different strains of mice. In allergic models the allergen is of course exogenous which allows the use of TCR transgenics recognizing model antigens such as ovalbumin (OVA).

One difficulty with translating antigen-induced tolerance regimens to human autoimmune disease is the lack of precise information on which T-cell epitopes are the key targets for the autoaggressive cells that drive pathology. For example, although candidate autoantigens are available for MS, type 1 diabetes and rheumatoid arthritis (RA), we currently do not know enough about the aetiology of these human diseases. This may underlie the lack of success with antigen-based trials in MS and RA for example [4]. Translating specific immunotherapy (SIT) has therefore been fastest and most successful in allergic diseases with well-defined allergens [5]. There are several routes of application – subcutaneous, intradermal, intramuscular, oral, intravenous, intraperitoneal and newer approaches including sublingual immunotherapy (SLIT), intranasal and intralymphatic injection. These generally deliver the antigen systemically to allow antigen exposure for all antigen-reactive T cells, which may be located in any of the lymphoid organs.

A drawback of using intact proteins for SIT in allergy is that the patient's pre-existing IgE can bind the antigen, leading to allergic reactions including anaphylaxis. This has driven the recent interest in peptide immunotherapy (PIT) [5, 13]. The peptides used contain T-cell epitopes, and so can provide T-cell tolerance but are devoid of antibody epitopes, negating the risk of anaphylaxis. Promising trials of PIT have been reported using pollen-, venom- and dander-allergic individuals [10, 14, 15], although the need to discern the exact mechanisms behind the induction of immunological tolerance remains. The basic paradigm for the therapeutic induction of immune tolerance is that the systemic delivery of antigen (either intact protein or peptide) in the absence of pathogen-associated molecular patterns (PAMPS) or 'danger signals' leads to an abortive T-cell activation that, rather than driving full differentiation and expansion of an effector T-cell population, renders the recipient refractory to subsequent attempts to provoke an immune response to that antigen through immunization. A full discussion of the cellular and molecular basis for tolerance induction can be found elsewhere [4, 11]. There is evidence that each of the 'three pilllars' of immune tolerance: T-cell death, T-cell anergy/adaptation and T-cell regulatory function can play their part in therapeutic tolerance to antigen. Which pillar is dominant probably depends on the precise model studied, the affinity of the TCR expressed by the T cells under study and the dose and length of antigen exposure.

The phenotype of tolerance may or may not be dependent on the route of administration. For instance, it makes sense that oral delivery of antigen might provoke a TGF-β-producing Th3 population, or a Foxp3+ population, given that the gut mucosa and the associated lymphoid tissues are rich in the TGF-β needed to drive such a response [12]. In contrast, the long-held belief that inhaled proteins would provoke an antigen-reactive Th2 response most likely reflected contamination of the model antigens used with PAMPS. Use of purer antigen preparations, free of lipopolysaccharide leads to unresponsiveness, rather than Th2 responses. Whether standard antigen-based tolerance modalities can reliably provoke disease-protective regulatory populations in mouse models is still a matter of debate. However, accumulating data from studies of allergic humans undergoing SIT now suggest that this is possible.

Are Antigen-Based Therapies Expanding Tregs?

There is good evidence that tolerance induced with antigen may have a regulatory component. This stems from observations that tolerization with one antigen/epitope can reduce pathology provoked by immunization with a distinct antigen(s). For example we showed such 'bystander suppression' could be active in EAE because inducing tolerance with a single peptide from PLP could greatly reduce pathology seen after immunization either with the PLP epitope, or with either of two MBP epitopes [16]. The explanation for this phenomenon was therefore that we were expanding a PLP-reactive regulatory population that was active in the CNS once PLP became available for presentation because of tissue damage caused by the MBP-reactive T cells. Subsequent studies indicated that in the EAE models IL-10-producing T cells were key (this may be because IL-10 seems to have potent protective effects in the CNS). It appears that the peptide-induced regulatory IL-10 producers do not express Foxp3 [17], although IL-10 can clearly be produced by Foxp3+ cells in the CNS [7]. Normally, peptides are rapidly cleared such that peptide-MHC complexes are below detectable levels within hours of administration [11]. To date, the most convincing data indicating that peptides can be used in vivo to convert Foxp3– cells into Foxp3+ cells comes from the use of implanted mini-pumps delivering a constant low dose of peptide [18]. The persistent stimulation this gives may be an important factor. We have encountered difficulties in generating Foxp3+ populations by soluble peptide administration (using three TCR transgenic systems). The only situation in which we have achieved this is when using an altered peptide ligand (APL) modified at an MHC-binding residue to provide an extremely stable interaction, with peptide-MHC complexes detectable in vivo for at least 7 days after peptide administration [S.M.A., unpubl. observations].

In an allergic airway model induced with HDM extract, PIT to Der p 1 reduced recall lymph node proliferative responses and the level of eosinophil infiltration to the lung, an effect that could be transferred by splenocytes from peptide-treated mice [19]. Using an OVA-reactive TCR transfer system, the authors reported an expansion of CD4+CD25+ and IL-10+ transferred cells following the peptide treatment regimen. However, the 3- to 4-fold increase in the percentage of transferred CD4+ cells expressing CD25+ or IL-10 was matched by a 3- to 4-fold drop in the absolute numbers of cells (it is likely that many of the transferred cohort died as a result of abortive activation in response to the peptide). Therefore, from these data, it is not clear that peptide administration actively expanding the putative regulatory population, or whether their increased frequency reflected a selective resistance to death. A note of caution should also be added when considering such studies showing an effect on pathology induced with a 'real' antigen (in this case HDM) and then using a different antigen (OVA) TCR transgenic system to predict what is happening in the pathologic setting. Using a single TCR system is very different from studying the response of a polyclonal population which will contain a heterogeneous TCR repertoire with a range of affinities

for the peptide-MHC complex of interest. This is difficult enough when using a single peptide, but we cannot assume that the same dose of two peptides from different antigens will affect the immune response in the same way. They may show drastically different affinity for MHC binding which can greatly influence the ability to induce tolerance and the form it may take [20].

A low dose of peanut extract given orally can prevent subsequent sensitization to the extract when given in alum. Anti-CD25 treatment overcame this, restoring IL-4, IL-5, IL-13 and IgE. Thus there was a requirement for Treg during the tolerization process [21]. However, this does not prove an expansion of peanut-reactive Tregs, but may rather indicate that in their absence tolerance cannot be established. Importantly the authors found that simply depleting of Tregs during oral dosing was not sufficient to produce a sensitized animal. This suggests that there is more to the natural prevention of allergic immunity than the control that is imposed by Tregs.

Transfer of naive, lung-derived CD4+CD25+ cells prior to sensitization could limited pathology in an OVA-induced allergic airway model [22]. Interestingly, this only worked if the cells were given intratracheally and not intravenously. Also, if these cells were sourced from an IL-10-deficient mouse, protection could only be transferred if the cells were first cultured in the presence of IL-10. The protective function correlated with increased TGF-β production in the lung. These interesting data suggest that exposure to IL-10 is important in the generation of a regulatory population that then protects against lung inflammation through a TGF-β-dependent mechanism.

Evidence is now accumulating that SIT/PIT can expand regulatory populations in allergic individuals, with reports of IL-10 producing T cells [14, 23, 24], which sometimes appear to be CD4+CD25+ [23]. PIT using peptides from the cat allergen Fel d 1 reduced PBMC proliferative and IL-5 responses, but increased IL-10 production in cat-allergic asthmatic individuals [15]. This study also developed a flow cytometric assay for antigen-specific suppression. CD4-negative cells taken pretreatment were stored. Co-culture with CD4+ cells isolated after PIT showed that these cells could limit the Fel d 1-induced division of the pretreatment cells. Bohle et al. [25] followed patients undergoing daily SLIT with birch pollen Bet v 1. Four weeks after initiation of treatment, PBMC showed reduced proliferative capacity and IL-4 production to Bet v 1 compared with the levels seen prior to starting treatment. The reduced proliferation correlated with increased IL-10 production and Foxp3 expression (real-time PCR after culture with Bet v 1) and could be reversed by removal of CD25+ cells prior to assay. Interestingly, although Bet v 1-induced proliferative capacity and IL-4 production remained suppressed at the 52-week follow-up, enhanced IL-10 and Foxp3 levels were no longer evident. Instead, Bet v 1-induced IFN-γ expression was markedly increased. Importantly, the patients showed a clinical improvement that was maintained at 52 weeks. Does this mean that a short phase of 'regulatory activity' is sufficient to dampen a deleterious Th2 response, allowing the system to re-set towards a less dangerous type 1 response? This may also happen in other human situations. Intriguingly, it is not impossible that the T cells making IFN-γ at 52 weeks are also those (or the descendents of those) T cells that were making IL-10 at 4 weeks. It is known that the same T cell can be produce both IFN-γ and IL-10 (IL-10 was originally identified in a Th1 clone) and that expression of these two cytokines may have differing temporal regulation [26].

New Directions

Even when using PIT, it is possible that pre-existing antibodies could cause anaphylaxis by binding the peptide. For example, anti-peptide antibodies are often evident in EAE [4]. This is most likely only an issue when the mice are actively immunized with peptide. Nevertheless, it has prevented analysis of whether PIT could be established in immune mice because fatal anaphylaxis developed upon peptide application. Using EAE induced with MOG peptide, we have developed an APL that does not bind the anti-peptide antibodies (and therefore does not provoke anaphylaxis), whilst still interacting with the TCR. This APL was highly tolerogenic in pre-immune mice and could dramatically reverse clinical signs of EAE [27]. Although the molecular and cellular basis for the tolerance induced remains to be defined, this is the first study to use APL to avoid antibody-peptide binding, which may have application in an allergic situation in which the antibody-epitope and T-cell epitope are inseparable.

There are several outstanding questions over whether/how SIT/PIT can promote Treg function (table 1, fig. 1). An important question is what provokes Treg accumulation into the inflamed organ? A recent study reported that intratracheal delivery of a histamine receptor 4 (H4R) led to reduced pathology in an OVA-induced allergic airway model [28]. This correlated with an increased number of Foxp3+ cells in the lung. Translating to humans, the H4R agonist could preferentially attract CD4+CD25+Foxp3+ cells in a transmigration assay. Thus, Tregs that can control allergic inflammation may be specifically attracted to the site through release of inflammatory mediators. Another question is whether Treg expansion requires presentation by a particular antigen presenting cell. Subcutaneous administration of very low doses of a nucleosomal histone peptide can delay development of nephritis in lupus-prone mice through the generation of TGF-β-producing regulatory T cells (either CD4+CD25+ or CD8+). A recent report suggests that the generation of these cells involves plasmacytoid dendritic cells (pDC) that produce large quantities of TGF-β, but little IL-6, which might also explain the reduced Th17 expansion

Table 1. Outstanding questions over whether/how SIT/PIT can promote Treg function

What is the key site for Treg function (lymphoid organs or target organ)?
Which chemokines attract Tregs to inflammatory sites and which cytokines stimulate their proliferation during inflammation?
Do Tregs regulate immune pathology by directly suppressing T cells, B cells, plasma cells (reduced IgE is seen in allergic models), or innate immune cells?
Do Tregs and effector T cells recognize the same epitopes?
Are there specific 'Treg epitopes'?
Can Foxp3– cells be converted to Foxp3+ Tregs using antigen-based therapies?
What is the best protocol to expand Tregs? (Persistent antigenic stimulation?)

seen in the protected mice [29]. Of note, this might be an unusual situation as the activation of the pDC by TLR-9 ligation by the nucleosomal antigen seemed crucial. This may not be the case in other immunopathological situations.

There is a key need to develop precise techniques to identify the expansion of regulatory populations in response to antigen treatment and equally importantly, which epitopes within an antigen might act as targets for regulatory cells. Nagato et al. [30] identified a peptide from Bet v 1 (residues 141–156) that appears to be a promiscuous MHC binder (binding to DR4, DR9, DR11, DR15 and DR53). Notably, the authors were able to generate two 'Treg clones' by in vitro priming of PBMC from Bet v 1-allergic individuals with the peptide. These clones expressed CD25, GITR and Foxp3 and suppressed the in vitro activation of other cells in a cell contact dependent, IL-10- and TGF-β-independent manner. Although not perfect (the need to clone cells takes us some way from the in vivo reality) this report suggests that we may be able to develop better assays that allow ex vivo screening for potential 'Treg epitopes'. Of note, we have recently reported a novel methodology for identifying antigen-reactive Foxp3+ Tregs. Classically, such cells are anergic when stimulated in vitro (they do not proliferate in response to antigen unless provided with exogenous IL-2).

However, we have found that Tregs sampled from the inflamed CNS during EAE will incorporate BrdU in response to antigen in vitro. This allows a flow cytometric assay in which we counterstain with anti-Foxp3 to quantitate the frequency of Tregs responding to the antigen of interest [31]. Whether this is a peculiarity of Tregs sampled from inflammatory sites is unclear (although the assay also works on lymph nodes draining the site of immunization). If we can translate this to work with human peripheral blood, it will allow us (a) to track the number of Tregs recognizing a defined protein/peptide during treatment that antigen, and (b) to use peptide libraries to screen for 'Treg epitopes' in an allergen or an autoantigen (which would thus far have not been revealed by standard assays). If such Treg epitopes exist it will allow us to design new peptide vaccines to specifically expand Tregs without running the risk of inadvertently hyperactivating the antigen-reactive T cells that are already driving pathology.

Acknowledgements

Work in the authors' laboratory is supported by grants form the Medical Research Council (UK), the Wellcome Trust and the UK Multiple Sclerosis Society. S.M.A. is a MRC Senior Research Fellow and holds a RCUK Fellowship in Translational Medicine.

References

1 Bettelli E, Oukka M, Kuchroo VK: Th17 cells in the circle of immunity and autoimmunity. Nat Immunol 2007; 8:345–350.

2 Romagnani S: The role of lymphocytes in allergic disease. J Allergy Clin Immunol 2000;105:399–408.

3 Perkins C, Wills-Karp M, Finkelman FD: IL-4 induces IL-13-independent allergic airway inflammation. J Allergy Clin Immunol 2006;118:410–419.

4 Miller SD, Turley DM, Podojil JR: Antigen-specific tolerance strategies for the prevention and treatment of autoimmune disease. Nat Rev Immunol 2007;7:665–677.

5 Larche M, Wraith DC: Peptide-based therapeutic vaccines for allergic and autoimmune diseases. Nat Med 2005;11: S69–76.

6 Sakaguchi S: Naturally arising Foxp3-expressing CD25+CD4+ regulatory T cells in immunological tolerance to self and non-self. Nat Immunol 2005;6: 345–352.

7 McGeachy MJ, Stephens LA, Anderton SM: Natural recovery and protection from autoimmune encephalomyelitis: contribution of CD4+CD25+ regulatory cells within the central nervous system. J Immunol 2005;175: 3025–3032.

8 Leech MD, Benson RA, deVries A, Fitch PM, Howie SEM: Resolution of Der p 1-induced allergic airway inflammation is dependent on CD4+ CD25+ Foxp3+ regulatory cells. J Immunol 2007;179:7050–7058.

9 Masteller EL, Warner MR, Tang Q, Tarbell KV, McDevitt H, Bluestone JA: Expansion of functional endogenous antigen-specific CD4+CD25+ regulatory T cells from nonobese diabetic mice. J Immunol 2005;175:3053–3059.

10 Oldfield WL, Larche M, Kay AB: Effect of T-cell peptides derived from Fel d 1 on allergic reactions and cytokine production in patients sensitive to cats: a randomised controlled trial. Lancet 2002;360:47–53.

11 Hochweller K, Sweenie CH, Anderton SM: Immunological tolerance using synthetic peptides – basic mechanisms and clinical application. Curr Mol Med 2006;6:631–643.

12 Faria AM, Weiner HL: Oral tolerance and TGF-β-producing cells. Inflamm Allergy Drug Targets 2006;5:179–190.

13 Larche M, Akdis CA, Valenta R: Immunological mechanisms of allergen-specific immunotherapy. Nat Rev Immunol 2006;6:761–771.

14 Akdis CA, Blesken T, Akdis M, Wuthrich B, Blaser K: Role of interleukin-10 in specific immunotherapy. J Clin Invest 1998;102:98–106.

15 Verhoef A, Alexander C, Kay AB, Larche M: T cell epitope immunotherapy induces a CD4+ T cell population with regulatory activity. PLoS Med 2005;2:e78.

16 Anderton SM, Wraith DC: Hierarchy in the ability of T cell epitopes to induce peripheral tolerance to antigens from myelin. Eur J Immunol 1998;28: 1251–1261.

17 Nicolson KS, O'Neill EJ, Sundstedt A, Streeter HB, Minaee S, Wraith DC: Antigen-induced IL-10+ regulatory T cells are independent of CD25+ regulatory cells for their growth, differentiation, and function. J Immunol 2006;176:5329–5337.

18 Kretschmer K, Apostolou I, Hawiger D, Khazaie K, Nussenzweig MC, von Boehmer H: Inducing and expanding regulatory T cell populations by foreign antigen. Nat Immunol 2005;6:1219–1227.

19 Zuleger CL, Gao X, Burger MS, Chu Q, Payne LG, Chen D: Peptide induces CD4+CD25+ and IL-10+ T cells and protection in airway allergy models. Vaccine 2005;23:3181–3186.

20 McCue D, Ryan K, Wraith DC, Anderton SM: Activation thresholds determine susceptibility to peptide-induced tolerance in a heterogeneous myelin-reactive T cells repertoire. J Neuroimmunol 2004;156:96–106.

21 Van Wijk F, Wehrens EJ, Nierkens S, Boon L, Kasran A, Pieters R, Knippels LM: CD4+CD25+ T cells regulate the intensity of hypersensitivity responses to peanut, but are not decisive in the induction of oral sensitization. Clin Exp Allergy 2007;37:572–581.

22 Joetham A, Takeda K, Taube C, Miyahara N, Matsubara S, Koya T, Rha YH, Dakhama A, Gelfand EW: Naturally occurring lung CD4+CD25+ T cell regulation of airway allergic responses depends on IL-10 induction of TGF-β. J Immunol 2007;178:1433–1442.

23 Gardner LM, Thien FC, Douglass JA, Rolland JM, O'Hehir RE: Induction of T 'regulatory' cells by standardized house dust mite immunotherapy: an increase in CD4+ CD25+ interleukin-10+ T cells expressing peripheral tissue trafficking markers. Clin Exp Allergy 2004;34:1209–1219.

24 Tarzi M, Klunker S, Texier C, Verhoef A, Stapel SO, Akdis CA, Maillere B, Kay AB, Larche M: Induction of interleukin-10 and suppressor of cytokine signalling-3 gene expression following peptide immunotherapy. Clin Exp Allergy 2006;36:465–474.

25 Bohle B, Kinaciyan T, Gerstmayr M, Radakovics A, Jahn-Schmid B, Ebner C: Sublingual immunotherapy induces IL-10-producing T regulatory cells, allergen-specific T-cell tolerance, and immune deviation. J Allergy Clin Immunol 2007;120:707–713.l

26 O'Garra A, Vieira P: Th1 cells control themselves by producing interleukin-10. Nat Rev Immunol 2007;7:425–428.

27 Leech MD, Chung C-Y, Culshaw A, Anderton SM: Peptide-based immunotherapy of CNS autoimmune disease without anaphylaxis. Eur J Immunol 2007;37:3576–3581.

28 Morgan RK, McAllister B, Cross L, Green DS, Kornfeld H, Center DM, Cruikshank WW: Histamine 4 receptor activation induces recruitment of FoxP3+ T cells and inhibits allergic asthma in a murine model. J Immunol 2007;178:8081–8089.

29 Kang HK, Liu M, Datta SK: Low-dose peptide tolerance therapy of lupus generates plasmacytoid dendritic cells that cause expansion of autoantigen-specific regulatory T cells and contraction of inflammatory Th17 cells. J Immunol 2007;178:7849–7858.

30 Nagato T, Kobayashi H, Yanai M, Sato K, Aoki N, Oikawa K, Kimura S, Abe Y, Celis E, Harabuchi Y, Tateno M: Functional analysis of birch pollen allergen Bet v 1-specific regulatory T cells. J Immunol 2007;178:1189–1198.

31 O'Connor RA, Malpass KH, Anderton SM: The inflamed central nervous system drives the activation and rapid proliferation of Foxp3+ regulatory T cells. J Immunol 2007;179:958–966.

Stephen M. Anderton
University of Edinburgh, Institute of Immunology and Infection Research
School of Biological Sciences, Kings Buildings
West Mains Road, Edinburgh EH9 3JT (UK)
Tel. +44 131 650 5499, Fax +44 131 650 6564, E-Mail steve.anderton@ed.ac.uk

Blaser K (ed): T Cell Regulation in Allergy, Asthma and Atopic Skin Diseases.
Chem Immunol Allergy. Basel, Karger, 2008, vol 94, pp 211–219

Stem Cell Transplantation in Genetically Linked Regulatory T-Cell Disorders

Shalini Shenoy

St. Louis Children's Hospital, St. Louis, Mo., USA

Abstract

T-regulatory disorders are a heterogenous group characterized by autoimmune and allergic manifestations of varying onset, severity, and progression. The advent of sophisticated molecular and immunologic diagnostic techniques has resulted in accurate elucidation of etiopathogenesis of many immunoregulatory disorders previously clubbed under the autoimmune umbrella. The severity of presentation and progression, early morbidity and mortality, poor quality of life, and frequent refractoriness to immunosuppressive therapy has prompted studies of stem cell transplantation in many immunoregulatory disorders. The benefits of autologous or allogeneic transplantation are related to either suppression and reprogramming of the immune system (autologous transplant) or replacement of missing elements of immune regulation (allogeneic transplants). Transplant methods have steadily improved through a series of studies and trials to have the benefits of this approach outweigh the risks of procedure-related toxicities. This article summarizes the current status and the future goals of stem cell transplantation for T-cell immunoregulatory disorders and reviews advances in disease detection, targeted transplant strategies and novel approaches, and the pros and cons of transplant in this field.

Stem cell therapy is aimed at replacing, supplementing, repairing or reprogramming defective systems or cells in patients with immune system disorders after conditioning the host to accept and engraft the incoming cells. These goals are pursued either in the autologous or allogeneic transplant setting depending on the end result desired, the pathogenesis of the disorder in question, and weighing the risks and benefits of each procedure in afflicted patients.

The applicability of hematopoietic stem cell transplantation (SCT) has expanded significantly as molecular and immunologic mechanisms of previously ill-understood disorders are unraveled by new and advanced investigative techniques. Simultaneously, transplant trials have sought to achieve safety and success by using targeted methods of conditioning, stem cell source selection, and post-transplant care and intervention. This is work in progress, and continually improved transplant outcomes are a testament to well-planned study questions making inroads toward safe and successful transplants.

These events have led to an expansion of transplant trials for immunoregulatory disorders as the benefits of transplant continue to outweigh the risks. This review will focus on SCT for T-cell regulatory disorders and address the advantages and limitations of the same.

Stem Cell Therapy Perspectives

Stem cell therapy involves infusion of specialized cells utilized to perform specific functions. The traditional use of cell therapy includes harvest and cryopreservation of autologous hematopoietic cells either from the bone marrow (old approach) or mobilization and pheresis of hematopoietic stem cells from peripheral blood using stem cell-mobilizing cytokines such as hematopoietic colony-stimulating factors (G-CSF, GM-CSF) or chemokine inhibitors (AMD-3100). A more recent stem cell source is umbilical cord blood that has rich pleuripotent potential and can engraft at lower doses than bone marrow or mobilized peripheral blood stem cells.

The infusion and engraftment of stem cells allows patients to undergo chemoablative or immunoablative therapy targeted at their disease followed by autologous stem cell infusion to 'rescue' the ablated immunohematopoietic system. The advent of HLA typing allowed this process to be extended to allogeneic SCT with the replacement of the host hematopoietic and/or immune system by that from a normal donor. Since the advent of allogeneic transplantation three decades ago, stem cell therapy has come a long way and includes sophisticated methods of developing engineered cells targeted against disease or infection, or directed toward replacement of critical cell compartments. These include donor lymphocyte infusions, lymphokine-activated killer cells, tumor-infiltrating cells, virus-specific T cells (EBV, CMV), anti-cancer cytotoxic T cells, regulatory mesenchymal stem cells, and CD4+CD25+ regulatory T cells [1].

In general, immunosuppression, expansion of regulatory cells, costimulatory blockade, or promotion of a Th2 cytokine milieu is considered to be supportive of disease control in T-cell regulatory disorders such as autoimmune disease and graft-versus-host disease (GvHD) [2]. In contrast, killer cells, a Th1 cytokine milieu, or activated lymphocyte infusions support control of malignancy and infections. Maintaining a balance between the two

arms of the immune system is critical to the well-being of the patient and serves to avoid the morbidity and mortality associated with SCT. SCT studies are thus directed at targeting diseases with safe and effective conditioning regimen, successfully achieving engraftment of infused cells, and facilitating early immune reconstitution.

Pros and Cons of SCT

Autologous SCT provides a method of reprogramming the regulatory immune system in autoimmune disorders where dysregulation which often has genetic and additional multifactorial pathogenesis is responsible for damage and destruction of specific target organs. This approach proved beneficial initially in severely debilitating disorders such as systemic lupus erythematosus (SLE) and systemic sclerosis where myeloablation with high-dose chemoradiotherapy followed by stem cell rescue using cryopreserved autologous stem cells resulted in improvement in disease parameters. However, the toxicities of the conditioning regimen were high due to their intensity and side effects and compromised outcomes despite improvement in disease parameters [3]. More recently, myeloablation has been replaced with reduced intensity regimen that provides immunosuppression and lymphoablation but are designed to avoid major toxicities and achieve immune system reprogramming goals. The disorders where there is currently a rationale for SCT are listed in figure 1. SCT approaches are reviewed in a disease-specific fashion below to detail benefits and outcomes.

The field of allogeneic transplantation was initially targeted at the treatment of hematologic malignancies. However, as defective molecular and signaling pathways were described for disorders of immune regulation, it was apparent that successful engraftment of normal allogeneic donor cells could provide missing links in the immune system and normalize function. Thus, allogeneic transplantation for immune regulatory disorders is

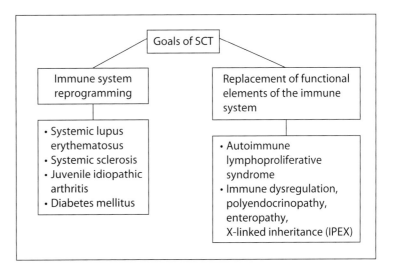

Fig. 1. Algorithm for SCT for immunoregulatory disorders.

rapidly evolving. Allogeneic transplants are limited by the availability of adequately HLA-matched donor sources, the risks of graft rejection and GvHD, infections, and early and late toxicities of conditioning regimen. Each of these complications adds to the morbidity and mortality associated with the procedure. In general, fully HLA-matched sibling donors, adequate numbers of stem cells, well-tolerated conditioning regimen, and the prevention of GvHD in the face of donor cell engraftment present the best scenario for success and cure. Conversely, mismatched unrelated donors, inadequate stem cell numbers, intense and toxic conditioning regimen, GvHD, invasive infections, and graft loss result in significant transplant-related toxicities and are often fatal. It is essential to consider the risk-benefit ratio of the procedure for therapy of the disease involved.

Progress in all aspects of transplant care such as improved HLA-matching, expansion of stem cell sources such as double cord blood products and CD34-selected stem cells, graft manipulation, safer non-ablative or reduced intensity conditioning regimen, and vastly improved care for GvHD and infections have made allogeneic transplants a feasible option for several immune regulatory disorders. Advances in transplant methods are listed in figure 2. These interventions have supported SCT trials with the goal of achieving either a cure or disease control for disorders that were previously fatal or morbid autoimmune disorders. Ongoing research seeks to achieve successful transplantation when indicated, with minimum toxicity.

Immune Regulatory Disorders Targeted by Stem Cell Transplantation

In the absence of distinct molecular or signaling abnormalities or genetic mutations, autoimmunity is likely propagated by disrupted balance between activated effector CD4+ T lymphocytes and tolerizing regulatory CD4+ T lymphocytes which produce anti-inflammatory cytokines. Familial predisposition often suggests as yet unidentified genetic and environmental influences. 'Reprogramming' the immune system to tolerate self antigens by autologous transplant includes removal of the offending activated autoreactive lymphocytes and promoting differentia-

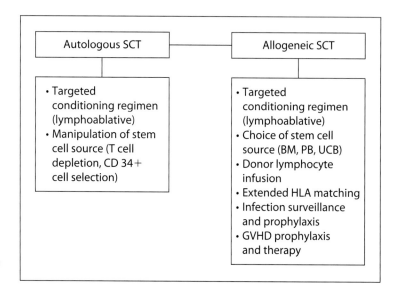

Fig. 2. Advances in SCT – increasing safety and efficacy.

tion and maturation of newly engrafted precursor cells in the presence of autoantigens to induce remission from autoimmunity. As in all chronic disorders, the long-term benefits and sustainability of improvement following transplant need prolonged follow-up. Many transplant studies are still young precluding conclusive statements regarding long-term efficacy of this treatment modality. However, it is clear that important advances are made with each study providing opportunities to build upon existing experience.

Autoimmune disorders that are a result of missing or defective immune molecules and pathways will not respond to autologous 'resetting' of the immune system and will need allogeneic transplants for cure. However, allogenicity itself is a harbinger of autoimmunity following donor cell engraftment in an allogeneic environment and often presents as GvHD and in this setting. In allogeneic SCT the balance between safe and effective transplants and transplant-related complications add another layer of complexity to evaluating outcomes.

Systemic Lupus Erythematosus

SLE is a heterogenous autoimmune disorder with a debilitating chronic course. Equivalent morbidity and mortality is also attributed to treatment (prolonged and intense immunosuppression) as to disease pathogenesis. Based on the observation that remission was induced in SLE patients transplanted for other indications, antigenic tolerance was sought with autologous SCT for SLE. A retrospective review of autologous SCT for SLE showed that it was useful for induction of remission (66%) but was not curative (relapse rate 32% at 6 months) and was likely to be toxic (treatment-related mortality 12% and more in those with longer duration disease) to patients with significant preexisting morbidity [3]. A prospective single-center study of non-myeloablative SCT (cyclophosphamide and antithymocyte globulin) in the treatment of refractory SLE patients improved upon previous experience. Treatment-related mortality (TRM) was 4% and the probability of disease-free survival at 5 years was 50%

[4]. Autoimmune complications were frequently part of post-transplant care (partial remission status) but were of lowered intensity. Targeted emerging lowered intensity therapy may help to maintain remission post transplant.

Systemic or Polyarticular Rheumatoid Arthritis

Progressive polyarticular or systemic juvenile idiopathic arthritis is a progressive debilitating disorder of chronic joint inflammation resulting in poor quality of life and early deaths. T-cell dysregulation is blamed based on disease response to cytokine inhibitory therapy. Myeloablation with high-dose cyclophosphamide with autologous stem cell rescue proved beneficial in a retrospective registry outcome analysis [5]. Long-term follow-up (median period 80 months) is reported on 22 patients with juvenile idiopathic arthritis who received autologous stem cells following treatment with low-dose total body irradiation, cyclophosphamide and antithymocyte globulin and a slow steroid taper. The probability of disease-free survival at 5 years was 36% while the majority of others relapsed between 2 and 16 months [6]. Of note, all patients on this trial were refractory to standard therapy supporting a benefit for SCT in refractory disease. While TRM was 9% (2 deaths), infections were a frequent complication in others, a reflection of the prolonged and profound lymphopenia (low naive CD4+CD45RA+ cells for 6 months) induced by SCT and the need for continued monitoring and support for infectious complications. T-cell immunosuppression is believed to have caused the 2 deaths; patients developed fatal macrophage activation syndrome following documented infection. Interestingly, with efforts to deplete grafts of autoreactive T cells prior to transplant (CD34+ stem cell selection), no correlation was detected between T-cell depletion and disease remission post transplant.

Systemic Sclerosis

A disease of complex pathogenesis, systemic sclerosis is characterized by autoimmunity, small vessel vasculopathy and progressive organ fibrosis resulting in early morbidity and mortality. Total body irradiation and myeloablative regimen were promising for disease control but resulted in high TRM rates and secondary malignancies [7]. This has prompted transplants with a non-myeloablative approach using cyclophosphamide and ATG that achieves lymphoablation, and has been used successfully without regimen-related deaths [8]. Of 10 patients studied, 9 improved within 12 months. Two recurred between 1 and 2 years. Thus, patients tolerated non-ablative transplants better. The jury on efficacy is still out as slowly progressive autoimmune disorders such as systemic sclerosis need prolonged follow-up to determine the consistency and duration of treatment benefit.

Type 1 Diabetes Mellitus

Type 1 diabetes mellitus (DM) is a result of cell-mediated autoimmunity against pancreatic β cells and is associated with vascular complications, organ damage, need for lifelong hormone, and impaired quality of life [9]. Immunosuppression has previously reduced insulin needs likely due to inhibition of β-cell destruction. These data as well as clinical improvement in autoimmunity described for other immune regulation disorders have prompted recent trials of non-ablative autologous transplants in patients with type 1 DM [10]. Chemotherapy and cytokine mobilized peripheral blood stem cells were infused following cyclophosphamide and ATG conditioning in 15 newly diagnosed patients with DM. Of note, established diabetic ketoacidosis was a contraindication due to increased toxicity. At a median follow-up of 18 months, 14 of the 15 patients became insulin free for variable periods of time ranging from 1 to 35 months, and there was no associated mortality after the procedure. These promising results have prompted the development of further trials and investigation into other stem cell sources such as umbilical cord blood cells.

Autoimmune Lymphoproliferative Syndrome

Autoimmune lymphoproliferative syndrome (ALPS) is characterized by lymphadenopathy, splenomegaly, autoimmune hematologic cytopenias, and a wide spectrum of organ dysfunctions secondary to autoimmune organ destruction ranging from the kidney to the brain [11, 12]. Clinical manifestations are variable within families though they inherit the same mutation suggesting additional genetic or antigen-mediated influences in disease pathogenesis. The associated lymphoproliferation is associated with the development of lymphomas in several affected kindred. The pathogenesis of this disease has been traced to inherited mutations in the gene encoding Fas, a death receptor critical for lymphocyte apoptosis. This regulatory mechanism is necessary to prevent overexpansion of activated lymphocytes that mediate autoimmunity. In the event of severe disease or progression to a lymphomatous presentation, autologous transplantation is not indicated as in other regulatory disorders, as it would fail to correct the underlying defect in lymphocyte apoptosis. Albeit rare, recognition of severe cases of ALPS, accurate and timely diagnosis, and intervention if necessary with SCT would be critical for disease control. Successful myeloablative allogeneic transplantation from an unrelated donor is described in a child with ALPS that progressed to cardiorespiratory failure and lymphoma-like extensive lymphoproliferation despite immunosuppression and cytotoxic therapy [13]. The post-transplant course was complicated by significant GvHD necessitating further immunosuppression.

Immune Dysregulation, Polyendocrinopathy, Enteropathy, and X-Linked Inheritance

The genetic basis of immune dysregulation is always an exciting discovery and results from careful investigation of patients or kindred with similar manifestations. A recently described severe and often fatal autoimmune disorder called immune dysregulation, polyendocrinopathy, enteropathy, and X-linked inheritance (IPEX) or X-linked autoimmunity-allergic disregulation syndrome, is one such advance in understanding the ravages caused by immune dysregulation. Mutations in FoxP3 results in the loss of regulatory CD4+CD25+ T-cell function that is critical for the regulation of autoimmunity on antigen exposure [14, 15]. Patients develop life-threatening diarrhea and hypersensitivity to food, eczema, failure to thrive, and destruction of endocrine organs (hypothyroidism, adrenal insufficiency, DM), presumably following specific immune activation followed by targeted autoimmunity. A rare milder phenotype has been described resulting in decreased levels of FoxP3 protein in T cells and the development of late-onset autoimmune colitis, arthritis, nephritis, etc. The dramatic phenotype of rapid onset of allergy, diarrhea and endocrinopathy is more common making this one of the most severe immunoregulatory disorders that is associated with early mortality.

Allogeneic stem cell transplant can provide normal donor-derived regulatory T cells and halt the disease process. Myeloablative conditioning can support engraftment but associated toxicities especially in a decompensated host remain tough problems [16]. Non-ablative conditioning is well tolerated but graft rejection rates are high in immunocompetent hosts depending on graft source and host factors. We have previously reported the largest experience with reduced intensity allogeneic transplants for IPEX that was well tolerated, supported sustained engraftment, and demonstrated normalization of FoxP3+ T-cell numbers [17]. The observation that FoxP3 expression was highest post transplant in the memory phenotype CD4+ T-cell compartment, even after 2 years following allogeneic peripheral blood SCT (instead of from host thymus educated naive CD45RA+ cells), has raised questions about their durability long-term [18]. Clinically, allergic manifestations and chronic diarrhea are reversed by transplant. However, preexisting organ damage such as endocrinopathy is permanent. Infections and GvHD early post transplant demand more supportive care than in the autologous transplant setting. This severe and ultimately fatal autoimmune disorder requires allogeneic SCT on an emergent basis upon detection to avoid irreversible organ damage.

Discussion

SCT for immunoregulatory disorders have come a long way since they were first attempted. Improvements in the various facets of transplant such as stem cell sources and graft manipulation, targeted and safer conditioning regimen, improved monitoring and supportive care, and new interventions to prevent or treat GvHD have been instrumental in increasing the availability of this procedure for more diseases. This has resulted in an expansion of SCT indications especially in the realm of non-malignant disorders where transplant can provide an option for disease control or cure. In the younger age groups, as many as 30% of transplants are performed for non-malignant disorders. Immunoregulatory disorders are a large subgroup of this non-malignant population as transplant provides a method of setting the immune system in the right direction.

SCT includes autologous and allogeneic transplants and the choice is dependent on the end result desired as well as the risks and benefits of each procedure. Autologous transplants after immunoablative therapy function on the premise of T-cell suppression versus clonal deletion as a cause of tolerance induction in autoimmunity.

This immune 'resetting' is sought to increase naive T cells that are tolerogenic and enhance recovery of a diverse T-cell receptor repertoire while decreasing autoreactive memory T cells. It is notable that B cell compartments and the humoral response are not predictive of clinical response to SCT for autoimmune disorders. Allogeneic transplants in immunoregulatory disorders serve to replace absent or mutated regulatory elements of the immune system with normal functional donor cells. Studies of allogeneic transplantation are likely to increase as disease mechanisms are better elucidated and transplant methods become targeted and safer.

Allergy and autoimmunity were previously considered separated by etiology and pathogenesis. The description of the IPEX syndrome closely linked the two. Alloantigen stimulation in the presence of immune dysregulation and absence of regulatory T-cell function results in severe and often life-threatening manifestations of allergy in affected individuals. Subsidence of allergic manifestations with the correction of this immune regulatory defect suggests that there are likely additional targets of immune system defects related to allergy that are awaiting discovery. We will likely see an increasing connection between these areas of investigation and intervention in the future.

Transplant and allergy also intersect in indirect ways. Acute chest syndrome is a frequent complication in patients with sickle cell disease and has been recently reported to be exacerbated or precipitated by asthma and respiratory allergies. Since SCT can halt this pulmonary destruction process, ongoing investigation at our and other institutions is focused on determining genetic and cytokine pathways and modulators for asthma in sickle cell disease.

Work is in progress to overcome disease and transplant-related barriers. It is a challenge for the immunologist or rheumatologist to identify patients at an early stage of their disease and commit them to SCT before the development of major organ damage that affects SCT outcome. The time from diagnosis to transplant is critical – the earlier the intervention, and the younger the patient, the better the outcome. Often, in contrast to SCT for malignant disorders, the development of major disease-related organ toxicity promotes consideration for transplant in immunoregulatory disorders and this approach is often justified given the variability of disease manifestations within the same disease cohort. A lack of long-term follow-up studies that establish true benefit from SCT for slowly progressive and intermittently remitting disorders often preclude consideration of transplant.

From the transplant perspective, autologous transplants have gradually moved away from the high-dose chemo/radiotherapy approach to the immuno/lymphoablative reduced intensity approach in an effort to limit early and late toxicities. These include irreversible damage to organs and growth, endocrine function defects, performance problems, quality-of-life issues, and a predisposition to the development of secondary malignancies. Targeted use of medications that support selective depletion of immune cell compartments such as rituximab, alemtuzumab, ATG, helped to reduce the intensity of conditioning while achieving transplant goals. For consideration of allogeneic transplants, the benefits in immunoregulatory disorders should consistently outweigh the risks of mortality, infection, graft rejection, and GvHD.

Transplant safety has improved steadily over time with the use of graft sources enriched for stem cell numbers and extensively matched for HLA phenotypes, conditioning regimen changes, and excellent prophylaxis and monitoring for GvHD and infections. The advantages and disadvantages of using HLA-matched family members that may be potential carriers of disease and manifest disease symptoms in the future remains controversial due to the variability in disease onset and manifestations.

In conclusion, SCT for immunoregulatory T-cell disorders remains an exciting area of investigation in terms of defining efficacy, safety, and long-term outcomes. SCT is likely to benefit a carefully identified subset of patients with the potential for severe disease manifestations. In the future, this subset may be identified by genetic patterns or early disease markers that herald poor outcome either for survival or quality of life. Current studies support a role for SCT in an increasing number of T-regulatory disorders in an effort to achieve either disease control or cure. Transplant advances in the future based on current experimental efforts include advanced conditioning techniques, genetic modification of autologous stem cells, taking advantage of the pleuripotency and cryopreservability of autologous umbilical cord blood cells, and in vitro expansion of hematopoietic stem cells prior to infusion to benefit transplant outcomes.

References

1   Slavin S, Morecki S, Weiss L, Or R: Donor lymphocyte infusion: the use of alloreactive and tumor-reactive lymphocytes for immunotherapy of malignant and non-malignant disease in conjunction with allogeneic stem cell transplantation. J Hematother Stem Cell Res 2002;11:265–276.
2   Schwartz R: Natural regulatory T cells and self-tolerance. Nat Immunol 2005;6: 327–330.

3   Jayne D, Passweg J, Marmont A, et al: Autologous stem cell transplantation for systemic lupus erythematosus. Lupus 2004;13:168–176.
4   Burt R, Traynor A, Statkute L, et al: Non-myeloablative hematopoietic stem cell transplantation for systemic lupus erythematosus. JAMA 2006;295: 527–535.

5   Snowden J, Passweg J, Moore J, et al: Autologous hematopoietic stem cell transplantation in severe rheumatoid arthritis: a report from the EBMT and ABMTR. J Rheumatol 2004;31: 482–488.
6   Brinkman D, de Kleer I, ten Cate R, et al: Autologous stem cell transplantation in children with severe progressive systemic or polyarticular juvenile idiopathic arthritis. Arthritis Rheum 2007;56:2410–2421.

7 Ades L, Guardiola P, Socie G: Second malignancies after allogeneic hematopoietic stem cell transplantation: new insight and current problems. Blood Rev 2002;16:135–146.

8 Oyama Y, Barr W, Statkute L, et al: Autologous non-myeloablative hematopoietic stem cell transplantation in patients with systemic sclerosis. Bone Marrow Transplant 2007;40:549–555.

9 Couri C, Foss M, Voltarelli J: Secondary prevention of type 1 diabetes mellitus: stopping immune destruction and promoting β-cell regeneration. Braz J Med Biol Res 2006;39:1271–1280.

10 Voltarelli J, Couri C, Stracieri A, et al: Autologous nonmyeloablative hematopoietic stem cell transplantation in newly diagnosed type 1 diabetes mellitus. JAMA 2007;297:1568–1576.

11 Infante A, Britton H, DeNapoli T, et al: The clinical spectrum in a large kindred with autoimmune lymphoproliferative syndrome caused by a Fas mutation that impairs lymphocyte apoptosis. J Pediatr 1998;133:629–633.

12 Shenoy S, Arnold S, Chatila T: Response to steroid therapy in autoimmune lymphoproliferative syndrome secondary to ALPS. J Pediatr 2000;3:101–109.

13 Sleight B, Prasad V, DeLaat C, et al: Correction of autoimmune lymphoproliferative syndrome by bone marrow transplantation. Bone Marrow Transplant 1998;22:375–380.

14 Gambineri E, Torgerson T, Ochs H: Immune dysregulation, polyendocrinopathy, enteropathy, and X-linked in heritance (IPEX) a syndrome of systemic autoimmmunity caused by mutations of FoxP3, a critical regulator of T-cell homeostasis. Curr Opin Rheumatol 2003;15:430–435.

15 Chatila T, Blaeser F, Ho N, et al: JM2, encoding a fork head-related protein is mutated in X-linked autoimmunity-allergic disregulation syndrome. J Clin Invest 2000;106:R75–R81.

16 Baud O, Goulet O, Canioni D, et al: Treatment of the immune dysregulation, polyendocrinopathy, enteropathy, X-linked syndrome (IPEX) by allogeneic bone marrow transplantation. N Engl J Med 2001;344:1758–1762.

17 Rao A, Kamani N, Filipovich A, et al: Successful bone marrow transplantation for IPEX syndrome after reduced-intensity conditioning. Blood 2007;109:383–385.

18 Zhan H, Sinclair J, Adams S, et al: Immune reconstitution and recovery of FoxP3 (forkhead box P3)-expressing T cells after transplantation for IPEX (immune dysregulation, polyendocrinopathy, enteropathy, X-linked) syndrome. Pediatrics 2008;121:e998–e1002.

Shalini Shenoy, MD
St. Louis Children's Hospital
660 S. Euclid Avenue, Campus Box 8116
St. Louis, MO 63110 (USA)
Tel. +1 314 454 6018, Fax +1 314 454 2780, E-Mail shenoy@wustl.edu

Author Index

Akdis, C.A. 67, 158
Akdis, M. 67
Aktas, E. 48
Anderton, S.M. 201
Apostolou, I. 8

Bedke, T. 29
Boussiotis, V.A. 178

Cavani, A. 93
Chatila, T.A. 16
Chattopadhyay, S. 138
Cone, R.E. 138

Deniz, G. 48

Elkord, E. 150
Enk, A.H. 29
Erten, G. 48

Finotto, S. 83

Hammad, H. 189
Holt, P.G. 40

Jutel, M. 67, 158

Karakhanova, S. 29
Kretschmer, K. 8

Lambrecht, B.N. 189
Leech, M.D. 201
Li, L. 178

Mahnke, K. 29
Maizels, R.M. 112

O'Rourke, J. 138

Puccetti, P. 124

Ring, S. 29
Romani, L. 124

Schmidt-Weber, C.B. 1
Shenoy, S. 211
Stassen, M. 58
Strickland, D.H. 40

Taube, C. 58
Turner, D.J. 40

Verginis, P. 8
von Boehmer, H. 8

Werfel, T. 101
Wikstrom, M.E. 40
Wittmann, M. 101

Yazdanbakhsh, M. 112

Subject Index

Stem cell transplantation (SCT) (continued)
   immune dysregulation, polyendocrinopathy,
      enteropathy X-linked syndrome 216, 217
   prospects 217, 218
   rationale 213, 214
   rheumatoid arthritis 215
   systemic lupus erythematosus 214, 215
   systemic sclerosis 215
goals 212, 213
overview 211, 212
safety and efficacy 213, 214
Systemic lupus erythematosus (SLE), stem cell
   transplantation therapy 214, 215
Systemic sclerosis, stem cell transplantation therapy
   215

Tacrolimus, atopic dermatitis management 195
T-box expressed in T-cells (T-bet), deficiency in
   asthma 87, 89
Th1 cell
   cytokine profile 1, 2
   differentiation 4, 5, 88
   functional overview 2, 3
   fungal infection response 128, 129
Th2 cell
   cytokine profile 1, 2
   differentiation 4, 5, 88
   functional overview 2, 3
   fungal infection response 128, 129
   Treg interactions in asthma 85, 86
Th17 cell
   atopic dermatitis role 107
   cytokine profile 2
   differentiation 4, 5, 88
   fungal infection response 129, 130
   inflammation role 4
   Treg interactions in asthma 86, 87
Thymic stromal lymphopoietin (TSLP)
   inflammatory response in allergic diseases 183
   lung dendritic cell maturation role 193, 194
Toll-like receptors (TLRs)
   fungal infection 126, 127, 134
   Treg activity induction with ligands 154, 155
Transforming growth factor-β (TGF-β)
   delayed-type hypersensitivity suppression by
      ocular-induced CD8+ Treg mediation 146,
      147
   T-cell anergy role 181, 182

Treg
   airway hyperresponsiveness
      inhibition role 44
      respiratory tolerance role 40
      roles 44, 45
   allergen-specific immunotherapy mediation
      activity induction 153, 154, 205–208
      CD4+CD25+ cells 164, 165
      clinical relevance 168, 169
      histamine receptors 170, 171
      miscellaneous cells 165
      suppression mechanisms 166–168
      Th3 cells 164
      Tr1 cells 163, 164
   allergic disease inhibition
      induction of Treg activity
         allergen-specific immunotherapy 153, 154
         Toll-like receptor ligands 154, 155
      mechanisms 151–153
      mouse models 151
      therapeutic prospects 155, 156
   allergy role 3, 4
   antigen-presenting cell interactions
      B-cells 34, 35
      dendritic cells
         allergic and inflammatory reactions 35–37
         maturation status and Treg induction poten-
            tial 29, 30
         maturation suppression by Tregs 30–33
      macrophages 32–34
   atopic dermatitis role 107, 108
   contact hypersensitivity modulation 94–97
   development 9–12, 17, 18, 88, 150, 151
   Foxp3
      expression 8, 9
      mutation and disease 22, 24, 96
      roles
         development 18
         function 17
      transcriptional regulation
         Foxp3 22
         Treg transcriptome 18–21
   functional overview 2, 9, 12, 13
   fungal infection and dampening of inflammation
      and allergy 130–133
   heritable disorders 22, 24
   histamine effects 74–76
   lung dendritic cell control 192

natural resolution of autoimmune and allergic
    inflammation 202–204
natural versus induced cells 21, 22, 43, 44, 182
ocular-induced CD8+ Tregs
    afferent and efferent mechanisms 141–143
    anterior chamber-associated immune deviation
    141
    delayed-type hypersensitivity suppression
        animal studies 140, 141
        antigen specificity 143, 144
        interferon-γ mediation 145, 146
        Qa-1^b restriction 144, 145

transforming growth factor-β mediation
    146, 147
overview 138, 139
suppressor activity 139, 140
products 2, 16
subtypes 83, 150
Th2 cell interactions 85, 86
therapeutic interventions 24
Tumor necrosis factor-α (TNF-α), inflammatory
    response in allergic diseases 182, 183

VAF347, dendritic cell effects in allergic disease 196